Interdisciplinary Perspectives on Genetic Syndromes and Human Development

Dimitra V. Katsarou
https://orcid.org/0000-0001-8690-0314
University of the Aegean, Greece

Assimina Tsibidaki
https://orcid.org/0000-0001-6430-2436
University of the Aegean, Greece

IGI Global
Scientific Publishing
Publishing Tomorrow's Research Today

Vice President of Editorial	Melissa Wagner
Director of Acquisitions	Mikaela Felty
Director of Book Development	Jocelynn Hessler
Production Manager	Mike Brehm
Cover Design	Jose Rosado

Published in the United States of America by
IGI Global Scientific Publishing
701 East Chocolate Avenue
Hershey, PA, 17033, USA
Tel: 717-533-8845 | Fax: 717-533-7115
Website: https://www.igi-global.com E-mail: cust@igi-global.com

Library of Congress Cataloging-in-Publication Data

LCCN: 2026938751 (CIP Data Pending)
ISBN13: 9798337384856
Isbn13Softcover: 9798337384863
EISBN13: 9798337384870

British Cataloguing in Publication Data
A Cataloguing in Publication record for this book is available from the British Library.

Table of Contents

Detailed Table of Contents

The proposed model integrates principles from developmental psychopathology, neuroconstructivism, and developmental systems theory, viewing development as a dynamic process shaped by interactions among biological, cognitive, and environmental factors over time. Genetic syndromes are conceptualized not as fixed conditions but as influences that bias developmental processes, leading to diverse outcomes. Concepts such as equifinality and multifinality highlight variability in developmental trajectories. Early differences in attention, perception, and motor exploration can produce cascading effects across domains, shaping later cognitive and socio-emotional development. Environmental contexts and interventions interact with these processes, potentially altering developmental pathways. Overall, the model emphasizes longitudinal, process-oriented perspectives for understanding atypical development and informing assessment and intervention.

Educational transitions represent critical junctures for students with genetic syndromes, requiring coordinated support addressing communication and cognitive development. This chapter examines evidence-based school interventions across

Families of children with rare genetic syndromes are confronted with complex challenges that extend beyond medical management and substantially affect family functioning, emotional well-being, and everyday life. This chapter presents a systematic review of sixteen recent primary research projects examining the quality of life (QoL) of families of children with rare genetic syndromes, with the aim of synthesizing evidence on QoL dimensions, reported levels, associated factors, and methodological approaches. The findings indicate reduced family QoL, particularly in emotional well-being and family dynamics, with overall levels ranging from low to moderate and varying across dimensions. Family cohesion and access to social and material support emerged as key protective factors. Implications are discussed with a particular focus on family-centered psychosocial interventions that conceptualize the family as a dynamic and cohesive system, capable, when adequately supported, of constructing meaning, strengthening resilience, and functioning in ways that promote well-being.

Autism has been recorded as a particularly common coexisting health condition in individuals diagnosed with certain genetic syndromes. Researchers collected data from 114 parents of children with autism aged 4–25 to examine their perceived quality of life and stress levels, as well as the relationship between these variables, while considering selected demographic characteristics. The complexity of care needs in chronic health conditions makes it necessary to systematically study parenting experience. The results showed a strong and statistically significant negative relationship between stress and quality of life, with stress explaining a significant proportion of the variation in quality of life. Differences were found in terms of gender, educational level and marital status. Findings highlight the importance of psychosocial support for parents of children with autism.

Preface

INTRODUCTION

As editors of *Interdisciplinary Perspectives on Genetic Syndromes and Human Development*, we are pleased to present a volume that brings together diverse voices across disciplines to address a shared and pressing concern: how to better understand and support individuals with genetic syndromes throughout the course of their lives. This book emerges from the recognition that while scientific advances have expanded what we know about genetic conditions, meaningful integration of this knowledge into educational, developmental, and social contexts remains incomplete.

We invite readers into a dialogue that moves beyond disciplinary boundaries. The chapters in this volume reflect an interdisciplinary commitment to bridging genetic science with developmental psychology, education, caregiving, and community practice. Collectively, they illuminate how genetic syndromes intersect with human development in complex ways, shaping learning, behavior, identity, and participation across environments and life stages.

Recent advances in genetics and neuroscience have led to earlier diagnoses, improved medical care, and increased life expectancy for individuals with conditions such as Down syndrome, Fragile X syndrome, Williams syndrome, Prader–Willi syndrome, Angelman syndrome, and Turner syndrome. Yet, despite these achievements, the broader developmental, psychosocial, and educational dimensions of these conditions have not received equivalent attention in scholarly and applied literature. This volume seeks to address that imbalance.

Grounded in biopsychosocial, ecological, and lifespan-oriented frameworks, the contributions in this book explore how genetic syndromes influence not only biological processes but also learning trajectories, family dynamics, social inclusion, and overall well-being. We have intentionally curated work that centers lived experiences alongside empirical research, recognizing that individuals and families are not merely subjects of study but active participants in shaping developmental pathways.

This volume aspires to serve as a comprehensive reference for researchers, educators, clinicians, therapists, caregivers, and policy makers. It combines theoretical rigor with practical insight, offering frameworks that inform inclusive education, therapeutic intervention, family support, and community engagement. In doing so, it underscores the importance of translating scientific knowledge into practices that enhance quality of life.

A central motivation for this book is the persistent gap between medical and neurobiological research and its application in real-world contexts. Contributors respond to this challenge by advancing integrated perspectives that bridge genetics with educational and developmental sciences, highlight the essential role of families and caregivers, and promote sustained interdisciplinary dialogue. Attention is also given to ethical considerations, cultural variability, and the need for approaches that remain responsive across the lifespan, including adolescence and adulthood.

We hope this volume will not only inform but also inspire—encouraging collaboration across fields, fostering inclusive practices, and supporting advocacy efforts that recognize the dignity and potential of every individual. We also welcome engagement from emerging scholars and practitioners, whose perspectives are vital to the continued evolution of this field.

In bringing together these contributions, we aim to advance a more holistic understanding of genetic syndromes and human development—one that is as attentive to complexity as it is committed to inclusion.

ORGANIZATION OF THE BOOK

In Chapter 1, the volume opens with a theoretically rich and integrative model that repositions genetic syndromes within a dynamic developmental framework. Drawing on developmental psychopathology, neuroconstructivism, and developmental systems theory, the chapter challenges static, deficit-oriented views by conceptualizing genetic syndromes as influences that shape—rather than determine—developmental pathways. The authors emphasize variability through the principles of equifinality and multifinality, illustrating how early differences in attention, perception, and motor engagement can cascade across domains over time. This process-oriented perspective underscores the importance of longitudinal analysis and highlights the powerful role of environmental contexts and interventions in redirecting developmental trajectories.

Chapter 2 turns to the critical issue of educational transitions, examining how communication and cognitive profiles associated with specific genetic syndromes require carefully coordinated, school-based supports. The chapter synthesizes evidence across multiple conditions, illustrating how distinct developmental profiles necessitate tailored interventions. From augmentative communication strategies and literacy-focused instruction to anxiety management and multidisciplinary coordination, the authors demonstrate how targeted supports can ease transitions and enhance educational participation. This contribution reinforces the need for responsive, individualized planning within inclusive educational systems.

In Chapter 3, the volume engages with the ethical terrain surrounding advances in genetic science. The authors critically examine the implications of genetic testing, diagnosis, and emerging interventions, raising important questions about privacy, informed consent, discrimination, and the psychological impact of genetic knowledge. The discussion extends to broader societal concerns, including equitable access to genetic services and the ethical boundaries of genome editing. By situating scientific progress within moral and social contexts, this chapter provides a necessary counterbalance, urging thoughtful and responsible application of genetic technologies.

Chapter 4 addresses the foundational role of early identification and intervention, emphasizing the transformative potential of timely developmental screening. The authors review contemporary diagnostic practices, including emerging technologies such as digital phenotyping and genomic workflows, and highlight how multidisciplinary collaboration enhances early detection. The chapter further explores evidence-based intervention models, particularly family-centered and naturalistic approaches, demonstrating how early support can significantly improve developmental outcomes and family well-being. This contribution underscores early childhood as a critical window for shaping long-term trajectories.

In Chapter 5, a detailed case-based analysis offers a nuanced view of family-centered intervention in the context of a rare genetic condition. Through an in-depth examination of a young child's developmental journey, the chapter illustrates how therapeutic goals can be embedded within everyday family routines to support communication, autonomy, and social participation. Particular attention is given to the reorganization of family roles, the involvement of siblings, and the realities of limited access to specialized services. This chapter powerfully highlights the central role of families as active agents in developmental support.

Chapter 6 expands the focus to the broader family system by synthesizing research on quality of life among families of children with rare genetic syndromes. The review reveals consistent challenges in emotional well-being and family dynamics, while also identifying key protective factors such as cohesion and access to support networks. The authors advocate for family-centered psychosocial interventions that recognize the family as a dynamic, meaning-making system capable of resilience. This chapter reinforces the importance of addressing not only individual outcomes but also the well-being of the family unit as a whole.

In Chapter 7, the relationship between parental stress and perceived quality of life is examined within the context of autism, a condition frequently co-occurring with genetic syndromes. Drawing on empirical data, the chapter demonstrates a strong inverse relationship between stress and quality of life, while also identifying demographic variables that shape parental experiences. The findings highlight the complex demands placed on caregivers and underscore the urgent need for targeted psychosocial support systems that address both stress reduction and well-being.

Chapter 8 provides an interdisciplinary overview of therapeutic interventions across the lifespan, focusing on occupational, physical, and recreational therapies. The chapter emphasizes person-centered and participation-oriented approaches, illustrating how coordinated interventions can support motor development, daily functioning, health, and social inclusion. By highlighting the importance of family involvement, environmental adaptations, and community engagement, this contribution advances a holistic vision of care that extends beyond clinical settings into everyday life.

Chapters 9 and 11 introduce innovative applications of artificial intelligence in the early detection and classification of neurodegenerative conditions, particularly Alzheimer's disease. Chapter 9 presents a deep learning framework utilizing residual neural networks to achieve highly accurate classification of disease stages from neuroimaging data, demonstrating the potential of advanced computational tools in diagnostic precision. Complementing this, Chapter 11 proposes a hybrid neural network model that integrates attention mechanisms and optimization strategies to enhance feature extraction and model performance. Together, these chapters illustrate how technological advancements can contribute to earlier and more reliable diagnosis, with implications for intervention and care planning.

Chapter 10 explores the biological underpinnings of neurodevelopmental and neurodegenerative conditions through the lens of oxidative stress and microbial dysbiosis. The authors examine how imbalances in oxidative and antioxidant systems contribute to neuronal damage and disease progression, situating these processes within broader physiological and environmental contexts. This chapter deepens the biological dimension of the volume, linking molecular mechanisms to functional outcomes and reinforcing the importance of integrative, multi-level approaches to understanding complex conditions.

Taken together, these chapters reflect the core mission of this volume: to integrate knowledge across disciplines, connect research with practice, and foreground the lived realities of individuals with genetic syndromes and their families.

CONCLUSION

As editors, we close this volume with a deep appreciation for the breadth, rigor, and humanity reflected across its chapters. *Interdisciplinary Perspectives on Genetic Syndromes and Human Development* has been shaped by a shared commitment to advancing understanding beyond disciplinary silos and toward a more integrated, responsive, and inclusive approach to research and practice. The contributions gathered here collectively affirm that genetic syndromes are not static clinical entities, but dynamic influences embedded within complex developmental systems that unfold over time and across contexts.

A central thread running through this volume is the recognition that meaningful progress lies not only in scientific discovery, but in its thoughtful translation into everyday practice. Whether through early identification and intervention, educational inclusion, family-centered care, ethical reflection, or technological innovation, the chapters illustrate the transformative potential of bridging knowledge with action. They also underscore that development is inherently relational—shaped by families, professionals, communities, and the broader social and cultural environments in which individuals live.

Importantly, this work calls attention to voices and perspectives that have too often remained at the margins. By foregrounding lived experiences alongside empirical evidence, the volume emphasizes dignity, agency, and participation as essential components of human development. It also highlights the resilience of individuals and families, while acknowledging the structural and systemic challenges that continue to shape their experiences.

Looking ahead, we see this volume not as a conclusion, but as an invitation. It invites continued interdisciplinary dialogue, deeper collaboration across research and practice, and sustained advocacy for policies and systems that support inclusion and quality of life across the lifespan. It also calls upon emerging scholars and practitioners to build upon this foundation, bringing new questions, methods, and perspectives to a field that is both evolving and urgently needed.

We hope that this book will serve as a meaningful resource and a catalyst for change—informing research, guiding practice, and ultimately contributing to a more inclusive and equitable understanding of human development in the context of genetic diversity.

Chapter 1
A Comprehensive Developmental Theoretical and Empirical Model for Genetic Syndromes as Developmental Conditions

Dimitra V. Katsarou
http://orcid.org/0000-0001-8690-0314
University of the Aegean, Greece

ABSTRACT

The proposed model integrates principles from developmental psychopathology, neuroconstructivism, and developmental systems theory, viewing development as a dynamic process shaped by interactions among biological, cognitive, and environmental factors over time. Genetic syndromes are conceptualized not as fixed conditions but as influences that bias developmental processes, leading to diverse outcomes. Concepts such as equifinality and multifinality highlight variability in developmental trajectories. Early differences in attention, perception, and motor exploration can produce cascading effects across domains, shaping later cognitive and socio-emotional development. Environmental contexts and interventions interact with these processes, potentially altering developmental pathways. Overall, the model emphasizes longitudinal, process-oriented perspectives for understanding atypical development and informing assessment and intervention.

DOI: 10.4018/979-8-3373-8485-6.ch001

INTRODUCTION

Genetic syndromes constitute a major category of neurodevelopmental conditions associated with chromosomal anomalies or gene mutations that influence multiple domains of development, including cognition, language, behavior, and adaptive functioning. Conditions such as Down syndrome, Williams syndrome, Fragile X syndrome, Angelman syndrome, and Prader–Willi syndrome illustrate how genetic variations can affect developmental pathways in complex and heterogeneous ways. Historically, research on genetic syndromes focused primarily on identifying behavioral phenotypes, that is, characteristic cognitive and behavioral patterns associated with specific syndromes. Although this descriptive approach contributed significantly to the understanding of syndrome-related characteristics, contemporary developmental research increasingly recognizes that these profiles are dynamic, developmentally sensitive, and subject to considerable variability across individuals (Karmiloff-Smith, 1998; Cicchetti, 2008). From this perspective, genetic syndromes are better understood not as fixed diagnostic entities but as developmental conditions that shape, but do not determine, developmental trajectories across the lifespan.

These ideas are consistent with contemporary theoretical approaches in developmental science, including developmental psychopathology, neuroconstructivism, and developmental systems theory, which conceptualize development as a dynamic, multilevel process emerging from interactions among genes, brain development, cognitive processes, and environmental experiences (Gottlieb, 2007; Johnson, 2011; Westermann et al., 2007). Such approaches highlight that developmental differences in genetic syndromes often arise from variations in developmental timing, learning opportunities, and environmental interactions, rather than from fixed deficits. Consequently, understanding the development of individuals with genetic syndromes requires integrative models that consider both biological mechanisms and contextual influences, including educational inclusion and early intervention practices (Katsarou, 2023; Katsarou et al., 2025a; Katsarou et al., 2025b; Katsarou & Andreou, 2017, 2022a, 2022b). This developmental perspective provides a foundation for examining genetic syndromes as evolving developmental trajectories, thereby offering new insights for research, clinical practice, and educational support.

The proposed Integrated Developmental Trajectories Model reconceptualizes genetic syndromes as developmental conditions rather than static diagnostic entities. Instead of viewing these syndromes as fixed *nosological labels* that inevitably produce stable cognitive or behavioral "profiles," the model conceptualizes them as biological starting points that bias the organization and timing of developmental processes. Through continuous interaction with environmental contexts, these processes give rise to emergent phenotypes.

The central assumption of the model is that phenotypic outcomes—including cognitive, socio-emotional, psychopathological, and adaptive functioning—are not direct expressions of underlying genetic causation. Rather, they represent the result of developmental pathways and transactions (including cascades) operating across multiple levels of organization: genes, biology, brain development, cognition, behavior, and environmental context. In this perspective, outcomes are products of dynamic developmental processes rather than linear causal expressions (Karmiloff-Smith, 1998; Gottlieb, 2007; Cicchetti, 2008).

This synthesis draws upon three major theoretical traditions which, despite their different conceptual vocabularies and priorities, converge on a shared meta-principle: development is dynamic, multilevel, and probabilistic, characterized by emergent properties and continuous feedback mechanisms.

First, developmental psychopathology provides the conceptual framework for understanding continuity and change across development, as well as the principles of equifinality (different pathways leading to similar outcomes) and multifinality (similar early conditions leading to different outcomes). It also emphasizes the interplay between risk and protective factors, as well as processes of resilience in developmental trajectories (Sroufe, 1997; Cicchetti, 2008; Cicchetti, & Rogosch, 1996).

Second, neuroconstructivism specifies the underlying mechanisms through which development unfolds. Within this framework, cognitive functions are not viewed as pre-specified modules. Instead, they emerge progressively through the specialization of neural networks, shaped by multiple biological and environmental constraints and by experiential input. Even small early deviations in fundamental mechanisms of learning or regulation may be amplified over time, producing developmental cascade effects (Karmiloff-Smith, 1998; Westermann et al., 2007; Johnson, 2011).

Third, developmental systems theory and dynamic systems approaches emphasize the principle of coaction in developmental causation and reject simplistic linear explanations based on the nature–nurture dichotomy. Genes, epigenetic processes, neural activity, family and cultural contexts, and developmental niches interact to co-produce the developing phenotype (Gottlieb, 2007; Griffiths & Gray, 1994; Thelen & Smith, 1994).

Empirical evidence from research on at least six genetic syndromes—Down syndrome, Fragile X syndrome, Williams syndrome and Prader–Willi syndrome,—consistently demonstrates that:

(a) similar levels of performance at a given age may reflect different underlying developmental processes;
(b) the timing and rate of developmental change (growth trajectories) are often more diagnostically informative than single cross-sectional measurements; and

(c) within-syndrome variability, including molecular subtypes and environmental transactions, substantially shapes developmental trajectories (Maeder et al., 2016; Olszewski et al., 2017; Sadhwani et al., 2023; Dykens et al., 2007; Mason-Apps et al., 2020).

DEFINITIONS AND CONCEPTUAL FRAMEWORK

The explanatory power and coherence of the model depend on clear conceptual definitions that are compatible with the three theoretical traditions on which it is based: developmental psychopathology, neuroconstructivism, and developmental systems theory.

Developmental pathways.

Developmental pathways refer to sequences of states and transformations in which each developmental state constrains or facilitates possible subsequent states through nonlinear feedback processes. Within the framework of developmental psychopathology, pathways are evaluated in relation to typical developmental trajectories and are examined through concepts such as continuity and change, risk and protective processes, equifinality, and multifinality (Cicchetti, 2008; Cicchetti & Rogosch, 1996; Sroufe, 1997).

Biasing of organization and timing.

Genetic variations—such as copy number variations (CNVs), trisomies, or single-gene mutations—do not determine a fully specified cognitive outcome. Rather, they bias developmental processes by influencing:

(a) which neural or physiological systems mature earlier;
(b) the rate of maturation of these systems;
(c) the capacity for reorganization and plasticity; and
(d) the types of experiences that are more likely to be sought, generated, or reinforced.

Within the neuroconstructivist framework, this principle is described in terms of developmental constraints, through which small initial differences may be progressively amplified, producing cascade-like developmental effects (Karmiloff-Smith, 1998; Westermann et al., 2007).

Emergent phenotypes.

Emergent phenotypes refer to observable patterns of behavior, cognitive functioning, or psychopathology that do not exist as predetermined entities but instead arise gradually through the interaction of multiple developmental levels. This concept is closely associated with:

(i) the principle of probabilistic epigenesis, and
(ii) models of progressive specialization or interactive specialization of neural circuits during development (Gottlieb, 2007; Johnson, 2011; Westermann et al., 2007).

In addition to these core concepts, two complementary notions function as supporting mechanisms within the model.

First, developmental cascades refer to processes whereby changes in one developmental domain (for example, attentional regulation) alter learning opportunities in other domains (such as linguistic interaction), producing cumulative developmental consequences over time (Masten & Cicchetti, 2010).

Second, transactional models emphasize the reciprocal and evolving interaction between the child and the environment. From this perspective, both risk and compensation are not static attributes but dynamic relational processes that unfold over time through ongoing interactions between individual characteristics and environmental contexts (Sameroff, 2009).

THEORETICAL SYNTHESIS

Developmental Psychopathology

Developmental psychopathology conceptualizes atypical development as a variation or deviation within general developmental principles, emphasizing patterns of continuity and discontinuity, mechanisms of risk and protection, and interactions across multiple levels of organization (Cicchetti, 2008; Sroufe, 1997). The application of this framework to genetic syndromes is direct: a syndrome may introduce significant biological risks, yet developmental outcomes depend on the individual's developmental history, including lived experiences, interventions, and broader social conditions.

The concepts of equifinality and multifinality provide a critical corrective to static descriptions of genetic syndromes. First, similar behavioral outcomes—such as social anxiety or language delay—may emerge through different developmental pathways across different syndromes. Second, individuals with the same genetic condition may diverge substantially in their developmental trajectories due to contextual influences, caregiving environments, comorbid conditions, and stochastic developmental processes (Cicchetti & Rogosch, 1996).

Neuroconstructivism

Neuroconstructivism proposes that cognitive development is a process of representational construction arising from interactions between brain plasticity and experience under multiple constraints operating across levels of organization (from cellular processes to neural systems, cognition, and social interaction). This perspective rejects the assumption that adult phenotypes directly correspond to innate, pre-specified cognitive modules (Karmiloff-Smith, 1998; Westermann et al., 2007).

A key contribution of this framework is its emphasis on early domain-general processes—such as attention, sensory processing, arousal regulation, and motor exploration—as gateways to experience. Consequently, even small differences in the ways infants and young children sample and engage with their environment may systematically alter the quality and quantity of learning opportunities. Over time, these differences can generate developmental cascade effects that shape the organization of cognitive and social systems (Johnson, 2011; Westermann et al., 2007).

Developmental Systems Theory and Dynamic Systems Approaches

Developmental systems theory (DST) and related dynamic systems approaches conceptualize causation as distributed across a network of developmental resources, including genetic, epigenetic, behavioral, ecological, and cultural processes that collectively sustain the life cycle. Within this framework, development is fundamentally epigenetic in the broad sense—organized through ongoing interactions rather than dictated by a unidirectional "genetic program" (Gottlieb, 2007; Griffiths & Gray, 1994; Moore, 2016).

From this perspective, a genetic syndrome should not be interpreted as a direct causal determinant in a narrow sense. Instead, it represents a factor that reshapes the developmental landscape, shifting developmental probabilities. The resulting phenotype emerges through the temporally extended interaction between the organism and its environment, rather than through a predetermined genetic blueprint (Gottlieb, 2007; Thelen & Smith, 1994).

CONVERGENCES AND TENSIONS

Despite their conceptual differences, the three traditions converge on four central principles:

(i) an emphasis on developmental trajectories rather than static snapshots,
(ii) multilevel causation,
(iii) the emergence of developmental outcomes through transactions and cascade processes, and

(iv) heterogeneity as an expected outcome of development rather than an anomaly (Cicchetti, 2008; Gottlieb, 2007; Karmiloff-Smith, 1998; Masten & Cicchetti, 2010).

Nevertheless, certain tensions remain, primarily at the methodological and conceptual levels. Developmental psychopathology often organizes research around risk, psychopathology, and normative comparisons. Neuroconstructivism places greater emphasis on mechanisms of representational change and neural specialization, frequently drawing on computational and neuroscientific models. Developmental systems theory, by contrast, adopts a more radically anti-reductionist stance, advocating conceptualizations in which notions such as "genetic risk" are reframed as relationships among developmental resources rather than intrinsic properties of genes.

These tensions, however, can be productive when they encourage more rigorous multilevel research designs and clearer hypotheses regarding when and how early deviations may become amplified into developmental cascades (Astle et al., 2022; Lenroot & Giedd, 2011).

Multilevel Mechanisms Over Time

Time-Sensitive Processes, Plasticity, and "Windows" of Vulnerability and Opportunity

The premise that genetic influences are interpreted differently across developmental stages presupposes the existence of sensitive periods and mechanisms of critical-period plasticity (Hensch, 2005; Knudsen, 2004). Developmental systems theory and developmental neuroscience further clarify that sensitive periods are properties of neural circuits and functional systems—for example, inhibitory networks, extracellular matrix (ECM) regulation, and synaptic pruning—rather than merely age-defined developmental phases (Hensch, 2005).

Within the integrated model, sensitive periods function as amplifiers of developmental bias. If a genetic syndrome shifts the timing of maturation of a particular system—for example, those involved in attentional regulation or motor exploration—then the child encounters the same environmental experiences at a different developmental stage, resulting in different developmental consequences. Consequently, intervention strategies should be considered fundamentally timing-sensitive, targeting specific developmental windows when plasticity is greatest (Knudsen, 2004; Lenroot & Giedd, 2011).

Epigenetics and the Regulation of Gene Expression by Experience

Epigenetics provides concrete mechanisms through which experience becomes biologically embedded. Molecular processes such as DNA methylation and chromatin modification can produce long-term changes in the expression of genes involved in neuroendocrine regulation and stress responsivity. A classic experimental paradigm demonstrates that variations in maternal caregiving are associated with differences in methylation of the glucocorticoid receptor gene promoter and corresponding alterations in the functioning of the hypothalamic–pituitary–adrenal (HPA) axis (Weaver et al., 2004).

Within the context of genetic syndromes, this evidence suggests that the genetic starting point interacts with lived experiences—such as medical hospitalizations, sensory processing differences, family stress, and access to intervention—thereby shaping neurodevelopment through epigenetic co-regulation. Causation, therefore, should not be conceptualized as a linear process of *gene outcome*, but rather as a dynamic system of interactions:

gene ↔ neural activity ↔ experience ↔ regulation of gene expression (Gottlieb, 2007; Lenroot & Giedd, 2011).

Gene–Environment Correlation and Interaction (rGE and G×E) in Developmental Conditions

The concept of gene–environment correlation (rGE) suggests that genotypes influence the environments individuals experience. Classical theoretical formulations distinguish between passive, evocative, and active forms of rGE. The influential model proposed by Scarr and McCartney (1983) describes how children actively contribute to the construction of their own developmental environments.

In genetic syndromes, rGE processes may be particularly pronounced because the phenotype—such as heightened social approach, hyperphagia, or regulatory difficulties—elicits specific responses from caregivers, educators, and social systems. These responses, in turn, influence the distribution and quality of developmental experiences available to the child.

Similarly, gene–environment interactions (G×E) indicate that environmental influences may vary in magnitude and direction depending on biological vulnerability. Psychiatric and developmental research increasingly emphasizes the need for mechanistic bridges between epidemiological findings and neuroscientific evidence in order to fully understand the developmental pathways underlying G×E processes (Caspi et al., 2005).

Stochastic Processes as a "Fourth Pillar" of Developmental Heterogeneity

Even when individuals share the same genotype and experience broadly similar environmental conditions, development involves an inherent degree of stochasticity in cellular and molecular processes. Gene expression itself is intrinsically noisy and probabilistic, with fluctuations occurring at the level of individual cells. These variations can influence cell differentiation, tissue organization, and functional outcomes during development (Raj & van Oudenaarden, 2008).

Furthermore, both theoretical and empirical evidence suggests that stochastic epigenetic variability can generate substantial phenotypic diversity, with important implications for both development and disease processes (Feinberg, 2010). Recent reviews in developmental biology emphasize that stochastic mechanisms may play a decisive role not only in pathological conditions but also in normal morphogenesis, shaping developmental trajectories through probabilistic biological processes (Jenkins et al., 2024; van Heyningen, 2024).

Within the proposed framework, stochasticity therefore constitutes a fourth pillar of developmental heterogeneity, complementing genetic variation, environmental influences, and developmental system interactions. It highlights that developmental outcomes cannot be fully predicted even when genetic and environmental conditions appear similar, reinforcing the importance of probabilistic and dynamic models of development.

EMPIRICAL EVIDENCE

The empirical literature most compatible with the present model has three common characteristics: it is longitudinal and trajectory-based, it employs multilevel measures (behavior, cognition, and neurobiology), and it assumes that syndrome specificity is often better understood in terms of developmental processes rather than final, fixed "profiles" (Astle et al., 2022; Karmiloff-Smith, 1998; Masten & Cicchetti, 2010;).

Table 1. Systematic comparative table of studies across at least six syndromes

Syndrome	Study	Sample	Ages	Methods / Instruments	Design	Main Findings (in Trajectory / Process Terms)	Effect Sizes	Main Limitations
Down syndrome	Mason-Apps et al. (2020)	DS $n = 18$, TD $n = 26$ (matched on NVMA)	DS approximately 17–36 months, TD approximately 9–24 months	Mullen (NVMA), PLS-4 (AC/EC), Reading CDI (RV/EV)	Longitudinal: 3 time points over 12 months + comparison at equivalent NVMA gain	When NVMA was taken into account, expressive communication and vocabulary were similar, whereas infants with DS showed a relative advantage in receptive language (RV/AC); this supports the view that the phenotype of "expressive weakness" emerges later in development.	Cohen's d values were reported for group comparisons (e.g., $d \approx 0.15$ for NVMA at TP1; additional comparisons also reported).	Follow-up covered only 1 year and a very early stage of language development; follow-up during the grammatical/ syntactic phase is needed.

continued on following page

Table 1. Continued

Syndrome	Study	Sample	Ages	Methods / Instruments	Design	Main Findings (in Trajectory / Process Terms)	Effect Sizes	Main Limitations
Fragile X syndrome	Martin et al. (2013)	FXS-O $n = 29$, FXS-ASD $n = 40$, DS $n = 34$, TD $n = 48$ (with attrition at V2/V3)	Chronological age approximately 3.1–17.9 years (depending on group/visit)	CASL (vocabulary/syntax/pragmatics), Leiter-R (nonverbal MA), ADOS (ASD)	Longitudinal: up to 3 visits; HLM / mixed models	Productive language profiles differed by syndrome and ASD status; within groups, vocabulary > pragmatics > syntax; findings indicate different pathways toward "language difficulty" (equifinality) and within-syndrome heterogeneity (multifinality).	No single Cohen's *d* is given in the abstract; *F* tests and HLM parameters are reported.	Boys only; sample attrition at V2/V3; limited ecological validity (standardized tasks versus natural interaction).

continued on following page

Table 1. Continued

Syndrome	Study	Sample	Ages	Methods / Instruments	Design	Main Findings (in Trajectory / Process Terms)	Effect Sizes	Main Limitations
22q11.2 deletion syndrome	Maeder et al. (2016)	22q11.2DS n = 95, controls n = 100 (55% with multiple time points)	6–26 years	CPT-II (attention/ impulsivity), Stroop ratio (inhibition), digit span backward (working memory), semantic verbal fluency + PPVT	Longitudinal with mixed models	Atypical trajectories were found in working memory and verbal fluency (plateau/ slowing with age), whereas inhibition showed a similar developmental shape but at lower levels; different executive-function trajectories were associated with negative symptoms.	p values and trajectory patterns are reported; standardized effect sizes are not presented consistently across the article.	Only a limited subset of executive functions was examined; possible divergence between laboratory EF measures and ecological functioning (e.g., BRIEF versus performance tasks).

continued on following page

integrate molecular, neural, cognitive, and ecological levels of analysis. This limits the capacity to rigorously test transactional and cascade-based developmental hypotheses (Astle et al., 2022; Lenroot & Giedd, 2011).

The most high-yield research priorities include the following:

1. Mapping Early "Developmental Gateways"

Which early mechanisms—such as attention, sensorimotor processing, and regulatory processes—predict later cascades in language and social cognition within specific syndromes? Which mechanisms are shared across syndromes (equifinality) and which are syndrome-specific? (McDuffie & Abbeduto, 2009; Westermann et al., 2007).

2. Mechanistic Integration of rGE and G×E in Rare Syndromes

How does evocative gene–environment correlation (rGE) shape learning opportunities by influencing how caregivers and environments respond to the child's phenotype? How do these processes interact with sensitive developmental periods to alter developmental trajectories? (Scarr & McCartney, 1983; Lenroot & Giedd, 2011).

3. Epigenetic and Stochastic Markers of Heterogeneity

To what extent does stochastic genetic or epigenetic variability explain differences in developmental trajectories among individuals with the same molecular subtype? (Jenkins et al., 2024; Raj & van Oudenaarden, 2008; Feinberg, 2010).

4. Linking Neurodevelopmental Trajectories with Clinical Risk

Which neurodevelopmental markers—for example, changes in brain morphology or plateaus in executive functioning—predict the emergence of psychotic or anxiety-related symptoms, and at which developmental windows might preventive interventions be most effective? (Maeder et al., 2016; Olszewski et al., 2017).

5. Translating Trajectory-Based Models into Intervention Outcomes

DISCUSSION

The Integrated Developmental Trajectories Model proposed in this work reframes genetic syndromes as dynamic developmental conditions rather than static diagnostic entities. By synthesizing insights from developmental psychopathology, neuroconstructivism, and developmental systems theory, the model highlights that phenotypic outcomes emerge through time-dependent interactions across multiple levels of organization, including genetic, neural, cognitive, behavioral, and environmental processes. This integrative perspective challenges traditional interpretations that treat syndromes as producing fixed cognitive or behavioral "profiles" and instead emphasizes developmental processes, timing, and probabilistic pathways.

A central implication of this perspective is that phenotypic expression is historically and developmentally situated. Empirical evidence across several genetic syndromes—including Down syndrome, Williams syndrome, Fragile X syndrome, Angelman syndrome, Prader–Willi syndrome, and 22q11.2 deletion syndrome—demonstrates that developmental outcomes cannot be adequately captured by cross-sectional comparisons or static characterizations. Rather, developmental differences frequently reflect variation in rates of change, timing of developmental transitions, or nonlinear trajectories, rather than qualitative differences in underlying mechanisms.

For instance, findings in Down syndrome indicate that infants may display a relative advantage in receptive language when nonverbal mental age is controlled, suggesting that the widely reported expressive-language difficulties associated with the syndrome may represent a later developmental divergence rather than an intrinsic early deficit. Similarly, research in Williams syndrome shows that standardized scores may decline over time even as raw scores increase, highlighting the importance of distinguishing developmental rate differences from actual loss of skill. These examples illustrate how reliance on standardized scores alone can lead to misleading interpretations if developmental trajectories are not considered.

The developmental trajectory perspective also provides a more coherent framework for interpreting heterogeneity within syndromes. Individuals sharing the same genetic alteration may show markedly different outcomes because their developmental pathways are shaped by gene–environment transactions, epigenetic regulation, stochastic biological processes, and differences in developmental timing. Consequently, heterogeneity should not be viewed as a methodological problem or noise in the data but rather as an expected property of complex developmental systems.

Another important implication concerns the role of developmental cascades. Early differences in foundational processes—such as attentional regulation, sensory processing, or motor exploration—may influence the quality and quantity of learning opportunities available to the child. Over time, these small early differences can produce cumulative effects across multiple domains, including language, executive functioning, and social cognition. This cascading logic aligns closely with neuroconstructivist accounts of development, which emphasize how early domain-general processes constrain and shape later specialization of neural and cognitive systems.

From a theoretical standpoint, the proposed model also highlights the importance of integrating biological and contextual levels of explanation. Developmental systems theory suggests that genes do not act as isolated causal agents but instead participate in networks of interactions involving neural activity, behavior, environmental input, and cultural practices. In this sense, genetic syndromes alter the probability landscape of development, but they do not determine specific outcomes. The resulting phenotype emerges through ongoing coaction between organism and environment across time.

Taken together, these considerations support a shift toward process-oriented, trajectory-based approaches in both research and clinical practice. Rather than asking what the phenotype of a given syndrome "is," researchers and clinicians should instead ask how the phenotype emerges, through which mechanisms, and at what developmental moments interventions may have the greatest impact.

FUTURE DIRECTIONS

Although the developmental trajectory framework provides a promising integrative perspective, several important research challenges remain. Addressing these challenges will require methodological innovation, interdisciplinary collaboration, and more comprehensive longitudinal data.

1. Dense Longitudinal and Multilevel Datasets

One of the most pressing priorities is the development of dense longitudinal datasets that integrate multiple levels of analysis, including genomic, neural, cognitive, behavioral, and environmental measures. Many existing studies still rely on limited numbers of time points, which restricts the ability to detect nonlinear trajectories, developmental plateaus, or shifts in developmental timing. Future research should prioritize multi-wave longitudinal designs beginning in early infancy, particularly in syndromes where diagnosis is possible shortly after birth.

2. Identification of Early Developmental Gateways

A key theoretical prediction of the model is that early differences in foundational processes, such as attention, sensorimotor integration, and arousal regulation, function as developmental gateways that shape later cognitive and social development.

Identifying these mechanisms is critical for understanding how developmental cascades unfold. Future research should aim to determine which early processes predict later outcomes across different syndromes and which represent syndrome-specific pathways.

3. Integration of Gene–Environment Transactions

Further research is needed to clarify how gene–environment correlations and interactions shape developmental trajectories in genetic syndromes. In particular, evocative gene–environment processes, whereby a child's phenotype elicits specific responses from caregivers and social environments, may play an important role in shaping developmental opportunities. Longitudinal designs that combine behavioral observation, environmental assessment, and biological markers will be necessary to fully understand these processes.

4. Epigenetic and Stochastic Sources of Heterogeneity

Emerging evidence suggests that epigenetic variability and stochastic biological processes may contribute substantially to phenotypic heterogeneity even among individuals with the same genetic mutation. Future studies should explore whether epigenetic profiles or molecular variability can predict differences in developmental trajectories, particularly within specific molecular subtypes of genetic syndromes.

5. Linking Neurodevelopmental Trajectories to Clinical Risk

Another important direction concerns the identification of neurodevelopmental markers that predict later psychiatric risk. Longitudinal neuroimaging and neurocognitive studies may help clarify how deviations in brain maturation trajectories are associated with outcomes such as anxiety, psychosis, or social dysfunction. Identifying such markers could enable earlier preventive interventions.

6. Trajectory-Based Outcome Measures in Intervention Research

Finally, intervention research should move beyond static outcome measures toward trajectory-based endpoints. Rather than evaluating success solely in terms of changes in standardized test scores, future studies should assess whether interventions alter the slope, timing, or stability of developmental trajectories. Such an approach would align clinical evaluation more closely with contemporary developmental theory.

CONCLUDING PERSPECTIVE

Overall, the Integrated Developmental Trajectories Model provides a conceptual framework for understanding genetic syndromes as dynamic developmental systems shaped by interactions among biology, experience, and time. By emphasizing trajectories, multilevel causation, and emergent phenotypes, the model offers a foundation for more precise research designs and more effective intervention strategies.

Advancing this framework will require continued efforts to bridge developmental theory, neuroscience, genetics, and clinical practice, ultimately leading to a more comprehensive understanding of how complex developmental conditions unfold across the lifespan.

REFERENCES

Astle, D. E., Holmes, J., Kievit, R., & Gathercole, S. E. (2022). Annual Research Review: The transdiagnostic revolution in neurodevelopmental disorders. *Journal of Child Psychology and Psychiatry, and Allied Disciplines*, *63*(4), 397–417. DOI: 10.1111/jcpp.13481 PMID: 34296774

Caspi, A., Moffitt, T. E., Cannon, M., McClay, J., Murray, R., Harrington, H., Taylor, A., Arseneault, L., Williams, B., Braithwaite, A., Poulton, R., & Craig, I. W. (2005). Moderation of the effect of adolescent-onset cannabis use on adult psychosis by a functional polymorphism in the catechol-O-methyltransferase gene: Longitudinal evidence of a gene X environment interaction. *Biological Psychiatry*, *57*(10), 1117–1127. DOI: 10.1016/j.biopsych.2005.01.026 PMID: 15866551

Chapman, R. S., Hesketh, L. J., & Kistler, D. J. (2002). Predicting longitudinal change in language production and comprehension in individuals with Down syndrome. *Journal of Speech, Language, and Hearing Research: JSLHR*, *45*(5), 902–915. DOI: 10.1044/1092-4388(2002/073) PMID: 12381048

Cicchetti, D. (2008). A multiple-levels-of-analysis perspective on research in developmental psychopathology. In Cicchetti, D., & Cohen, D. (Eds.),; 2nd ed., Vol. 1, pp. 27–57). Developmental psychopathology. Wiley.

Cicchetti, D., & Rogosch, F. A. (1996). Equifinality and multifinality in developmental psychopathology. *Development and Psychopathology*, *8*(4), 597–600. DOI: 10.1017/S0954579400007318

Dykens, E. M., Maxwell, M. A., Pantino, E., Kossler, R., & Roof, E. (2007). Assessment of hyperphagia in Prader-Willi syndrome. *Obesity (Silver Spring, Md.)*, *15*(7), 1816–1826. DOI: 10.1038/oby.2007.216 PMID: 17636101

Feinberg, A. P. (2010). Epigenomics reveals a functional genome anatomy and a new approach to common disease. *Nature Biotechnology*, *28*(10), 1049–1052. DOI: 10.1038/nbt1010-1049 PMID: 20944596

Fidler, D. J. (2005). The emerging Down syndrome behavioral phenotype in early childhood: Implications for practice. *Infants and Young Children*, *18*(2), 86–103. DOI: 10.1097/00001163-200504000-00003

Gottlieb, G. (2007). Probabilistic epigenesis. *Developmental Science*, *10*(1), 1–11. DOI: 10.1111/j.1467-7687.2007.00556.x PMID: 17181692

Griffiths, P. E., & Gray, R. D. (1994). Developmental systems and evolutionary explanation. *The Journal of Philosophy*, *91*(6), 277–304. DOI: 10.2307/2940982

Hensch, T. K. (2005). Critical period plasticity in local cortical circuits. *Nature Reviews. Neuroscience*, *6*(11), 877–888. DOI: 10.1038/nrn1787 PMID: 16261181

Jenkins, D., Chubb, J. R., & Galea, G. (2024). Stochastic processes in development and disease. *Philosophical Transactions of the Royal Society B: Biological Sciences, 379*(1900).

Johnson, M. H. (2011). Interactive specialization: A domain-general framework for human functional brain development? *Developmental Cognitive Neuroscience*, *1*(1), 7–21. DOI: 10.1016/j.dcn.2010.07.003 PMID: 22436416

Karmiloff-Smith, A. (1998). Development itself is the key to understanding developmental disorders. *Trends in Cognitive Sciences*, *2*(10), 389–398. DOI: 10.1016/S1364-6613(98)01230-3 PMID: 21227254

Katsarou, D. (2023). Difficulties in locating discrete diagnostic categories: The examples of Down Syndrome and Williams Syndrome and Developmental Language Disorders and Dyslexia. In Katsarou, D. (Ed.), *Developmental Language Disorders in Childhood and Adolescence* (pp. 31–46). IGI Global. DOI: 10.4018/979-8-3693-0644-4.ch003

Katsarou, D., & Andreou, G. (2017). Receptive and Expressive Semantic Skills in Children with Down Syndrome. *International Education and Research Journal*, *3*(3), 135–136.

Katsarou, D., & Andreou, G. (2022a). Phonological patterns in Greek language in toddlers and children with Down Syndrome and language impairment. *British Journal of Special Education*, *49*(3), 420–237. DOI: 10.1111/1467-8578.12410

Katsarou, D., & Andreou, G. (2022b). Morphosyntactic abilities in young children with Down Syndrome: Evidence from the Greek language. *International Journal of Language & Communication Disorders*, *57*(5), 937–947. DOI: 10.1111/1460-6984.12730 PMID: 35689466

Katsarou, D., Argyriadis, A., Sofologi, M., Argyriadi, A., Kougioumtzis, G., Megari, K., Mantsos, E., & Theodoratou, M. (2025a). Edwards Syndrome: Neurocognitive and linguistic profile, diagnosis, overlaps and treatment. *Polski Merkuriusz Lekarski*, *54*(4), 540–545. DOI: 10.36740/Merkur202504116 PMID: 40929546

Katsarou, D., Theodoratou, M., Sofologi, M., Kougioumtzis, G., Efthymiou, E., Argyriadis, A., Patsiaouras, A., Mantsos, E., Argyriadi, A., & Papadopoulou, S. (2025b). Angelman Syndrome: Neurocognitive and linguistic profile, overlaps, interventions and quality of life. In Megari, K. (Ed.), *Clinical applications of pediatric neuropsychology from infancy to adolescence* (pp. 143–156). IGI Global. DOI: 10.4018/979-8-3693-9689-6.ch007

Knudsen, E. I. (2004). Sensitive periods in the development of the brain and behavior. *Journal of Cognitive Neuroscience, 16*(8), 1412–1425. DOI: 10.1162/0898929042304796 PMID: 15509387

Lenroot, R. K., & Giedd, J. N. (2011). Annual research review: Developmental considerations of gene by environment interactions. *Journal of Child Psychology and Psychiatry, and Allied Disciplines, 52*(4), 429–441. DOI: 10.1111/j.1469-7610.2011.02381.x PMID: 21391998

Maeder, J., Schneider, M., Bostelmann, M., Debbané, M., Glaser, B., Menghetti, S., Schaer, M., & Eliez, S. (2016). Developmental trajectories of executive functions in 22q11. 2 deletion syndrome. *Journal of Neurodevelopmental Disorders, 8*(1), 10. DOI: 10.1186/s11689-016-9141-1 PMID: 27018204

Martin, G. E., Losh, M., Estigarribia, B., Sideris, J., & Roberts, J. (2013). Longitudinal profiles of expressive vocabulary, syntax and pragmatic language in boys with fragile X syndrome or Down syndrome. *International Journal of Language & Communication Disorders, 48*(4), 432–443. DOI: 10.1111/1460-6984.12019 PMID: 23889838

Mason-Apps, E., Stojanovik, V., Houston-Price, C., & Eadie, P. (2020). Early language development in Down syndrome: A longitudinal study. *Journal of Child Language, 47*(3), 543–569.

Masten, A. S., & Cicchetti, D. (2010). Developmental cascades. *Development and Psychopathology, 22*(3), 491–495. DOI: 10.1017/S0954579410000222 PMID: 20576173

McDuffie, A., & Abbeduto, L. (2009). Language disorders in children with mental retardation of genetic origin: Down syndrome, Fragile X syndrome, and Williams syndrome. *Handbook of child language disorders*, 44-66.

Mervis, C. B., & Klein-Tasman, B. P. (2004). Methodological issues in group-matching designs: A levels for control variable comparisons and measurement characteristics of control and target variables. *Journal of Autism and Developmental Disorders, 34*(1), 7–17. DOI: 10.1023/B:JADD.0000018069.69562.b8 PMID: 15098952

Molenaar, P. C. M. (2004). A manifesto on psychology as idiographic science. *Measurement*, *2*(4), 201–218.

Moore, D. S. (2016). *The developing genome: An introduction to behavioral epigenetics* (2nd ed.). Oxford University Press.

Olszewski, A. K., Kikinis, Z., Gonzalez, C. S., Coman, I. L., Makris, N., Gong, X., Rathi, Y., Zhu, A., Antshel, K. M., Fremont, W., Kubicki, M. R., Bouix, S., Shenton, M. E., & Kates, W. R. (2017). The social brain network in 22q11. 2 deletion syndrome: A diffusion tensor imaging study. *Behavioral and Brain Functions : BBF*, *13*(1), 4. DOI: 10.1186/s12993-017-0122-7 PMID: 28209179

Raj, A., & van Oudenaarden, A. (2008). Nature, nurture, or chance: Stochastic gene expression and its consequences. *Cell*, *135*(2), 216–226. DOI: 10.1016/j.cell.2008.09.050 PMID: 18957198

Sameroff, A. J. (2009). *The transactional model of development: How children and contexts shape each other*. American Psychological Association. DOI: 10.1037/11877-000

Scarr, S., & McCartney, K. (1983). How people make their own environments: A theory of genotype–environment effects. *Child Development*, *54*(2), 424–435. PMID: 6683622

Sroufe, L. A. (1997). Psychopathology as an outcome of development. *Development and Psychopathology*, *9*(2), 251–268. DOI: 10.1017/S0954579497002046 PMID: 9201444

Thelen, E., & Smith, L. B. (1994). *A dynamic systems approach to the development of cognition and action*. MIT Press. DOI: 10.7551/mitpress/2524.001.0001

van Heyningen, V. (2024). Stochasticity in genetics and gene regulation. *Philosophical Transactions of the Royal Society B: Biological Sciences, 379*(1900).

Weaver, I. C., Cervoni, N., Champagne, F. A., D'Alessio, A. C., Sharma, S., Seckl, J. R., Dymov, S., Szyf, M., & Meaney, M. J. (2004). Epigenetic programming by maternal behavior. *Nature Neuroscience*, *7*(8), 847–854. DOI: 10.1038/nn1276 PMID: 15220929

Westermann, G., Mareschal, D., Johnson, M. H., Sirois, S., Spratling, M. W., & Thomas, M. S. (2007). Neuroconstructivism. *Developmental Science*, *10*(1), 75–83. DOI: 10.1111/j.1467-7687.2007.00567.x PMID: 17181703

Chapter 2
School-Based Support and Educational Transitions:
Communication and Cognition in Genetic Syndromes

Deepak Gupta
http://orcid.org/0000-0003-3929-1362
Institute of Technology and Management, Gwalior, India

Khujamkulova Iroda
Termez University of Economics and Service, Uzbekistan

Ismagilova Madina Faridovna
Urgench State Pedagogical Institute, Urgench, Uzbekistan

Muborak Hamidova
Kimyo international university in Tashkent, Uzbekistan

Khujayev Muminjon
Alfraganus University, Tashkent, Uzbekistan

Muxlisov Sodiqjon Saidjonovich
Bukhara State University, Bukhara, Uzbekistan

Zuxra Babayeva
Mamun University, Khiva, Uzbekistan

ABSTRACT

Educational transitions represent critical junctures for students with genetic syndromes, requiring coordinated support addressing communication and cognitive development. This chapter examines evidence-based school interventions across five genetic conditions: Down syndrome, Fragile X syndrome, Williams syndrome, Angelman syndrome, and autism spectrum disorder. Systematic analysis reveals syndrome-specific profiles demanding tailored educational approaches.

DOI: 10.4018/979-8-3373-8485-6.ch002

Down syndrome students benefit from augmentative communication systems and literacy-focused interventions. Fragile X syndrome requires early pharmacological consideration alongside behavioral supports. Williams syndrome students need anxiety management during transitions despite strong verbal abilities. Angelman syndrome presents unique communication challenges necessitating multidisciplinary coordination.

1. INTRODUCTION

Educational environments serve as primary developmental contexts for children with genetic syndromes, yet these settings present unique challenges requiring specialized support systems. The intersection of communication abilities and cognitive functioning fundamentally shapes educational experiences and outcomes for students with neurodevelopmental differences. As our understanding of genetic syndromes has expanded beyond purely medical conceptualizations, educational research has increasingly recognized the necessity of syndrome-specific interventions that address distinctive cognitive-linguistic profiles (Reilly et al., 2015).

This chapter synthesizes current evidence on school-based support mechanisms and educational transition strategies for students with five prevalent genetic conditions: Down syndrome, Fragile X syndrome, Williams syndrome, Angelman syndrome, and autism spectrum disorder. While each syndrome manifests distinct neurobiological underpinnings and phenotypic presentations, commonalities emerge in the educational challenges faced and the structural supports required for successful school participation. The dual focus on communication and cognition reflects their interdependent relationship in educational contexts, where linguistic competence enables access to curriculum while cognitive abilities shape learning trajectories.

Educational transitions—whether from early intervention to formal schooling, between educational levels, or toward post-secondary outcomes—represent periods of heightened vulnerability requiring coordinated support. These transitions demand not only academic preparation but also social-emotional readiness, environmental adaptation, and systemic coordination among stakeholders. Contemporary educational frameworks increasingly emphasize inclusive practices, yet implementation remains inconsistent, particularly for students with complex support needs (Boundy et al., 2023). This chapter addresses this implementation gap by examining evidence-based practices across syndrome-specific and transdiagnostic contexts.

1.1 Rationale and Scope

The genetic syndromes examined in this chapter were selected based on three criteria: prevalence in educational settings, availability of intervention research, and distinct cognitive-communicative profiles offering instructive contrasts. Down syndrome, occurring in approximately 1 in 700 births, represents the most common chromosomal condition and benefits from extensive educational research. Fragile X syndrome affects approximately 1 in 4,000 males and 1 in 8,000 females, constituting the most prevalent inherited cause of intellectual disability. Williams syndrome, though rarer at 1 in 7,500 births, presents a unique dissociation between verbal and visuospatial abilities that challenges conventional educational approaches (Palikara et al., 2018).

Angelman syndrome, occurring in 1 in 12,000 to 20,000 births, exemplifies severe communication impairment requiring alternative communication systems. Autism spectrum disorder, while genetically heterogeneous, shares neurodevelopmental features with other conditions examined and affects approximately 1 in 36 children, making school-based support critically important. Together, these conditions represent a spectrum of educational needs while highlighting syndrome-specific considerations essential for effective intervention.

This chapter adopts an interdisciplinary perspective, integrating insights from special education, speech-language pathology, psychology, and genetics. Rather than providing exhaustive syndrome descriptions, the focus remains on actionable educational strategies supported by empirical evidence. The organizational structure progresses from syndrome-specific profiles through intervention approaches to transdiagnostic transition planning, ultimately synthesizing implications for educational practice and policy.

1.2 Theoretical Framework

Educational support for students with genetic syndromes draws upon multiple theoretical frameworks that together inform comprehensive intervention. Bronfenbrenner's ecological systems theory provides a foundational lens, recognizing that student development occurs within nested contexts—microsystem (classroom), mesosystem (home-school connections), exosystem (educational policies), and macrosystem (cultural values)—all influencing educational experiences (Wongkittirungrueang & Cheausuwantavee, 2025). This ecological perspective emphasizes that effective interventions must address multiple system levels simultaneously rather than focusing exclusively on individual student characteristics.

Figure 1. Ecological systems framework for educational transitions

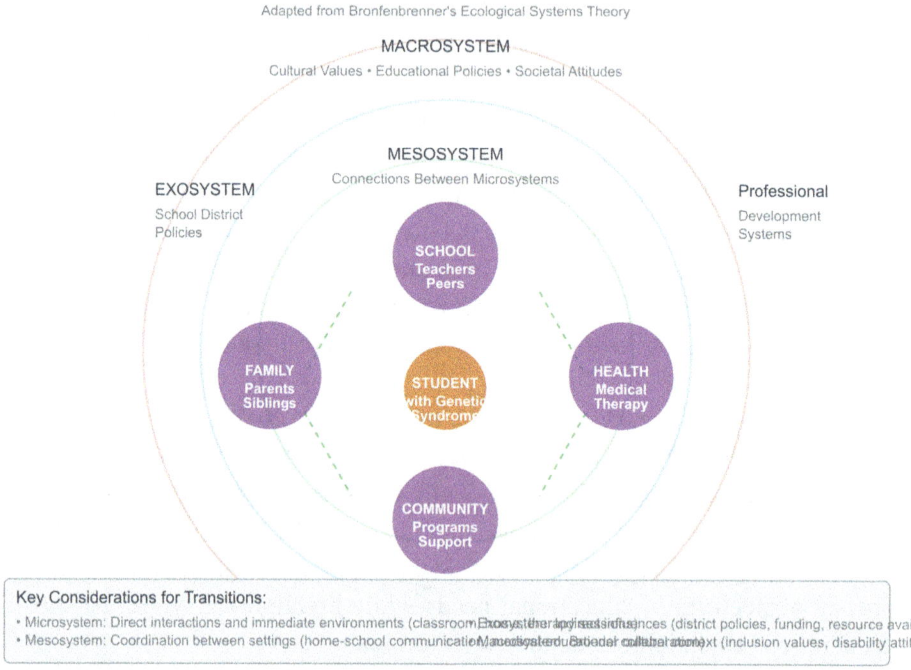

Figure 1 illustrates the multiple nested systems that influence educational experiences and transitions for students with genetic syndromes, based on Bronfenbrenner's Ecological Systems Theory. The framework shows: (1) Macrosystem - cultural values, educational policies, and societal attitudes; (2) Exosystem - school district policies and professional development systems; (3) Mesosystem - connections between microsystems; (4) Microsystem - immediate environments including school, family, healthcare, and community; and (5) Individual student at the center. This visual emphasizes the need for coordinated support across all system levels.

Social constructivist learning theory, particularly Vygotsky's concept of the zone of proximal development, underscores the importance of scaffolded instruction tailored to individual readiness levels. For students with genetic syndromes, identifying appropriate instructional zones requires understanding syndrome-specific developmental trajectories and cognitive profiles. The social dimension of learning proves particularly relevant given that many genetic syndromes affect social cognition and peer relationships, necessitating explicit instruction in skills typically acquired through social observation.

Universal Design for Learning principles offer practical application of these theoretical foundations, advocating for multiple means of representation, expression, and engagement to accommodate learner variability. For students with genetic syndromes, UDL approaches prove especially valuable in addressing diverse cognitive-linguistic profiles without requiring complete curricular modifications. Additionally, the Response to Intervention framework provides systematic structures for identifying students requiring additional support and implementing tiered interventions, though adaptation remains necessary for students with known genetic conditions whose needs may not align with typical RTI trajectories.

2. SYNDROME-SPECIFIC COGNITIVE-COMMUNICATIVE PROFILES

Understanding the distinctive cognitive and communicative profiles associated with specific genetic syndromes provides essential foundation for designing targeted educational interventions. While individual variability exists within each syndrome, recognizable patterns emerge that inform instructional approaches, accommodation strategies, and support structures. This section examines five conditions, highlighting their educational implications while acknowledging the complexity of genotype-phenotype relationships.

Figure 2. Syndrome-specific cognitive-communicative profiles

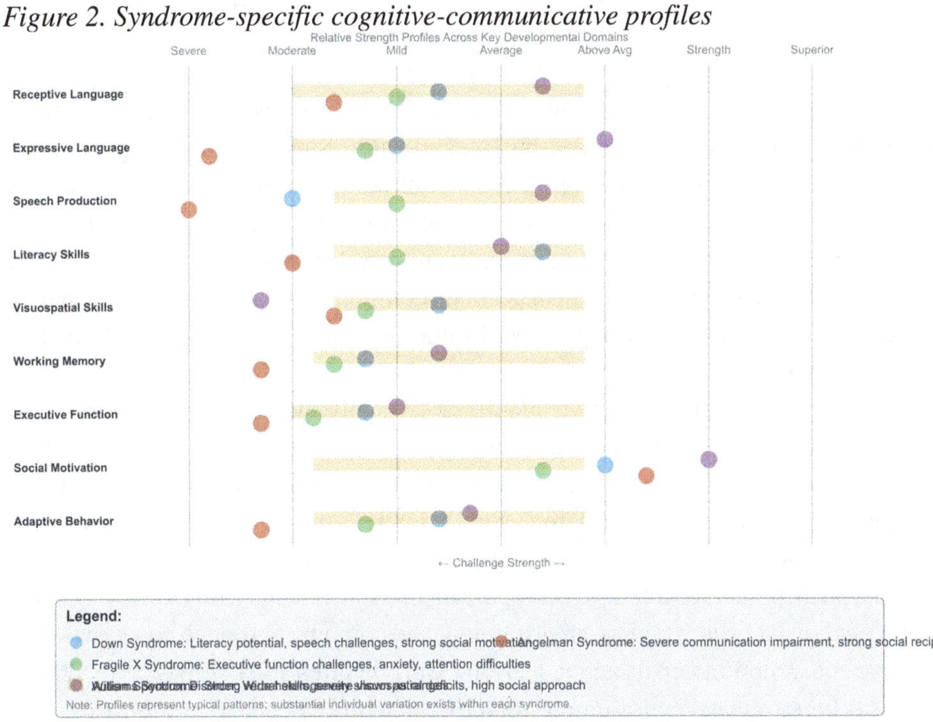

Figure 2 presents a comparative visualization of relative strengths and challenges across nine developmental domains for five genetic syndromes: Down syndrome, Fragile X syndrome, Williams syndrome, Angelman syndrome, and autism spectrum disorder. Domains assessed include: receptive language, expressive language, speech production, literacy skills, visuospatial skills, working memory, executive function, social motivation, and adaptive behavior. The visualization highlights distinctive profiles that inform educational intervention approaches, with particular attention to the substantial heterogeneity in autism spectrum disorder shown as ranges rather than single points. This figure helps educators understand syndrome-specific patterns while recognizing individual variability.

2.1 Down Syndrome: Literacy Potential Despite Speech Challenges

Down syndrome, resulting from trisomy 21, presents a characteristic profile wherein speech production abilities often lag behind receptive language and reading potential. Recent research challenges historical underestimations of literacy capacity in individuals with Down syndrome, revealing that reading abilities may exceed spoken language competence when appropriate instruction is provided (Buckley et al., 2024). This dissociation between speech production difficulties and literacy potential has profound implications for educational programming.

Speech production challenges in Down syndrome stem from multiple factors including motor planning difficulties, anatomical differences affecting the oral mechanism, and auditory processing weaknesses. Studies employing acoustic analysis reveal that speech intelligibility remains compromised even when speakers attempt clear or loud speech modifications, suggesting that simple behavioral cueing proves insufficient without systematic intervention (Darling-White & Jaeger, 2024). Educators must therefore distinguish between comprehension abilities—which may be relatively stronger—and expressive limitations that do not necessarily reflect cognitive capacity.

The cognitive profile in Down syndrome typically includes strengths in visual processing and social understanding alongside challenges with verbal working memory, executive function, and sequential processing. These patterns suggest educational approaches emphasizing visual supports, routine-based instruction, and explicit teaching of organizational strategies. Technology integration shows particular promise, with parents and caregivers reporting that individuals with Down syndrome engage extensively with tablets, smartphones, and computers, though concerns about passive consumption versus active learning warrant attention (Morris et al., 2024).

Early literacy intervention emerges as critical, with evidence suggesting that reading instruction should commence early and leverage visual-orthographic strengths.

Social communication interventions targeting pragmatic skills, turn-taking, and conversational participation demonstrate feasibility and preliminary efficacy in young children with Down syndrome, particularly when implemented by trained parents in naturalistic contexts (Stojanovik et al., 2024). The combination of parent-mediated interventions and school-based literacy programming offers comprehensive support addressing both oral and written language development.

2.2 Fragile X Syndrome: Behavioral and Pharmacological Considerations

Fragile X syndrome results from a CGG repeat expansion in the FMR1 gene, leading to reduced or absent FMRP protein production. This molecular disruption affects synaptic plasticity and neural connectivity, manifesting in intellectual disability, attention difficulties, social anxiety, and autism-like features. The neurobehavioral phenotype creates distinctive educational challenges requiring coordinated medical, behavioral, and instructional interventions (Protic et al., 2022).

Cognitive abilities in Fragile X syndrome span a wide range, though most affected males experience moderate intellectual disability while females demonstrate milder impairment due to X-inactivation patterns. Executive function deficits, particularly in working memory and inhibitory control, significantly impact academic performance. Visual-spatial processing and mathematics prove particularly challenging, contrasting with relatively stronger verbal abilities in some individuals, though language development typically shows delays. School-aged girls with Fragile X syndrome demonstrate cognitive abilities and adaptive behavior that, while below typical expectations, often exceed their academic achievement, suggesting that educational programming may not fully capitalize on existing capacities (Jordan et al., 2023).

Behavioral characteristics including social anxiety, sensory sensitivities, attention difficulties, and autism spectrum features fundamentally shape educational experiences. The Fragile X syndrome behavioral phenotype includes gaze aversion, hand-flapping, and perseverative speech patterns that may interfere with classroom participation and peer relationships. Understanding these behaviors as neurobiologically based rather than volitional proves essential for appropriate intervention. Sensory modifications to classroom environments—reducing auditory and visual stimulation, providing movement breaks, offering fidget tools—often prove more effective than behavioral contingencies alone.

Early intervention combining behavioral therapy with targeted pharmacological treatment shows promise in optimizing developmental trajectories. Medications addressing attention, anxiety, and mood dysregulation may enhance educational access, though medication alone proves insufficient without appropriate instructional modifications (Winarni et al., 2012). Neurodevelopmental research increasingly emphasizes critical periods during which interventions may exert maximal effects, with early childhood representing an optimal window for plasticity-based interventions (Milla et al., 2023). Educational teams must therefore maintain close collaboration with medical providers, recognizing that pharmacological management may influence attention, behavior regulation, and learning capacity.

2.3 Williams Syndrome: Verbal Strengths Contrasting Visuospatial Weaknesses

Williams syndrome, caused by a microdeletion on chromosome 7q11.23, presents one of the most striking cognitive dissociations in neurodevelopmental syndromes: relatively preserved verbal abilities alongside severely impaired visuospatial construction. This distinctive profile challenges educators to provide appropriately differentiated instruction that neither underestimates linguistic competence nor overestimates nonverbal reasoning abilities (Palikara et al., 2018). Individuals with Williams syndrome typically demonstrate sociable, gregarious personalities with strong interest in social engagement, yet this social approach orientation paradoxically co-occurs with difficulties interpreting social cues and managing peer relationships.

Language abilities in Williams syndrome often exceed expectations based on nonverbal IQ, with particular strengths in vocabulary and grammatical complexity. However, pragmatic language—the social use of language in context—frequently proves challenging. Individuals may demonstrate verbose, tangential speech with difficulty maintaining conversational topics or reading listener interest. Educational programming must therefore address both the form and function of language, ensuring that strong structural language skills translate into effective communication.

Visuospatial construction deficits manifest across tasks requiring integration of parts into wholes, spatial relationships, and motor planning. Mathematics proves particularly challenging, with difficulties extending beyond calculation to include spatial aspects of number concepts, geometry, and graphical representation. Educational approaches must provide extensive concrete manipulatives, verbal mediation of spatial concepts, and recognition that rote verbal learning may not reflect conceptual understanding.

Anxiety represents a pervasive concern in Williams syndrome, with specific fears often developing around sounds, animals, heights, and social evaluation. These fears significantly impact educational functioning, potentially limiting participation in physical education, assemblies, field trips, and other school activities. Novel therapeutic approaches incorporating play and humor demonstrate promise in addressing specific fears while maintaining engagement (Klein-Tasman et al., 2023). Educational transitions prove particularly anxiety-provoking, with students with Williams syndrome showing elevated anxiety during the transition from primary to secondary school despite their social interests (Sideropoulos et al., 2024).

Despite growing clinical recognition of Williams syndrome, educational research remains limited compared to more prevalent conditions. Intervention studies demonstrate concerning lack of diversity in participants, predominantly including White individuals with limited representation of other racial and ethnic groups (Shin et al., 2024). This homogeneity in research samples raises questions about generalizability and highlights the need for more inclusive research practices. Recent neuroscience research utilizing virtual reality assessments reveals complex social cognition profiles, suggesting that traditional assessments may incompletely capture the social processing abilities and challenges in Williams syndrome (Urgesi et al., 2024).

2.4 Angelman Syndrome: Severe Communication Impairment and Alternative Systems

Angelman syndrome results from loss of function of the maternally inherited UBE3A gene on chromosome 15q11-q13, leading to severe intellectual disability, absent or minimal speech, motor difficulties including ataxia, and a characteristic behavioral phenotype featuring frequent laughter and happy demeanor. The severity of communication impairment in Angelman syndrome necessitates early implementation of augmentative and alternative communication systems and requires coordinated multidisciplinary intervention (Duis et al., 2022).

Communication abilities in Angelman syndrome vary with genetic mechanism, with deletion cases typically showing more severe impairment than uniparental disomy or imprinting center mutations. Most individuals develop little or no functional speech, though receptive language typically exceeds expressive abilities. Alternative communication systems—including sign language, picture exchange communication systems, and electronic speech-generating devices—prove essential for functional communication. Educational programming must prioritize communication access as foundational for all other learning.

The cognitive profile includes severe intellectual disability with particular strengths in visual matching and social reciprocity. Attention difficulties, hyperactivity, and sleep disturbances frequently interfere with educational participation. Motor difficulties, particularly ataxia and tremor, affect fine motor skills necessary for writing and other academic tasks, reinforcing the necessity of alternative communication modalities. Genotype-phenotype correlations demonstrate that deletion cases show more severe neurodevelopmental outcomes across domains compared to other genetic mechanisms, though all individuals require substantial support (Mertz et al., 2014).

Educational programming for students with Angelman syndrome requires specialized expertise in severe/profound intellectual disability and alternative communication. Consensus standards emphasize multidisciplinary assessment and intervention addressing communication, motor development, behavioral supports, and medical management including seizure control (Duis et al., 2022). School-based teams must coordinate closely with medical providers, particularly given the high prevalence of epilepsy requiring medication management that may affect alertness and learning.

Overlap between Angelman syndrome and autism spectrum disorder, particularly in communication and social domains, has led to autism diagnoses in some individuals with Angelman syndrome. However, the distinct genetic etiology and behavioral phenotype warrant syndrome-specific intervention approaches rather than autism-focused programming alone (Peters et al., 2004). Educational teams must understand both the similarities and differences between these conditions to provide appropriate support.

2.5 Autism Spectrum Disorder: Heterogeneous Profiles Requiring Individualization

Autism spectrum disorder represents a genetically and phenotypically heterogeneous neurodevelopmental condition characterized by differences in social communication and restricted, repetitive behaviors or interests. Unlike the monogenic conditions previously discussed, autism involves complex polygenic inheritance with hundreds of contributing genetic variants. This heterogeneity demands highly individualized educational programming, as cognitive abilities range from intellectual disability to superior intelligence, and language abilities span nonspeaking to hyperlexia.

Communication profiles in autism vary extensively. Some autistic individuals remain nonspeaking throughout life, requiring robust alternative communication systems. Others develop functional speech but demonstrate pragmatic language difficulties affecting conversational reciprocity, narrative coherence, and perspective-taking. Still others exhibit advanced structural language with challenges in social-emotional language understanding. Educational assessment must therefore evaluate multiple dimensions of communication competence rather than relying on general language scores.

Cognitive profiles similarly demonstrate wide variability. While earlier estimates suggested that approximately 70% of autistic individuals had co-occurring intellectual disability, more recent research indicates that many individuals previously classified as having intellectual disability were inadequately assessed using measures inappropriate for autistic cognition. Some autistic individuals show spiky profiles with significant scatter across cognitive domains, performing exceptionally in specific areas while showing delays in others. Executive function challenges affecting planning, organization, and flexibility appear common across the autism spectrum regardless of overall intellectual ability.

Educational transitions present particular challenges for autistic students. Difficulty with change, need for predictability, sensory sensitivities, and social-communicative differences can make transitions between educational settings, grade levels, or activities stressful. Systematic transition planning proves essential, requiring coordination among sending and receiving educational settings, families, and students themselves. Research on transition to school for young autistic children emphasizes the importance of environmental preparation, social skill development, and individualized support planning (Marsh et al., 2017).

3. SCHOOL-BASED INTERVENTION APPROACHES

Effective school-based interventions for students with genetic syndromes integrate evidence-based practices addressing communication, cognition, and academic access. This section examines intervention approaches organized by primary focus area, recognizing that comprehensive programming requires integration across domains. Interventions range from syndrome-specific protocols to transdiagnostic approaches applicable across conditions. Implementation fidelity, family partnership, and cultural responsiveness emerge as critical factors mediating intervention effectiveness.

3.1 Communication Interventions: From Augmentation to Social Pragmatics

Communication interventions must address both form (phonology, morphology, syntax) and function (pragmatics, social use), with emphasis shifting based on individual profiles. For students with Down syndrome, augmentative communication approaches including speech-generating devices and visual supports enhance expressive communication while literacy instruction proceeds. Parent-implemented augmented communication interventions show promise with young children with Down syndrome, though effects demonstrate individual variability requiring careful monitoring and adjustment (Romski et al., 2023).

Early social communication intervention focusing on prelinguistic skills, joint attention, and gesture use demonstrates feasibility for young children with Down syndrome when delivered by trained parents in everyday contexts. Results from feasibility randomized controlled trials indicate that families can implement interventions with fidelity, though recruitment and retention challenges highlight the need for accessible, low-burden approaches (Stojanovik et al., 2024). School-based extensions of parent-mediated approaches require systematic training for educational staff and ongoing consultation.

For students with Williams syndrome, pragmatic language intervention targeting conversation skills, topic maintenance, and audience awareness addresses the dissociation between structural language strength and functional communication challenges. Explicit instruction in social communication rules, combined with video modeling and peer-mediated interventions, shows promise. Given the elevated anxiety in Williams syndrome, communication interventions must incorporate emotional regulation strategies and gradual exposure to socially challenging situations.

Students with Angelman syndrome and minimally speaking autistic students require robust alternative and augmentative communication systems implemented comprehensively across settings. Research supports starting AAC early rather than waiting for prerequisite skills, as communication access facilitates rather than impedes development. High-tech speech-generating devices offer advantages of voice output and expandability, while low-tech systems including picture exchange and sign language provide backup communication modalities. Educational teams must commit to total communication approaches ensuring all adults in the student's environment can both model and respond to alternative communication.

3.2 Cognitive and Academic Interventions: Targeted Support for Learning

Cognitive interventions target executive functions, working memory, attention, and processing speed—abilities foundational for academic learning. Given that many genetic syndromes affect these domains, explicit instruction and environmental supports prove essential. Strategy instruction teaching students how to approach tasks systematically, self-monitor, and organize information demonstrates effectiveness across syndromes. Visual supports including schedules, checklists, and graphic organizers scaffold cognitive demands and reduce working memory load.

Literacy instruction for students with Down syndrome should capitalize on relative strengths in whole-word reading and visual processing while addressing phonological awareness deficits. Balanced approaches combining sight word instruction with systematic phonics, explicit comprehension strategy instruction, and abundant reading practice optimize outcomes. Technology-based reading programs show promise, particularly when they incorporate speech synthesis allowing students to hear text read aloud, though effectiveness varies individually (Morris et al., 2024).

Mathematics instruction must address syndrome-specific cognitive profiles. For students with Williams syndrome, mathematics presents particular challenges given visuospatial deficits. Interventions should minimize spatial demands initially, use verbal mediation extensively, provide concrete manipulatives with explicit teaching about their symbolic meaning, and recognize that rote calculation may exceed conceptual understanding. For students with Fragile X syndrome, mathematics anxiety and avoidance prove common, requiring systematic desensitization, explicit teaching of anxiety management strategies, and celebrating small incremental progress.

For autistic students, Universal Design for Learning principles prove particularly relevant, providing multiple means of representation (visual and auditory information), expression (demonstrating knowledge through various modalities), and engagement (connecting to special interests). Special interests can be leveraged as motivational tools, entry points to curriculum, and contexts for developing academic skills. However, balance must be maintained between capitalizing on interests and expanding the repertoire of topics and activities.

3.3 Behavioral and Social-Emotional Interventions

Behavioral interventions address challenging behaviors interfering with learning and social participation. For students with Fragile X syndrome, antecedent-based interventions modifying environmental triggers prove more effective than consequence-based approaches alone. Sensory modifications, providing warning before transitions, reducing demands during periods of dysregulation, and teaching replacement behaviors demonstrate effectiveness. Parent-mediated therapy incorporating behavioral principles while respecting family priorities and cultural contexts shows promise across genetic syndromes (Alfieri et al., 2022).

Social skills interventions must balance skill development with environmental modification and peer education. Teaching neurotypical peers about genetic syndromes, modeling accepting interactions, and facilitating structured social opportunities creates inclusive environments while explicit social skills instruction addresses specific deficits. For students with Williams syndrome, despite superficial sociability, explicit instruction in friendship skills, conflict resolution, and safety awareness proves necessary given vulnerability to exploitation.

Anxiety interventions prove critical across syndromes. Cognitive-behavioral approaches adapted for developmental level, graduated exposure to feared situations, teaching physiological regulation strategies, and environmental accommodations reducing anxiety triggers demonstrate effectiveness. Novel approaches incorporating play and humor show particular promise for children with Williams syndrome, making exposure therapy more engaging and less threatening (Klein-Tasman et al., 2023). For autistic students, anxiety often relates to sensory overwhelm, unpredictability, or social demands, requiring targeted environmental modifications rather than solely individual-focused interventions.

3.4 Technology-Mediated Interventions: Promise and Considerations

Technology offers powerful tools for supporting students with genetic syndromes, from augmentative communication devices to educational software and artificial intelligence systems. Survey research indicates high rates of technology use by individuals with Down syndrome, particularly tablets and smartphones, though parents express concerns about passive versus active engagement (Morris et al., 2024). Educational applications must be carefully selected based on learning objectives rather than entertainment value, with active involvement preferred over passive consumption.

Artificial intelligence systems specifically designed for individuals with Down syndrome represent an emerging area, though systematic review reveals limited empirical evaluation of effectiveness. Qualitative synthesis emphasizes the importance of social approaches to AI development, involving individuals with Down syndrome and families throughout design processes to ensure systems meet actual needs and respect user autonomy (Dellunde & Moyà-Köhler, 2025). Educational applications of AI must balance technological capabilities with meaningful human interaction essential for social-emotional development.

Virtual reality technologies show promise for assessment and intervention across genetic syndromes. VR environments allow controlled presentation of social scenarios, spatial navigation tasks, and anxiety-provoking situations while maintaining safety and control. Recent research demonstrates that VR-based social cognition assessments reveal nuanced patterns in Williams syndrome not captured by traditional measures (Urgesi et al., 2024). However, implementation barriers including cost, technical expertise requirements, and potential sensory overwhelm must be addressed before widespread educational adoption.

Table 1. Syndrome-specific educational challenges, evidence-based interventions, and transition planning considerations

Syndrome	Key Educational Challenges	Evidence-Based Interventions	Transition Planning Considerations
Down Syndrome	• Speech production difficulties • Verbal working memory deficits • Executive function challenges • Sequential processing weaknesses	• Early literacy instruction leveraging visual strengths • Augmentative communication systems • Parent-mediated communication interventions • Technology-supported learning	• Ensure AAC systems transfer across settings • Emphasize inclusive placement with supports • Address independence and self-advocacy skills • Consider post-secondary education options
Fragile X Syndrome	• Social anxiety and gaze aversion • Attention difficulties and hyperactivity • Sensory sensitivities • Mathematics challenges • Executive function deficits	• Early intervention with pharmacological support • Sensory environmental modifications • Antecedent-based behavioral interventions • Structured routines and visual supports • Anxiety management strategies	• Gradual exposure to new environments • Coordinate with medical providers • Maintain consistent behavioral supports • Address sensory needs in new settings
Williams Syndrome	• Severe visuospatial deficits • Mathematics difficulties • Pragmatic language challenges • Specific fears and anxiety • Social vulnerability	• Verbal mediation of spatial concepts • Concrete manipulatives for mathematics • Pragmatic language intervention • Play-based exposure therapy for fears • Social safety instruction	• Proactive anxiety management during transitions • Extended familiarization periods • Address safety awareness and vulnerability • Support peer relationship development
Angelman Syndrome	• Absent or minimal speech • Severe intellectual disability • Motor difficulties (ataxia) • Attention and hyperactivity issues • Seizure management	• Comprehensive AAC implementation • Multidisciplinary coordination • Total communication approaches • Motor skill support for communication access • Functional skill emphasis	• Ensure all staff trained in AAC systems • Coordinate medical and educational services • Focus on functional independence skills • Plan for ongoing significant support needs
Autism Spectrum Disorder	• Social communication differences • Restricted interests and repetitive behaviors • Sensory processing differences • Executive function challenges • Variable cognitive-language profiles	• Universal Design for Learning approaches • Visual supports and schedules • Special interest integration • Explicit social skills instruction • Highly individualized programming	• Early and comprehensive transition planning • Environmental preparation and familiarization • Student-centered goal setting • Address predictability and change management • Systematic post-secondary planning

4. EDUCATIONAL TRANSITIONS: CRITICAL JUNCTURES REQUIRING COORDINATED SUPPORT

Educational transitions represent pivotal periods requiring heightened attention and coordinated support. Transitions occur at multiple points—from early intervention to preschool, preschool to elementary school, between grade levels, elementary to middle school, middle to high school, and high school to post-secondary outcomes. Each transition presents unique challenges while sharing common support needs. For students with genetic syndromes, successful transitions require planning that extends beyond academic readiness to encompass social-emotional preparation, environmental familiarization, and systemic coordination.

Figure 3. Transition timeline & support intensity

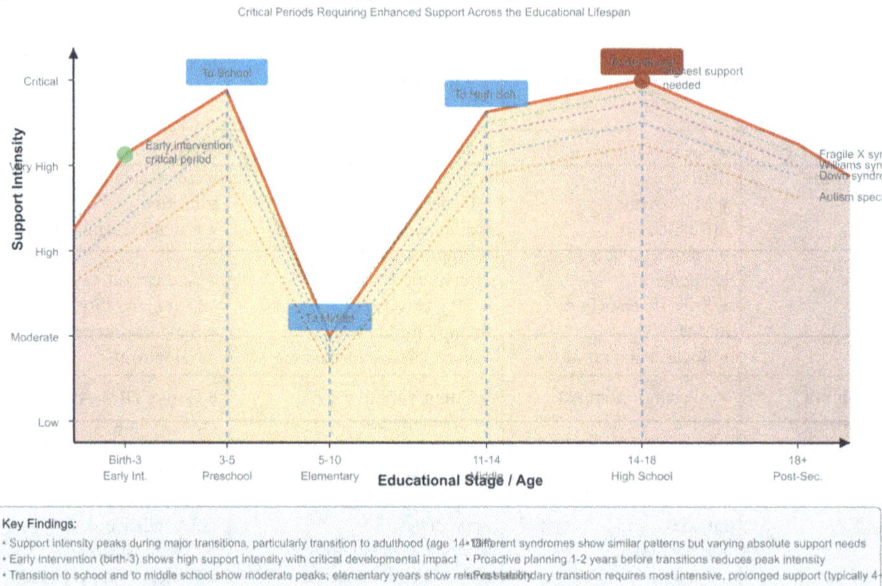

Figure 3 Depicts the trajectory of Support intensity required across the educational lifespan for students with genetic syndromes, highlighting critical transition periods demanding enhanced coordination and resources.

4.1 Transition to School: Establishing Foundations

The transition from early intervention or preschool to formal schooling marks a significant milestone involving new routines, expectations, and social demands. For autistic children, this transition has received particular research attention, revealing that preparation must address multiple domains including social skills, communication, self-regulation, and adaptive behavior (Marsh et al., 2017). Successful transitions involve both preparing the child for school and preparing the school for the child—modifying environments, training staff, and establishing support systems before school entry.

Environmental familiarization proves critical. Pre-transition visits allowing children to experience the school building, meet teachers, and practice routines reduce anxiety and increase predictability. Visual schedules, social stories, and video modeling can prepare students for new expectations. For students with Williams syndrome or Fragile X syndrome, gradual introduction to larger, noisier environments helps manage sensory and social anxieties. Schools must gather detailed information about individual needs, including communication systems, sensory preferences, behavioral supports, and medical considerations.

Cross-system collaboration between early intervention providers and schools ensures continuity of effective strategies. Information sharing should include not just formal assessment results but practical insights about what works—communication approaches, behavioral antecedents and responses, motivational strategies, and family preferences. Families serve as primary sources of expertise about their children and must be positioned as equal partners in transition planning rather than passive recipients of services.

4.2 Between-Level Transitions: Navigating Increased Complexity

Transitions between educational levels—particularly from primary to secondary school—involve substantial environmental and expectational changes. Secondary schools typically feature larger campuses, multiple teachers, increased academic demands, and more complex social hierarchies. For neurodivergent students, these changes prove particularly challenging. Research specifically examining the primary-to-secondary transition for neurodivergent children, including those with Williams syndrome and autism, reveals elevated anxiety levels during this period (Sideropoulos et al., 2024).

Preparation for secondary school should begin well before the actual transition, ideally a full school year in advance. Students benefit from explicit teaching about new school structures including class schedules, locker use, cafeteria procedures, and expectations for independence. For students with Down syndrome or Angelman syndrome requiring significant support, careful planning ensures that communication systems, assistive technology, and personal care needs can be met in the new environment. Middle and high school personnel require training in syndrome-specific characteristics and evidence-based supports, as secondary teachers often have limited special education preparation.

Maintaining inclusive placement during transitions proves challenging but important. Research examining educator perspectives on inclusion for students with Down syndrome reveals that successful inclusion requires adequate resources, appropriate training, collaborative relationships among staff, and administrative support (Boundy et al., 2023). Without these structural supports, transitions may result in more restrictive placements rather than continued inclusion with enhanced supports.

4.3 Transition to Adulthood: Post-Secondary Outcomes and Planning

The transition from high school to adult life represents the most consequential educational transition, determining long-term outcomes in employment, independent living, community participation, and quality of life. Federal legislation in many countries mandates transition planning for students with disabilities, yet implementation quality varies substantially. For autistic adolescents, research examining individualized education programs reveals that transition planning often begins late, includes limited student and family input, and emphasizes compliance over individualized goal-setting (Hughes et al., 2023).

High-quality transition planning requires several components. First, assessment must extend beyond academic skills to include vocational interests, independent living skills, community participation abilities, and self-determination. Second, planning must begin early—ideally by age 14—allowing time for skill development and exploration of options. Third, students must be centered in their own planning, with supports provided for meaningful participation including communication accommodations and decision-making scaffolds. Fourth, family involvement must be cultivated while respecting student autonomy and recognizing cultural variations in family roles.

Transition planning quality proves particularly variable for autistic students. Analysis of IEPs reveals that many lack measurable post-secondary goals, comprehensive present levels of performance addressing all transition domains, or coordinated activities linking school programming to post-school outcomes (Ruble et al., 2022). Improving transition planning requires systematic IEP review protocols, training for IEP team members, student and family education about transition processes, and accountability mechanisms ensuring implementation of written plans.

Ecological systems theory provides valuable framework for transition planning, emphasizing that successful transitions require addressing multiple system levels simultaneously. In Thailand, systematic application of Bronfenbrenner's ecological model to transition planning for autistic youth emphasizes family support, school-community collaboration, policy development, and cultural considerations (Wongkittirungrueang & Cheausuwantavee, 2025). This multi-level approach recognizes that individual skill development alone proves insufficient without supportive environments and systems facilitating adult participation.

4.4 Continuity and Coordination: Essential Elements Across Transitions

Regardless of specific transition type, certain elements prove universally important. Information transfer between settings must be comprehensive, timely, and accessible. Written reports alone prove insufficient; face-to-face meetings allowing dialogue, question-asking, and relationship-building facilitate more effective knowledge transfer. Families should be encouraged to create transition portfolios documenting effective strategies, preferences, and histories that can be shared with new educational teams.

Consistency in key supports—particularly communication systems and behavioral interventions—must be maintained across transitions. Discontinuity in augmentative communication approaches, for example, can result in communication regression and frustration. When changes in approaches prove necessary, they should be introduced gradually with training provided to all relevant parties. Peer relationships should be supported through transitions when possible, as familiar peers provide social continuity and support amid other changes.

Ongoing monitoring following transitions proves essential, as difficulties may emerge only after initial adjustment periods. Scheduled check-ins with families, systematic data collection on academic and behavioral progress, and willingness to modify supports based on emerging needs demonstrate responsive educational practice. Transitions should be conceptualized not as discrete events but as processes extending before and after the actual change in setting.

5. INDIVIDUALIZED EDUCATION PROGRAMS: QUALITY INDICATORS AND IMPLEMENTATION

Individualized Education Programs serve as foundational documents guiding educational services for students with disabilities, yet IEP quality varies substantially. High-quality IEPs demonstrate several characteristics: comprehensive present levels of performance synthesizing formal and informal assessment data; measurable annual goals addressing priority areas; specification of evidence-based services and supports; clear articulation of least restrictive environment considerations; and meaningful family and student participation in development. For students with genetic syndromes, IEPs must incorporate syndrome-specific knowledge while maintaining individualized focus.

5.1 Present Levels of Performance: Foundation for Programming

Present levels of academic achievement and functional performance must provide comprehensive pictures of student strengths and needs across domains relevant to educational participation. For students with genetic syndromes, this requires assessment addressing communication (receptive and expressive language, pragmatics, alternative communication), cognition (attention, memory, executive function, processing speed), academic skills (reading, mathematics, written expression), adaptive behavior (self-care, social skills, independent functioning), and behavioral/emotional regulation.

Assessment approaches must be culturally and linguistically appropriate, consider syndrome-specific characteristics, and include multiple methods beyond standardized testing. Dynamic assessment examining learning potential with supports, curriculum-based measurement tracking progress in actual instructional materials, behavioral observation in natural contexts, and family and student input all contribute to comprehensive understanding. Syndrome-specific assessment considerations prove important; for example, standard IQ tests may underestimate abilities in autistic students or those with significant motor impairments like Angelman syndrome.

Present levels should describe not just deficits but strengths and preferences that can be leveraged in instruction. For students with Williams syndrome, present levels should acknowledge both strong verbal skills and visuospatial challenges. For students with Down syndrome, visual learning strengths and literacy potential should be documented alongside speech production difficulties. The relationship between present levels and goals must be clear, with goals addressing priority needs identified through comprehensive assessment.

5.2 Goals and Objectives: Measurable and Meaningful

IEP goals must be measurable, allowing objective determination of progress, and meaningful, addressing skills that enhance educational access and functional independence. Goals should specify the skill to be developed, conditions under which performance will occur, criteria for success, and timeline for achievement. For students with genetic syndromes, goals must balance syndrome-specific needs with individual priorities and family values.

Communication goals for minimally speaking students should prioritize functional communication—making requests, sharing information, asking questions, expressing preferences—using appropriate alternative modalities. For students with Down syndrome, goals might address both speech intelligibility and use of supplementary AAC systems. Academic goals should reference grade-level standards when appropriate while acknowledging that alternate achievement standards may be necessary for some students with more significant cognitive disabilities.

Transition goals become required at specified ages (typically 14 or 16 depending on jurisdiction) and must address post-secondary education/training, employment, and independent living when appropriate. Research on transition IEP quality reveals that many transition goals lack measurability or connection to student preferences and strengths (Ruble et al., 2022). High-quality transition goals should be derived from age-appropriate transition assessments, reflect student and family input, and connect to coordinated activities within the IEP.

5.3 Services and Supports: Specification and Intensity

IEPs must specify special education and related services with sufficient detail to ensure implementation fidelity. Service specifications should include frequency (how often), duration (how long), and location (where provided). Vague language like "as needed" or "consultation" without quantification proves insufficient for accountability. For students with genetic syndromes requiring multiple services—speech-language therapy, occupational therapy, physical therapy, behavioral support—careful coordination prevents scheduling conflicts and ensures integrated service delivery.

Related services should be educationally necessary rather than provided merely because they might be beneficial. For students with Angelman syndrome, physical therapy addressing motor skills affecting educational access (mobility within school, fine motor skills for communication device use) qualifies as educationally necessary. Decisions about service intensity should be data-based, with progress monitoring informing adjustments. Response to intervention frameworks can guide service intensification when students fail to make adequate progress with current supports.

Accommodations and modifications must be specifically described rather than listed generically. Extended time alone may prove insufficient for students with processing speed difficulties; specification of exactly how much additional time and under what conditions proves more actionable. For students with Williams syndrome experiencing mathematics difficulties, appropriate modifications might include reduced problem sets, calculators for computation allowing focus on concepts, and verbal explanation opportunities supplementing written responses.

5.4 Participation and Collaboration: Stakeholder Engagement

Meaningful family participation in IEP development requires more than technical compliance with notification requirements. Families should receive information in accessible formats and languages, be supported in understanding educational jargon and processes, and be positioned as equal team members whose expertise about their children proves essential. For culturally and linguistically diverse families, attention to cultural values regarding disability, family structure, and educational priorities proves critical for authentic partnership.

Student participation in IEP meetings should be encouraged and supported from early ages, with accommodations provided to enable meaningful involvement. For minimally speaking students, alternative communication systems must be available during meetings. For students with intellectual disabilities, preparation before meetings including pre-teaching vocabulary and concepts, visual supports during meetings, and focused agendas addressing priority topics facilitate participation. Self-advocacy skills including expressing preferences, identifying strengths and needs, and participating in goal-setting should be explicitly taught and practiced.

Collaboration among IEP team members must extend beyond annual meetings to ongoing communication and coordination. Regular communication between general and special educators, related service providers, and families ensures consistency and allows rapid problem-solving when difficulties arise. For students with genetic syndromes requiring medical management, communication with healthcare providers proves important, though careful attention to privacy regulations must be maintained.

6. INCLUSIVE EDUCATION: PRINCIPLES, PRACTICES, AND CHALLENGES

Inclusive education—the principle that students with disabilities should be educated alongside typically developing peers in general education settings to the maximum extent appropriate—has gained increasing international acceptance. However, philosophical commitment to inclusion often exceeds practical implementation capacity. For students with genetic syndromes, successful inclusion requires not just physical placement but meaningful participation, academic access, social belonging, and individualized support within general education contexts.

6.1 Foundations of Inclusive Practice

Effective inclusive education rests on several foundational elements. First, administrative leadership must actively support inclusion through resource allocation, professional development, and expectation-setting. Research examining inclusion for students with Down syndrome reveals that educator perceptions of their roles, available resources, and administrative support significantly influence inclusion success (Boundy et al., 2023). Without adequate resources and support, even well-intentioned educators struggle to implement inclusive practices effectively.

Second, collaborative relationships among general educators, special educators, and related service providers prove essential. Co-teaching models, where general and special educators share instructional responsibility, show promise but require careful planning, defined roles, mutual respect, and scheduled collaboration time. Consultation models, where special educators support general educators in implementing accommodations and modifications, require ongoing communication and problem-solving. Regardless of specific model, collaboration must be structured and supported rather than assumed to occur naturally.

Third, general education curriculum must be made accessible through Universal Design for Learning principles. Rather than creating entirely separate curricula for students with disabilities, UDL advocates for designing instruction with flexibility from the outset—providing multiple representations of content, multiple means for students to demonstrate learning, and multiple pathways for engagement. For students with genetic syndromes, UDL reduces need for extensive individualized modifications while supporting diverse learning needs.

6.2 Educator Preparation and Support

General education teachers often feel unprepared to support students with significant disabilities, particularly those with genetic syndromes they may have limited knowledge about. Professional development must address both general special education competencies and syndrome-specific information. Understanding that behaviors in Fragile X syndrome stem from neurobiological differences rather than willfulness, or that students with Williams syndrome may demonstrate strong verbal skills masking conceptual misunderstanding, proves critical for appropriate instruction.

Professional development should be ongoing rather than one-time, job-embedded rather than theoretical, and collaborative rather than lecture-based. Learning communities where educators share strategies, problem-solve together, and observe each other's practice prove more effective than traditional workshop formats. Access to consultation from syndrome specialists—medical professionals, syndrome-specific organizations, experienced educators—supplements general professional development.

Paraprofessional support proves critical for many students with genetic syndromes in inclusive settings, yet paraprofessionals typically receive minimal training.

Comprehensive paraprofessional preparation addressing communication systems, behavioral supports, data collection, and ethical considerations enhances effectiveness. Importantly, paraprofessional support must be implemented thoughtfully to avoid inadvertent segregation within inclusive settings—hovering proximity, excessive assistance, and interference with peer interactions can isolate students despite physical inclusion.

6.3 Peer Relationships and Social Inclusion

Academic inclusion without social inclusion proves incomplete. Students with genetic syndromes may experience social isolation even when physically present in general education classrooms. Peer relationships require intentional facilitation through multiple strategies. Disability awareness programs educating typically developing students about differences and similarities reduce stigma and promote acceptance. Structured peer support programs pairing students with disabilities with peer buddies create opportunities for relationship development, though care must be taken to avoid patronizing dynamics.

Cooperative learning structures requiring interdependent collaboration can facilitate peer interactions while supporting academic goals. Assigning meaningful roles to students with disabilities within cooperative groups—rather than creating artificial participation—demonstrates respect and provides authentic contribution opportunities. For students with communication difficulties, ensuring all group members can understand and respond to their communication systems proves essential for genuine participation.

Social skills instruction must address both individual skill development and environmental modification. Teaching students with Williams syndrome to recognize unsafe social situations or helping autistic students navigate unstructured social times addresses individual needs, while educating peers about communication differences and modeling inclusive interactions modifies environments. The most effective social interventions combine these approaches rather than placing full responsibility on students with disabilities to adapt.

6.4 Balancing Inclusion and Specialized Services

The principle of least restrictive environment requires that students be educated with nondisabled peers to the maximum extent appropriate, with removal occurring only when the nature or severity of disability prevents satisfactory achievement in general education even with supplementary aids and services. However, determining what constitutes "appropriate" and when specialized services necessitate separate settings proves complex. For students with genetic syndromes, these decisions must be individualized rather than categorical.

Some specialized services can be delivered within inclusive contexts. Speech-language therapy can occur in classroom settings with peers benefiting from language-rich activities. Occupational therapy addressing fine motor skills can be embedded in art or writing activities. However, some intensive interventions—such as discrete trial training for students with autism or systematic phonics instruction for students with Down syndrome—may require focused pull-out sessions to maximize instructional intensity and minimize distractions.

The key consideration should be whether students are making meaningful progress toward IEP goals rather than adherence to ideological positions about inclusion. Ongoing data collection documenting academic, social, and behavioral outcomes should inform placement decisions. When students struggle in inclusive settings despite appropriate supports, team discussions should examine whether additional supports might enable success or whether alternative placements might better meet needs. Conversely, when students make excellent progress in specialized settings, teams should regularly consider increasing inclusive opportunities.

7. FAMILY PARTNERSHIP AND CULTURAL RESPONSIVENESS

Families represent the constant in children's lives as educational settings, providers, and priorities change over time. Authentic family-school partnerships prove essential for supporting students with genetic syndromes, yet achieving such partnerships requires intentional effort, cultural humility, and recognition of families as experts on their children. This section examines principles and practices for cultivating meaningful family engagement while attending to cultural and linguistic diversity.

7.1 Family-Centered Practices: Beyond Compliance

Family-centered practice positions families as equal partners in decision-making rather than passive recipients of professional expertise. This approach recognizes that families possess invaluable knowledge about their children's histories, strengths, preferences, and needs that cannot be captured through formal assessment. Educational professionals must actively solicit family input, value family priorities, and recognize that families make decisions within complex contexts balancing multiple demands and resources.

Parent-mediated interventions represent one form of family partnership, training parents to implement specific strategies supporting their children's development. Research on parent-mediated therapy for children with Fragile X syndrome and

Williams syndrome demonstrates feasibility and preliminary effectiveness, though careful attention to family burden and cultural appropriateness proves essential (Alfieri et al., 2022). Parent training should be offered as an option based on family interest rather than an expectation, recognizing that some families may not have capacity or desire to serve as primary interventionists.

Communication between home and school must be ongoing, bidirectional, and accessible. Daily communication logs, email updates, phone calls, and home visits allow information exchange and problem-solving. Technology facilitates communication, with apps allowing photo and video sharing of student activities, though digital access disparities must be recognized. Communication should emphasize strengths and positive developments alongside challenges, avoiding deficit-focused narratives that position children primarily as problems to be solved.

7.2 Cultural and Linguistic Diversity: Responsive Practices

Cultural values regarding disability, family structure, educational goals, and professional authority vary substantially across cultures. Educational professionals must approach cultural differences with humility and curiosity rather than assumptions. What constitutes appropriate family involvement, acceptable intervention targets, or valued outcomes may differ based on cultural background. For example, collectivist cultures may prioritize family harmony and conformity over individual self-advocacy, requiring educators to respect these values while also ensuring student voices are heard.

Linguistic diversity requires more than translated documents. Professional interpreters should be provided for all meetings with families whose primary language differs from the school language, and interpreters should be trained in educational terminology and special education processes. Written materials should be provided in families' primary languages, using clear language without jargon. However, interpretation and translation alone prove insufficient without cultural responsiveness attending to communication styles, decision-making processes, and relationship-building.

Systematic reviews of intervention research reveal concerning homogeneity in participant samples, with limited inclusion of racially, ethnically, and linguistically diverse families. Research on Williams syndrome interventions, for instance, predominantly includes White participants (Shin et al., 2024). This lack of diversity in research samples raises questions about whether evidence-based practices generalize across cultural contexts and highlights the need for culturally responsive research and practice.

7.3 Supporting Family Well-Being

Raising children with genetic syndromes presents unique challenges and stressors alongside joys and rewards. Families may experience heightened stress related to medical concerns, financial pressures, time demands, and worry about their children's futures. Educational systems can support family well-being through multiple mechanisms. Connecting families with parent support groups, syndrome-specific organizations, and community resources reduces isolation and provides practical assistance. Respite care, counseling services, and financial assistance programs, while often outside direct educational purview, represent critical supports that educational professionals can facilitate access to.

Schools can reduce rather than add to family stress by minimizing bureaucratic burden, communicating clearly and respectfully, responding promptly to concerns, and demonstrating flexibility when possible. Scheduling meetings at times accessible to working families, providing childcare during meetings, and offering virtual participation options demonstrate respect for family constraints. Most importantly, educators should recognize family expertise and resilience rather than approaching families from deficit perspectives assuming dysfunction or pathology.

8. FUTURE DIRECTIONS AND RESEARCH NEEDS

While substantial progress has been made in understanding educational needs of students with genetic syndromes and developing effective interventions, significant gaps remain. This section identifies priority areas for future research and practice development, organized around themes emerging from the synthesis of current evidence.

8.1 Longitudinal Research on Developmental Trajectories

Most research examining students with genetic syndromes employs cross-sectional designs capturing single time points. Longitudinal research following individuals across developmental periods would illuminate trajectories, identify predictors of outcomes, and reveal critical periods for intervention. Understanding how educational supports influence long-term outcomes in employment, independent living, and quality of life would strengthen evidence for specific approaches and justify resource investments.

Cohort studies examining educational experiences and outcomes across successive birth cohorts could reveal effects of changing practices, such as increased inclusion or earlier intervention access. Natural experiments when policies change—such as implementation of new transition requirements—offer opportunities to examine policy effects. Large-scale registry studies linking genetic, medical, educational, and outcome data could address questions impossible to answer with smaller samples.

8.2 Implementation Science: From Efficacy to Effectiveness

Many evidence-based practices demonstrate efficacy in controlled research settings but encounter implementation challenges in real-world schools. Implementation science frameworks could guide systematic examination of factors facilitating or impeding adoption of effective practices. Research addressing training needs, resource requirements, organizational barriers, and sustainability would support scaling of interventions beyond research contexts.

Pragmatic trials conducted in typical school settings with usual practitioners would provide more realistic estimates of intervention effects and implementation feasibility. Hybrid effectiveness-implementation designs examining both intervention outcomes and implementation processes simultaneously would efficiently answer multiple questions. Partnership with educational agencies implementing interventions at scale could produce actionable evidence while improving practice.

8.3 Technology and Innovation

Emerging technologies offer promising possibilities for supporting students with genetic syndromes while raising important questions requiring empirical investigation. Artificial intelligence systems personalized to individual learning patterns could provide adaptive instruction, though careful evaluation of effectiveness, accessibility, and potential biases proves essential (Dellunde & Moyà-Köhler, 2025). AI-powered approaches to student assessment — including automated feedback and personalized evaluation tools — are increasingly being explored in inclusive higher education contexts, with early evidence suggesting meaningful gains in accuracy and responsiveness to individual learner needs (Agrawal et al., 2026a). Complementary work on reimagining assessment frameworks through inclusive design principles and digital innovation highlights the importance of aligning evaluation practices with the diverse capabilities of all learners, including those with genetic conditions (Gupta et al., 2026a). Modern pedagogical approaches specifically tailored to empower students with disabilities, encompassing differentiated instruction and assistive technology integration, provide a further evidence-informed foundation for inclusive practice in higher education settings (Agrawal et al., 2026b). Digital leadership frameworks are likewise playing an increasingly important role in shaping institutional contexts that enable these inclusive educational innovations to take root and scale (Gupta et al., 2026b). Virtual and augmented reality applications for social skills training, spatial skill development, and anxiety exposure warrant rigorous evaluation.

Wearable technology monitoring physiological arousal could enable real-time anxiety management support for students with Williams syndrome or Fragile X syndrome. Brain-computer interfaces might eventually offer communication access for individuals with severe motor impairments affecting traditional AAC use. However, technological innovation must be guided by identified needs and empirically evaluated outcomes rather than uncritical adoption of novel technologies.

8.4 Diversity and Equity in Research and Practice

Systematic examination of diversity in research samples reveals concerning homogeneity, with limited representation of racially, ethnically, linguistically, and socioeconomically diverse participants. This homogeneity threatens generalizability and may perpetuate inequities if interventions prove differentially effective across populations. Intentional recruitment of diverse samples, community-engaged research approaches, and examination of cultural adaptation needs would address these gaps.

Intersectionality—recognition that individuals hold multiple identities that interact to shape experiences—requires attention in both research and practice. A student with Down syndrome who is also Black, from a low-income family, and an English learner faces distinct challenges and strengths compared to a White, middle-class, monolingual English-speaking student with Down syndrome. Educational responses must attend to this complexity rather than assuming syndrome diagnosis alone determines needs and appropriate supports.

9. CONCLUSION

Educational support for students with genetic syndromes has advanced substantially, moving from exclusion and low expectations to inclusive practices grounded in evidence-based interventions and high expectations for meaningful participation and learning. This chapter has synthesized current knowledge regarding school-based support and educational transitions across five genetic conditions—Down syndrome, Fragile X syndrome, Williams syndrome, Angelman syndrome, and autism spectrum disorder—highlighting both syndrome-specific considerations and transdiagnostic principles applicable across conditions.

Several themes emerge from this synthesis. First, understanding distinctive cognitive-communicative profiles associated with specific genetic syndromes informs appropriately tailored interventions while recognizing substantial individual variability within syndromes. Students with Down syndrome benefit from literacy-focused interventions capitalizing on visual strengths and reading potential. Students with Fragile X syndrome require behavioral supports addressing anxiety and attention alongside academic instruction. Students with Williams syndrome need interventions addressing the dissociation between verbal and visuospatial abilities while managing anxiety. Students with Angelman syndrome require robust alternative communication systems and multidisciplinary coordination. Autistic students need highly individualized approaches reflecting heterogeneous profiles.

Second, educational transitions represent critical junctures requiring coordinated support extending before and after the actual change in setting. Transition planning must begin early, involve students and families as central participants, address multiple outcome domains, and ensure continuity of effective supports. Quality varies substantially in current transition planning, particularly for post-secondary transitions, highlighting the need for systematic improvement efforts.

Third, inclusive education requires not just philosophical commitment but structural supports including administrative leadership, collaborative relationships among educators, professional development, and attention to both academic access and social belonging. Implementation quality proves more important than placement location, with ongoing monitoring of student progress informing individualized decisions about least restrictive environments.

Fourth, authentic family partnership proves essential, requiring cultural responsiveness, recognition of family expertise, and attention to family well-being alongside student support. Educational systems must move beyond compliance-focused family involvement to genuine partnership positioning families as equal decision-makers.

Technology offers promising tools for supporting communication, learning, and assessment, though careful evaluation of effectiveness and attention to equity in access prove necessary. Emerging technologies including artificial intelligence and virtual reality warrant investigation while maintaining focus on meaningful outcomes and human relationships.

Despite progress, significant challenges remain. Research samples lack diversity, limiting generalizability and potentially perpetuating inequities. Implementation gaps exist between evidence-based practices and typical practice. Longitudinal research examining trajectories and long-term outcomes remains limited. Educational systems often inadequately support successful transitions, particularly to post-secondary outcomes.

Addressing these challenges requires coordinated effort among researchers, practitioners, policymakers, and families. Research must prioritize questions with direct practice implications, include diverse samples, employ rigorous designs, and attend to implementation considerations. Practitioners require access to high-quality professional development, adequate resources, and supportive organizational contexts enabling evidence-based practice. Policies must ensure adequate funding, maintain high standards while allowing flexibility, and hold systems accountable for outcomes.

Ultimately, effective educational support for students with genetic syndromes reflects fundamental educational principles: knowing students as individuals, maintaining high expectations while providing necessary supports, partnering authentically with families, using evidence to guide practice, and committing to continuous improvement. As genetic knowledge expands and intervention approaches advance, these enduring principles provide foundation for supporting all students in reaching their potential while participating meaningfully in educational communities.

REFERENCES

Agrawal, A., Banerjee, A. R., Jhariya, M. K., Garg, N., Hashmi, I., Brar, V., Gupta, D., & Mishra, D. K. (2026a). AI-powered student assessment in higher education: Enhancing accuracy, feedback, and personalization. In Zaky, H. (Ed.), *Innovating assessment and evaluation in higher education: Inclusive practices and technological advancements* (pp. 177–202). IGI Global Scientific Publishing.

Agrawal, A., Bedekar, S., Bhadange, S., Sharma, T., Wagh, S., Mishra, R., & Gupta, D. (2026b). Modern pedagogical approaches to empower students with disabilities. In Salendab, F. (Ed.), *Teaching for inclusion in higher education: Pedagogies and digital practice* (pp. 41–66). IGI Global Scientific Publishing., DOI: 10.4018/979-8-2600-0976-5.ch002

Alfieri, P., Scibelli, F., Casula, L., Piga, S., Napoli, E., Valeri, G., & Vicari, S. (2022). Cooperative parent-mediated therapy in children with fragile X syndrome and Williams Beuren syndrome: A pilot RCT study of a transdiagnostic intervention—Preliminary data. *Brain Sciences*, *12*(1), 8. DOI: 10.3390/brainsci12010008 PMID: 35053752

Boundy, L., Hargreaves, S., Baxter, R., Holton, S., & Burgoyne, K. (2023). Views of educators working with pupils with Down syndrome on their roles and responsibilities and factors related to successful inclusion. *Research in Developmental Disabilities*, *142*, 104617. DOI: 10.1016/j.ridd.2023.104617 PMID: 37832326

Buckley, S., Burgoyne, K., & Loveall, S. (2024). Editorial: Speech, language, and literacy development in individuals with Down syndrome. *Frontiers in Psychology*, *14*, 1346494. DOI: 10.3389/fpsyg.2023.1346494 PMID: 38239463

Darling-White, M., & Jaeger, A. (2024). The impact of clear and loud speech cues on acoustic and perceptual features of speech production in adolescents with Down syndrome. *American Journal of Speech-Language Pathology*, *33*(6), 2768–2785. DOI: 10.1044/2024_AJSLP-24-00248 PMID: 39556033

Dellunde, P., & Moyà-Köhler, J. (2025). A social approach to artificial intelligence systems for people with Down syndrome: A qualitative systematic review. *International Journal of Developmental Disabilities*, *71*(1), 84–100. DOI: 10.1080/20473869.2025.2561165

Duis, J., Birch, R. M., Buchner, D. A., Segal, D., Miller, J., Tan, W.-H., & Bird, L. M. (2022). A multidisciplinary approach and consensus statement to establish standards of care for Angelman syndrome. *Molecular Genetics & Genomic Medicine*, *10*(3), e1843. DOI: 10.1002/mgg3.1843 PMID: 35150089

Gupta, D., Ashirova, A., Ilhom, J., Sanzhar, D., Giyosiddinov, M., Urozboev, K., & Nodira, E. (2026a). Digital leadership and educational transformation in ASEAN: Competencies, contexts, and strategic pathways. In Em, S. (Ed.), *Digital leadership and innovation in ASEAN education* (pp. 97–124). IGI Global Scientific Publishing., DOI: 10.4018/979-8-2600-1142-3.ch004

Gupta, D., Siddi, S., Jadeja, K., Rao, G. S., Vijayavadivu, V., & Ahire, P. (2026b). Beyond traditional testing: Reimagining assessment and evaluation through inclusive design and digital innovation. In Zaky, H. (Ed.), *Innovating assessment and evaluation in higher education: Inclusive practices and technological advancements* (pp. 1–40). IGI Global Scientific Publishing., DOI: 10.4018/979-8-3373-2130-1.ch001

Hughes, M. M., Kirby, A. V., Davis, J., Bilder, D. A., Patrick, M., Lopez, M., DaWalt, L. S., Pas, E. T., Bakian, A. V., Shaw, K. A., DiRienzo, M., Hudson, A., Schwenk, Y. D., Baroud, T. M., Washington, A., & Maenner, M. J. (2023). Individualized education programs and transition planning for adolescents with autism. *Pediatrics*, *152*(1), e2022060199. DOI: 10.1542/peds.2022-060199 PMID: 37345494

Jordan, T. L., Bartholomay, K. L., Lee, C. H., Lightbody, A. A., & Reiss, A. L. (2023). Cognition, academic achievement, and adaptive behavior in school-aged girls with fragile X syndrome. *Research in Developmental Disabilities*, *143*, 104622. DOI: 10.1016/j.ridd.2023.104622 PMID: 37939495

Klein-Tasman, B. P., Young, B. N., Levine, K., & Mohanty, E. (2023). Addressing fears of children with Williams syndrome: Therapist and child behavior in the context of a novel play-and humor-infused exposure therapy approach. *Frontiers in Psychology*, *14*, 1098449. DOI: 10.3389/fpsyg.2023.1098449 PMID: 37599735

Marsh, A., Spagnol, V., Grove, R., & Eapen, V. (2017). Transition to school for children with autism spectrum disorder: A systematic review. *World Journal of Psychiatry*, *7*(3), 184–196. DOI: 10.5498/wjp.v7.i3.184 PMID: 29043156

Mertz, L. G., Thaulov, P., Trillingsgaard, A., Christensen, R., Vogel, I., Hertz, J. M., & Østergaard, J. R. (2014). Neurodevelopmental outcome in Angelman syndrome: Genotype-phenotype correlations. *Research in Developmental Disabilities*, *35*(7), 1742–1747. DOI: 10.1016/j.ridd.2014.02.018 PMID: 24656292

Milla, L. A., Corral, L., Rivera, J., Zuñiga, N., Pino, G., Nunez-Parra, A., & Cea-Del Rio, C. A. (2023). Neurodevelopment and early pharmacological interventions in Fragile X syndrome. *Frontiers in Neuroscience*, *17*, 1213410. DOI: 10.3389/fnins.2023.1213410 PMID: 37599992

Morris, S., Farran, E. K., & Gilligan-Lee, K. A. (2024). Examining the prevalence and type of technology-use in people with Down syndrome: Perspectives from parents and caregivers. *Journal of Intellectual Disabilities*, *28*(3), 808–827. DOI: 10.1177/17446295231176121 PMID: 37201287

Palikara, O., Ashworth, M., & Van Herwegen, J. (2018). Addressing the educational needs of children with Williams syndrome: A rather neglected area of research? *Journal of Autism and Developmental Disorders*, *48*(9), 3256–3259. DOI: 10.1007/s10803-018-3578-x PMID: 29651682

Protic, D. D., Aishworiya, R., Salcedo-Arellano, M. J., Tang, S. J., Milisavljevic, J., Mitrovic, F., Hagerman, R. J., & Budimirovic, D. B. (2022). Fragile X syndrome: From molecular aspect to clinical treatment. *International Journal of Molecular Sciences*, *23*(4), 1935. DOI: 10.3390/ijms23041935 PMID: 35216055

Reilly, C., Senior, J., & Murtagh, L. (2015). A comparative study of educational provision for children with neurogenetic syndromes: Parent and teacher survey. *Journal of Intellectual Disability Research*, *59*(12), 1094–1107. DOI: 10.1111/jir.12210 PMID: 26780264

Romski, M., Sevcik, R. A., Barton-Hulsey, A., Fisher, E., King, S., Albert, A., Kaldes, L., & Walters, C. (2023). Parent-implemented augmented communication intervention and young children with Down syndrome: An exploratory report. *Frontiers in Psychology*, *14*, 1168599. DOI: 10.3389/fpsyg.2023.1168599 PMID: 37384179

Ruble, L. A., McGrew, J. H., Toland, M. D., & Findley, J. A. (2022). Individualized education program quality for transition-age students with autism. *Research in Autism Spectrum Disorders*, *91*, 101900. DOI: 10.1016/j.rasd.2021.101900 PMID: 35096138

Shin, E., Ravichandran, C., Renzi, D., Pober, B. R., McDougle, C. J., & Thom, R. P. (2024). Diversity of participants in Williams syndrome intervention studies. *Journal of Autism and Developmental Disorders*, *54*(10), 3888–3898. DOI: 10.1007/s10803-023-06088-2 PMID: 37584767

Sideropoulos, V., Palikara, O., Burchell, E., Ashworth, M., & Van Herwegen, J. (2024). Anxiety during transition from primary to secondary schools in neurodivergent children. *JCPP Advances*, *5*(2), e12262. DOI: 10.1002/jcv2.12262 PMID: 40519965

Stojanovik, V., Pagnamenta, E., Sampson, S., Jarrold, C., & Burgoyne, K. (2024). Evaluating an early social communication intervention for young children with Down syndrome (ASCEND): Results from a feasibility randomised control trial. *Pilot and Feasibility Studies*, *10*(1), 127. DOI: 10.1186/s40814-024-01551-y PMID: 39369246

Urgesi, C., Butti, N., Ferrari, E., Oldrati, V., Strazzer, S., Biffi, E., Gagliardi, C., Foti, F., Menghini, D., Finisguerra, A., Vicari, S., & Borgatti, R. (2024). New insights into social cognition in Williams syndrome from a comprehensive assessment and a virtual reality task. *Scientific Reports, 14*(1), 23562. DOI: 10.1038/s41598-024-79289-z

Winarni, T. I., Schneider, A., Borodyanskara, M., & Hagerman, R. J. (2012). Early intervention combined with targeted treatment promotes cognitive and behavioral improvements in young children with fragile X syndrome. *Case Reports in Genetics, 280813*, 1–4. Advance online publication. DOI: 10.1155/2012/280813 PMID: 23074686

Wongkittirungrueang, S., & Cheausuwantavee, T. (2025). Developing a systematic plan to enhance transitions for autistic youth in Thailand: Applying Bronfenbrenner's ecological systems theory. *Journal of Social Studies Education Research, 16*(1), 172–200. https://files.eric.ed.gov/fulltext/EJ1478321.pdf

KEY TERMS AND DEFINITIONS

Cognitive Support: Instructional strategies and tools designed to assist students with processing, memory, and problem-solving. This includes breaking down complex tasks into manageable steps, using visual aids, and providing repetitive practice to help learners with intellectual disabilities grasp and retain new information.

Communication Development: The gradual process by which children learn to understand, use, and manage language and non-verbal cues. In educational settings, this involves fostering the ability to express needs, follow instructions, and interact socially, often using assistive technology or speech therapy.

Down Syndrome: A genetic condition caused by an extra copy of chromosome 21. It typically results in mild-to-moderate intellectual disability and specific physical features. With early intervention and inclusive education, individuals can lead fulfilling lives and achieve significant milestones in their communities.

Educational Transitions: The pivotal periods when students move between different phases of schooling, such as starting kindergarten or entering high school. These shifts require careful planning to manage changes in environment, social expectations, and academic rigor, ensuring the student remains supported and engaged.

Genetic Syndromes: Conditions caused by abnormalities in an individual's genome, such as chromosomal alterations or gene mutations. These syndromes often result in distinct physical characteristics and varying degrees of cognitive or developmental challenges that require specialized medical and educational support throughout life.

School-Based Interventions: Specific programs or strategies implemented within the classroom to support students with diverse learning needs. These targeted actions—ranging from behavioral plans to specialized literacy coaching—aim to remove barriers to learning and help students achieve their individual academic and social goals.

Chapter 3
Moral and Ethical Challenges in Genetic Information, Diagnosis, and Medical Intervention

Sanjeev Kumar
http://orcid.org/0000-0002-7375-7341
Lovely Professional University, India

Pardeep Kumar
http://orcid.org/0000-0003-0308-7634
Lovely Professional University, India

ABSTRACT

Recent advances in the sphere of genetics and genomics have reinvented the system of medicine making it possible to generate early diagnosis, personalized treatment, and predictive care. However, these advancements have severe moral and ethical concerns of genetic information, diagnosis and medical intervention as well. Some of the problems that cause challenges to patients, medical professionals, and policy-makers include privacy, informed consent, potential discrimination, psychological impacts of genetic knowledge. The issue of genetic testing and the genome editing technology has become very popular and begs the question of the rationality of using such delicate information, the extent of medical practice, and what the society can expect after such human biology is fixed. The principles of personal freedom and the health goal of the community, the inequalities of access to genetic services, and their duty to their descendants in relation to hereditary risk are based on ethical concerns.

DOI: 10.4018/979-8-3373-8485-6.ch003

INTRODUCTION

The field of modern medicine has been revolutionized by the achievements of genetic and genomics and has given a unique possibility to understand human biology, pathology of illnesses and differences in the health outcomes in people. Since the human genome was sequenced, to the increased number of genome-wide association studies, the ability to investigate the genetic blueprint of an individual has changed the manner in healthcare is delivered, the way diseases are identified, and how interventions are developed. Genetic and genomic medicine has long since outgrown its former perception, and constitutes a phenomenally wide field of application, including predictive medicine to optimize drug treatment, pharmacogenomics to fine-tune drug treatment and genetic-based medicine to correct or suppress pathological processes. These inventions have assisted in changing the reactive medical records to preventive and proactive medical practice in which the clinicians have managed to utilize the genotype that is unique to the particular patient to diagnose and develop treatment plans (Clarke, 2014). The concept of personalized medicine is turning into a real one, which has led to the increased quality of the diagnosis, increased effectiveness of treatment and reduction of adverse effects. Such a genomic revolution implies vast potential benefits, but they are accompanied by several moral and ethical concerns, which are worth giving particular attention. As genetic technologies continue to be introduced in the clinical field, the questions about their usage, limitations, and position in the society have been brought up. Unlike the conventional diagnostic tests the genetic information is not only predictive but it is also very personal and in most cases it provides sensitive information about how a specific person is predisposed to a disease, how he would react to the treatment as well as whether he would even have the personality more than it is only his health to behavior, thinking and even his vulnerability to the changes in the environment (Cordeiro, 2014). The implications of such information can be devastating on both the individuals, families and communities. It can empower patients to possess information which will allow them to make informed decisions and assume responsibility of the management of their health however it can also lead to anxiety, stigmatization or discrimination in case of its abuse or misinterpretation. More to the point, genetic information is family-related and thus, the information on one person could have an impact on the other relatives who are the members of the same family and this presents a complex ethical concern regarding whether to reveal, consent and/or be accountable. The healthcare givers are thus faced with two problems of trying to maximize the value of genetic information that can be of benefit to the patients and yet safeguard the rights, privacy as well as health of their clients. A lot of clinical knowledge and the delicate feeling of legal regulations, social morals and moral principles are required to create a balance between these considerations (Kurnat-Thoma, 2020).

The recent explosion of genetic research and use in the sphere of medicine has also proven the imbalance of genetic services both in the country, and globally. The best genetic testing, counseling, and interventions tend to be concentrated in the areas that have more resources, disadvantaging the underprivileged population and contributing to the health disparities already present. This raises some pressing interrogatives to righteousness and justice in the administration of genomic medicine. The prospect of offering genetic advances to a few will be too good to be true since it will result in the social stratification of the world rather than cover it with better health outcomes (Kaye, 2023). The ethical frameworks in genetic medicine must therefore consider issues of equity, accessibility and cultural sensitivity as one of the ways in ensuring that the scientific development in genetic medicine can be enjoyed by every human being regardless of socioeconomic status, geographical location, and cultural orientation. Moreover, these frameworks also need to take into consideration the specifics of new technologies, such as genome editing, synthetic biology, and genetic analysis because of artificial intelligence, as they also introduce a new dimension of risk, uncertainty, and moral responsibility (Gainotti et al., 2018). The problem of informed consent is one of the greatest concerns of genetic medicine application. Unlike the traditional medical practice, genetic testing has enabled the creation of the information that has long term effect which is not deterministic but probabilistic and would be of interest not only to the person being tested but also to his/her family. In order to be confident that the patients are aware of the potential outcomes, constraints, and impacts of genetic testing, it is better to clarify the matter, offer concerned counseling, and concentrate on psychological and physical health. Informed consent in genetics is not just a formal requirement anymore; therefore, informed consent is a significant ethical practice that does not only respect patient autonomy but also promotes a better understanding and responsible decision making (Saulnier et al., 2018). This entails debating on the likelihood of incidental discoveries, explanation of variants of uncertain meaning and implication of predictive tests of late-onset conditions. The medical workers must address such dilemmas and make sure that they establish trust, empower their patients, and minimize harm. This can be detrimental to both therapeutic relationship and even to ethics of genetic medicine in general.

The problem of genetic medicine is a complex one in the society on top of the aspects of the individual. The genetic predispositions can also be predicted and this has repercussions in insurance, job, education and social relations which may yield to discrimination and prejudice. The policymakers, regulators and professional organizations have a role to play by coming up with rules and regulations that ensure that genetic information is not misused and at the same time encourage innovation and research. But again, this cannot always cause the same because legislation is usually a step behind science and there are still some loopholes in the saving which can compromise the rights of individuals or the confidence of the populace (Hachmeriyan et al., 2025). Moreover, the extent of social awareness about genetics is heterogeneous, and it is required to carry out educational campaigns, which will play their role in the formation of informed interests and the critical evaluation of ethical, social, and legal issues of genetic medicine. Scientific innovation and societal values discourse must be an ongoing process that must be open to the state of human right, dignity, and common good such that the genetics innovation can be oriented towards human rights, dignity and common good. The unethical concerns are also complicated by the fact that new powerful technologies such as CRISPR-mediated gene editing, gene therapy, and synthetic genomics have appeared. The interventions will cure hereditary diseases, prevent life threatening diseases, and even enhance human features, but could also go to the extremes that have been long ago laid down in the area of ethics and limitations to the manipulation of human biology. The ethical allowability of manipulation of the germline or the justifications of the medical intervention or not and the adverse effects to the future generations are issues, which raise concern. The fact that designer genes and human improvement may be possible raises the issue of what is the distinction between therapy and enhancement, what role can the process of genetic modification play in the society and what is the role of scientists, clinicians and governments to exercise caution and moral responsibility. As these technologies are being nurtured, there is a need to come up with frameworks that will provide bioethical principles, values of the people and regulation oversight to ensure that genetic interventions are carried out responsibly and fairly (on behalf of ESHG, ESHRE and EuroGentest2 et al., 2013).

Along with the technological and societal problems, there is the psychological concern of genetic knowledge that also needs to be mentioned. It is both anxiety and guilt-inducing and self-altering to learn that you have a genetic predisposition, and your life choices can be made in a completely different manner. Individuals must make complex decisions regarding reproductive planning, modifications in lifestyle, and long-term strategies of health care based on doubtful or probabilistic data. Genetic counseling is a very critical role as it is a connecting component which helps people in interpretation of results, weighing decision and handling feelings. Genuineness, cultural ability and awareness of the ethical intricacies that genetic data poses requires that a counselor is a skilled person. These arguments highlight the interdependence between the medical, ethical, and psychosocial dimensions of genomic medicine practice. Ethical concerns related to genetic medicine are important not only in the personal domain of care but also in the actions of research, the policy of the state, and the work of global health care (Bunnik et al., 2012). Research on human genetics needs to be performed following the principles of respect to persons, goodwill, and justice, and the research participant needs to be fully informed about it, the risks minimized, and the equal benefits distributed. On the same note, international collaboration in genomics should have put in place equal ethical standards to protect subjects, eliminate exploitation and improve equitable sharing of information. The policies ought to be directed at bio banking, sharing of information, intellectual property and cross borders research in which genetic information is not only a personal property but also a global resource. The practices will be developed with ethics in mind and thus the progress of science shall not outpace the respect of the morality and the benefits of the genomic medicine will be attained in a manner that will not jeopardize the dignity of the human (Hays, 2021).

GENETIC INFORMATION AND PRIVACY

Genetic medicine has resulted in proliferation of most sensitive personal information that has never existed in history. The genetic information has implications not only to the individual, but also to the relatives of the individual as compared to the traditional medical information whereby the implication is only of the individual. Such an anomaly renders the maintenance of confidentiality and protection of privacy graver. The problem of confidentiality when it is considered in reference to genetic information is not merely a question of professional professionalism, but also an essential condition of trust, good care, and acceptance of the existence of genomic technologies by the society. The more the patients are guaranteed that their personal information will remain confidential and no individual will misuse it, the more they will consent to undergo genetic testing and counseling (Clayton et al., 2018). The healthcare providers are therefore in a dilemma that they must use the genetic information to both diagnose and treat patients as well as ensure that they use the information as subtly as possible to prevent accidental exposure. The issues of genomics privacy are particularly challenging to maintain in the context of the digitalization of the healthcare system and the increasing popularity of huge databases, biobanks, and cloud computing services. Electronic health records plus genomic data result in opportunities of more personalized medicine and study, but simultaneously, exposes it to more vulnerability to data breach, hacking, and unauthorized transfer. Sometimes even de-identified data that is considered sufficient in the securing of privacy may be re-identified through cross-referencing with publicly accessible datasets. It implies that the clinicians are not the only ones who must uphold the integrity of genetic data, and this has been delegated to researchers, bioinformatical workers, data custodians, and institutional review boards. Ethics within the field implies strict data management measures, data storage measures, limited access and efficient measures of monitoring and auditing use. They should also include details on how they would use the data the patients will have and how this can be dangerous to share and also the rights of the patients to access or withdraw consent. It will require transparency in order to establish trust, especially where genetic information can be utilized to accomplish a bigger research or population study (Heath et al., 2016).

One of the greatest ethical concerns is the abuse of genetic information since it will lead to insurance, employment and social discrimination. The revelation of such information on genetic predisposition to certain diseases or conditions can be stigmatizing, can result in loss of opportunities, or even psychological pain, once disclosed in an inappropriate manner. An instance of this is that a person diagnosed to be carrying a gene with predisposing tendencies towards cancer may be denied health cover or be charged premiums. The possibility to base future performance or morbidity on genetic information may make employers tempted to utilize the genetic information to predict their future performance or morbidity, which raises some underlying equity, independence, and justice concerns. Besides ailment of an individual, improper use of genetic information can also ensure that structural injustices and endorse social prejudice persist even in a situation involving a complex genetic and environmental determinant trait (Li, 2016). These threats emphasize the necessity of ensuring that there is a consideration of critical ethical considerations, strong regulatory frameworks, and community education initiatives to avoid discrimination as useful applications of genetic information are also facilitated in relation to the healthcare and research endeavors. In order to counter such problems, numerous legal and regulatory mechanisms are put in place in countries of the world to safeguard genetic information. In the United States, a legal framework of protecting the rights of persons, including Genetic Information Nondiscrimination Act (GINA), has been put in place by enacting legislation on genetic information to discourage discrimination of the employers and health insurance companies on the genetic information of individuals, which forms a legal basis on the methods of protecting the rights of individuals (Prince & Roche, 2014). Similarly, European Union General Data Protection Regulation (GDPR) has also given special attention to the problem of data privacy and therefore, to use personal data, express consent is mandatory and has given the right to access, rectify or erase data. In the institutional level, it is also subject to ethical principles where application of that research with a genetic data should be in line with principles of confidentiality, informed consent, and minimization. To overcome the disadvantages of genetic information utility and privacy, genetic research programs and biobanks are inclined to design the governance systems that have oversight committees, anonymization procedures, and access management tools. Even despite these attempts, the issue persists and particularly in the global research environment whereby it is compounded by the various legal provisions and cultural demands making this practice more challenging

(Gerke et al., 2025). It is essential to reconcile laws, and, at the same time, live by the local norms to make sure that purity in ethics reigns, and that there is scientific advancement (De Groot, 2023).

Family consideration also borders on the considerations of ethical issues and genetic privacy. The question of disclosure is not typically a straightforward issue due to the nature of the genetic information which is shared among the relatives of a person. The effects of the genetic discoveries on the health of the siblings, the children or the other family members, are some of the moral dilemmas that patients may undergo in cases of genetic discoveries. Is it justifiable that a person discloses information about a hereditary disease even when the family members do not want to be informed? What should clinicians do in case of the ethical dilemma between the patient confidentiality and the potential of alerting at-risk family members? The responses to these questions suggest the complexity of the problem of genetic privacy and its impossibility to reduce it to the rules of non-disclosure. Ethical decision making in the given case will require being sensitive to the rights, preferences, and wellbeing of all parties involved and effective communicating and counseling to prevent potential conflicts. Privacy has some additional problems with the evolving environment of technology. The advances in genetic testing directly at the consumer, ancestry profiling and mobile health applications have made genetic information accessible to everyone, although they have opened up new avenues of data disclosure. Consumers may unwittingly give sensitive information to business entities, social networks or third-party researchers and this raises the issue of consent, ownership and responsibility of the information. Ethical practice must also be used within the community not just within the clinical context by educating the people, protecting consumers and establishing transparency and disclosure policies by the commercial providers. People should be aware of what genetic information usage means, and there should be a chance to secure the information, so that genetic science will not be misused, and there should be an overall faith in it.

Moreover, views on privacy are relative to cultural, social and ethical issues. Some of the concepts include autonomy, confidentiality and familial responsibility that vary in different societies and affect the genetic sharing, interpretation and action of genetic information. Such aspects as the way of making decisions in the family and the collective responsibility can be more emphasized in collectivist societies and less in the individualistic societies where the individual independency and privacy take greater priority. Such differences should be listened to by ethical principles and respect to the local values in the absence of violating some fundamental ethical principles of confidentiality, beneficence, and justice. Failure to deal with these cultural aspects could lead to certain ethical mistakes, misunderstandings and imbalances. The ethical management of genetic information is the most important in the ethical way of practicing genomic medicine. Clinicians, researchers, and policymakers are forced to keep confidentiality, prevent the risk of misuse, and fulfill legal and regulatory frameworks. Other than the necessity to conform, there is the moral necessity to explore the broader societal, family and cultural dimensions of genetic privacy. Protection of genetic information is not a technological or legal issue only, but one of the pillars of trust, respect and ethical standards in modern healthcare. As the genomic technologies continued to evolve, and be more actively used in clinical practice, the problem of genetic privacy protection would have to be carefully considered, the interdisciplinary cooperation would have to be given the first priority, and the formulation of the policies would have to be proactive. It is through these considerations and considerations that medical fraternity can reap the benefits of genetic information and minimize the risks by taking care of the issues in a very considered and holistic manner where equality will be promoted as well as the dignity and the rights of all individuals will be considered.

INFORMED CONSENT OF GENETIC ASPECT

Informed consent is a medical practice ethical principle, which assumes greater significance in genetic testing. As part of the comparison to the conventional diagnostic procedures the genetic tests often possess the implication, which stretches well beyond the immediate person, who is being assessed, to the biological relatives of the same person as well as the generations yet to come. The informed consent is based on the respect of patient autonomy because it is obligatory that the medical interventions to the health and well-being of a patient shall be taken by this individual as a voluntary and well-informed decision. In the example of genetics, it entails the complete reporting of the character of the test, chances, limitations, the uncertainties as well as the potential psychological, social or legal effects. Consent is not an administrative ceremony, but an on-going conversation, which allows patients to understand and bargain the complex ethical, medical and social issues of genetic information. The biggest tenet which would be identified as the background of informed consent in the genetic testing scenario is that individuals should be accorded with the freedom to make decisions based on precise, pertinent and comprehensible information (O'Neill, 2001). The patients must be informed of the purposes of the test: diagnostic, predictive, carrier screening or research study. They are expected to understand the possible outcomes that can be acquired, the extraneous facts that are not part of the initial reason of running the test, the degree of certainty of the findings. Most genetic tests are probabilistic in nature; having a gene version does not mean that one is more likely to develop a condition but it may be a predictor that one is at risk to develop the disease. The explanation of these uncertainties should be done in a proper manner using simple language omitting jargon that will cause confusion and scare to the patients. Clinicians are also expected to support the potential psychosocial impact such as anxiety, stress, or altered life planning implications or reproductive decision/long-term health monitoring implications (Vears et al., 2021).

The process of genetic risk communication is a tough one. The risk data tend to be probabilistic, complex and relies on a myriad of genetic and environmental factors. Depending on personal experience, cultural background or health literacy, risk may have different meanings and hence it may be challenging to take decisions. Considering the example that a particular person may consider a 30 percent chance of developing a condition within a lifetime something to freak out over, another person may identify it as something manageable. The healthcare providers are therefore supposed to communicate with the patient as per the level of understanding that the patient has and use visual tools, decision supporting tools and counseling techniques that increase the level of understanding and informed decision making (Lorenzo et al., 2023). Besides, the patients may not confront emotional responses (fear, guilt, or anxiety), which disturbs the process of information processing in the patients. The genetic counseling plays a crucial role in the process in taking care of these emotional elements of the process, and assisting the patients to weigh the potential benefits and harms of the testing, family implications, and make a decision based on their values and preferences. The question of informed consent on genetic testing is particularly problematic in regard to the minors and the vulnerable groups of people. Children and teenagers are not usually legally nor cognitively in a sound condition to give a fully-informed consent but testing may be required clinically to prevent or relieve health jeopardy. Most of these ethical principles indicate that unless there is immediate medical benefit, predictive or carrier testing in children is not to be conducted, and indicates the right of the child of an open future and future autonomy. As a rule, whenever some form of testing is carried out, consent is usually drawn by a parent or a guardian and in other instances when the consent can be drawn by the parent or a guardian, the consent of the child is also required (Bergner et al., 2014). Individuals who have cognitive impairment, mental illnesses or socioeconomic backgrounds are simply more vulnerable groups, and more difficult to ensure that the consent is actually informed and voluntary. It may be required as well to ensure that it is comprehended, including simplified explanations, protracted counseling sessions, and enabling decision-making model. Key Components and Challenges of Informed Consent in Genetic Testing are shown in Table 1.

Table 1. Key components and challenges of informed consent in genetic testing

Component	Description	Challenges	Ethical Considerations
Purpose of Test	Explains why the genetic test is being performed (diagnostic, predictive, carrier screening, research)	Patients may misunderstand the scope or type of test	Autonomy, clarity of information
Potential Outcomes	Results may include positive, negative, or uncertain findings; may reveal incidental information	Interpreting probabilistic or uncertain results	Non-maleficence, patient comprehension
Communication of Risk	Explaining probabilistic genetic risks and implications for health	Complexity of information, varying health literacy	Beneficence, accuracy, psychological support
Familial Implications	Results may affect siblings, parents, or extended family	Ethical dilemmas about disclosure to relatives	Confidentiality vs. duty to warn, respect for family autonomy
Consent for Minors	Obtaining parental/ guardian consent; seeking assent from children when appropriate	Balancing child's autonomy with parental responsibility	Right to an open future, protection of vulnerable populations
Consent for Vulnerable Populations	Individuals with cognitive or socio-economic limitations	Ensuring comprehension and voluntariness	Justice, inclusivity, equitable access
Direct-to-Consumer Testing	Genetic tests obtained outside clinical supervision	Limited counseling, potential misunderstanding	Responsibility, public education, transparency
Documentation	Written record of consent, including data usage and storage	Ensuring clarity and legal compliance	Accountability, ethical compliance
Ongoing Consent	Ability to withdraw or update consent over time	Patients may not fully understand evolving implications	Respect for autonomy, continuous engagement

ETHICAL ISSUES IN DIAGNOSIS AND PREDICTIVE TESTING

With the introduction of the genetic testing into clinical practice, the diagnosis of most diseases has undergone a metamorphosis with the prospects of an early diagnosis and active treatment. Despite the immense potential of these innovations in improving patient outcomes, they also have a spectrum of ethical concerns. The knowledge about the genetic predispositions may have great psychological, social and even ethical consequences on the person, and therefore, the policy-makers, clinician and even the genetic counselor must be acutely aware of this. Genetic testing may be empowering and overwhelming as compared to the conventional diagnostic tests that may present probabilistic information as regards to future health. The ethical issue in this respect must then come to a compromise between the good and the potential ill of predictive knowledge. Psychological impact on genetic knowledge can be regarded as one of the biggest problems of genetic testing in prediction and diagnosis. The realization that they carry a gene in their possession that predisposes them to disease can be anxiety-inducing, stressful, or depressing or in some cases this can lead to the change in planning of life or poor interpersonal relationship (Kothinti, 2024). Individuals may develop feelings of culpability due to the fact that there is a likelihood that the disease may be passed on to their children or they fear stigmatization in the social or workplace groups. Genetic risk is uncertain, and these emotional reactions become stiffer with the fact that individuals are not able to make decisions under uncertain conditions and attempt to assess possibilities. This affective load is the reason why pre- and post-test counseling are important in that trained professionals may go through the process of interpretation of their results, risk contextualization, and coping with patients (Andersson et al., 2016).

Predictive testing is associated with more complications due to immanent uncertainties. There are many genetic variations that predispose individuals to a condition but does not guarantee the occurrence of the condition. To give an example, a BRCA1 or BRCA2 mutation in the body can predispose the development of breast and ovarian cancer by a significant margin although not all of the carriers will actually get the illnesses. Similarly, the probability estimates obtained using polygenic risk scores of complex diseases, such as diabetes or cardiovascular, are influenced by lifestyle and environmental factors and the interaction of multiple genes. It is a very delicate kind of information to convey: patients may overconfidently eat in the outcomes, misjudge the risk (Ursin et al., 2021). This is one of the ethical considerations in predictive testing that the information should be clear, no coercion should take place and adequate support should be provided to make the decision. Regarding the autonomy, there is a necessity to make sure that the risks of misrepresentation or misuse of genetic knowledge are decreased. The other ethical dilemma is the need to create a balance between diagnosis and potential harm at an early stage. In a nutshell, preventive care, specification in the treatment and improved results of this health condition can be achieved through early disease diagnosis, yet people may be exposed to unnecessary stress, medicalization, or surgery.

Ethical considerations of diagnosis and predictive testing are even more challenging to families. Genetic information is also genetic as a result of which the test results of one person may influence other members of the family who may not have even agreed to be tested. This may create some dilemma to the clinicians on whether to share such information or not and/or how to share such to the at-risk family members to preserve patient privacy or perhaps the advantage of warning the family members about severe health risks. Ethical codes are inclined to adhere to the principle of voluntary disclosure which is supported with the help of counseling and education, yet in certain circumstances, disclosure can be ethically justified to prevent the existence of serious damages. These instances must be considered carefully, recorded and considered considering both legal and cultural provisions. Equity in genetic testing is another ethical issue. Diagnosis and prediction are often expensive and involve a high level of technology, and they are concentrated in big cities and densely populated regions, which limits access to underserved populations. Such disparity raises the issue of equality and balance where only certain parts of the society can be able to have the benefit of early diagnosis and tailor-made measures. Predictive testing should therefore be ethically practiced, but at a broader level that is outside the individual patient, yet to the society at large in order to ensure that policies that bring about fair access and curb health disparities are encouraged. These entail alleviation of financial crunch, upgrading of healthcare facilities and education and counseling that is culturally relevant to the culturally diverse communities. Informed consent and patient understanding is also complicated regarding the provision of predictive outcomes. Patients are also to be made aware of the possible medical, social, and insurance outcomes of the medical consequences. There may be misinterpretation of genetic risk and the lack of the necessity of interventions, changes in lifestyle, or social anxiety. The significant ethical work of the healthcare providers is to make sure that patients receive adequate support and education before the testing. Moreover, the introduction of direct-to-consumer genetic testing also brought about more confusion because patients were able to obtain predictive information without the aid of a professional, which would be even worse in the possibility of misinterpretation and psychological trauma.

The medical practitioners should devise mechanisms of addressing the medical, ethical, and social concerns when predictive testing is exercised in order to make sure that the medical test is exercised in a responsible, fair, and sensitive way to the need of different patients and families. As additional ethical issues arise in the development of the field of genetic medicine, new ethical considerations and policy developments, as well as educating the masses will be required to guide responsible use of diagnostic and predictive technology, so that the possibility of early diagnosis can generate health-related benefits of value and acceptable to the ethics. Key Ethical Issues in Diagnosis and Predictive Genetic Testing are shown in Table 2.

Table 2. Key ethical issues in diagnosis and predictive genetic testing

Ethical Issue	Description	Challenges	Considerations for Practice
Psychological Impact	Learning genetic risk can cause anxiety, stress, guilt, or altered life planning	Emotional distress, fear of stigma, misinterpretation of risk	Pre- and post-test counseling, psychosocial support, patient-centered communication
Uncertainty in Results	Many genetic results are probabilistic rather than definitive	Patients may overestimate or underestimate risk, leading to anxiety or poor decisions	Clear communication of probabilities, use of visual aids, repeated counseling
Early Diagnosis vs. Potential Harm	Early detection can improve outcomes but may also cause unnecessary stress or interventions	Testing for late-onset diseases with no cure (e.g., Huntington's, Alzheimer's)	Benefit-harm assessment, patient values, non-maleficence, ethical deliberation
Familial Implications	One person's results may affect biologically related family members	Confidentiality vs. duty to warn relatives	Encourage voluntary disclosure, provide guidance and counseling, consider ethical/legal frameworks
Equity and Access	Advanced testing may be limited to resource-rich populations	Health disparities, unequal access to care	Promote fair access, policy advocacy, culturally sensitive education
Informed Decision-Making	Patients may not fully understand complex genetic information	Misinterpretation of results, inappropriate health decisions	Comprehensive informed consent, plain language explanations, decision-support tools
Direct-to-Consumer Testing	Tests obtained outside clinical supervision may lack proper counseling	Misinterpretation, psychological harm, lack of follow-up	Public education, clear information from testing companies, availability of genetic counseling

MEDICAL INTERVENTION AND GENOME EDITING

With the introduction of the technological era of the gene therapy and genome editing technologies, the medical profession has entered a new stage, and genetic diseases can now be cured, prevented and even cured. The normal medical treatment of the illness in most cases is aimed at reducing the symptoms or slowing down the disease process; however, the gene-based treatment has an opportunity to correct the same causes of the diseases. Gene therapy is an initiative to correct or substitute the mutated genes or to restore the natural biological functions or inject fresh genes to dominate the disease mechanisms. At the same time, as the technology of genome editing, including CRISPR-Cas9, simplified and made it very accurate to mutate a specific set of DNA, it is a new age of human biology conquest. The technologies have transformed the paradigm of reactive care into the form of proactive, personalized and potentially curative care. However, among the potential benefits of such technologies, there is a multitude of ethical issues that place the conventional medical values, social principles, and rules in danger. The dilemma of possible good and harm is one of the major ethical issues of the application of gene therapy. The fact that the sphere of intervention is concentrated on the health improvement or restoration, however, the innovative character and complexity of the presented interventions make the situation rather unpredictable. These are the risks of genetic modification that should be considered like off-target genetic modification, immune response and other unwanted effects on other genes prior to the use of genetic modification to the vast population. Experimental processes can make part of the gene therapies as compared to the conventional therapies where decades of data have accumulated. This gray zone provides the clinicians and the researchers with the responsibility to assure the patients that they will be properly informed of the possible consequences, whether positive or negative, and that they will be provided with the actual informed consent which will indicate the complexity of the intervention. The following principles are involved in ethical practice, beneficence which is the maximization of a good, non-maleficence which is minimization of harm and transparency and honesty with patients on risks and uncertainty.

These ethical issues are enhanced with the emergence of genome editing, specifically the CRISPR technology. CRISPR renders the editing of the genome exceptionally precise e.g. potential of healing mutations which would lead to the development of extremely inherited diseases. It is, though, also allowing the editing of germline too i.e. the editing can be transferred to the future generations. This ability raises some serious ethical concerns about the ethicality to manipulate the human heredity, what could be the possible long-term consequence to the individual as well as the society and whether it has some undesirable consequence that can be actualized within a generation or so. Although the potential of germline editing to cure debilitating diseases like cystic fibrosis or Tay-Sachs disease may be correct, the ethical factor is beyond unbelievable. This is due to the fact that the unintended consequences might extend to the treated, the unborn generations and therefore, a careful approach that is thought provoking is taken. There are numerous ethical theories which advocate a conservative approach, which only allows any intervention to be made under forcefully medical grounds but not any enhancement end or electivity intervention until the safety, effectiveness and social acceptability of any intervention has been proven. Genome editing to improve human beings is one of the most controversial areas in medicine in as far as ethics is concerned. On top of the cure of diseases, there is an opportunity to edit physical strength, intelligence or even physical appearance with the assistance of the genome editing. Although all such applications are theoretically acceptable, they are contradictory to the established social norms, introduce issues of equality and equity, and may contribute to the further emergence of inequalities. The technologies of its enhancement will be provided to the largest possible number of people who could afford them, and this may result in genetic division that will proceed to generate the social stratified. Moreover, the improvement will culminate into commodification of human features, which are not the standards of perfection that cannot be achieved and avoidance of the natural diversity. The ethical consideration is devoted to the contrast between the treatment, which is meant to restore the normal functioning, and the non-medical ones, which are aimed at modifying the characteristics of a human being. Policies and guidelines that are acceptable application should also balance on scientific innovation, moral responsibility, equity and respect to the human dignity.

The ethical issues associated with the essence of gene therapies and genome editing technologies are equity and access. Cost and special infrastructural needs and concentration in urban or resource-intensive areas limit the availability to deliver inequalities in providing access to such life-changing interventions. The question of justice implies that medical innovations must be a prerogative of every person who can use them instead of the chosen ones. The solution to such imbalances can be viewed as a process of the narrowing of economic and geographical distance, as well as, provision of culturally sensitive education and communication. The health institutions and international organizations along with the policymakers could also help in the equitable distribution, access to treatments and mechanisms of funding and incentives distribution to aid in improving equity in healthcare delivery. Genome editing and gene therapy should also be done in a responsible and ethical way which should be controlled by the regulatory bodies. The pace of the technological change has been startlingly increased as well as the law and policy frameworks have failed to keep up with the change and have introduced a lack of governance and responsibility. The regulations ought to include all the principles of research, clinical study, data security, patient safety as well as long-term follow-up. The other consideration that can be made is to work with the international community since genetic research and practice do not observe the boundaries of country borders. To ensure that technology is used safely and responsibly, consistency in the monitoring systems and reporting of ethical issues should be implemented to ensure that the people do not lose trust. Genome editing has a social and cultural effect that makes ethical issues even harder.

Anxiety, hope, or ambivalence may be present in the patient in the context of gene therapy/genome editing in terms of his or her role in the experimentation. It brings in the element of the consideration complex as regards personal identity, responsibility and the morality of choice owing to the fact that, genome can be modified and this can be passed on to new generation. They need counseling and support structures, which should be provided to assist the patients to endure such tribulations hence making well-informed, voluntary, and value decisions. Additional ethical principles that are applied to the research ethics are clinical and social ethics. The research and trial of gene therapies should possess ethical concerns of high standards such as of respect of persons, beneficence and justice. A clinical trial should be utilized in a way that would reduce the risk, offer a fair participation in the trial besides ensuring that the participants were aware of the consequences of participating in the trial. This particular care is required on the case of vulnerable populations (e.g. children or individuals with limited consent capacity) so as to regulate autonomy and exploitation. Ethical principles of genetic research are transparency, peer review and accountability. The possibilities of the genome editing and the prospect of revolutionizing medicine with the help of gene therapy is enormous and it has given hope to the previous victims of the incurable diseases in which the genetics of the diseases holds no significance. Meanwhile, the quality of the ethical consideration in such technologies is extremely high to achieve the balance between the innovation and responsibility. Protection of patient safety, informed consent, equity, and the implications to the society and intergenerational is the highest to put into consideration. Ethical deliberation should be priori, interdisciplinary and interlayered and should encompass the contributions of scientists, clinicians, ethicists, policy makers and lay people.

The medical intervention and genome editing is a new healthcare benefit that is characterized by the enormous potential in science as well as an identical risk to the moral weight. Gene therapy and CRISPR technologies promise to cure and prevent genetic disorders, but they also have complicated issues of risk, consent, intergenerational impacts, enhancement and impacts to the society. Special attention to these problems should be paid, in particular, to the ethical standards, successful regulation control, fair access, cultural sensitivity, and sustained contact with the patients, their families, and the community. Only safe, responsible, and morally upright approach to implementing the transformative potential of the genome editing can bring the potential to a reality in a manner safe and responsible and ethical thought of the society.

GENETIC MEDICINE IMPLICATION ON THE FAMILY AND THE SOCIETY

Genetic medicine also enhances the power of influence on the family and the whole society in general by providing the incredible possibilities of preventing the diseases, revealing the diseases on their first stages and treating the maladies in a specific manner. Contrary to the traditional medical information, genetic information is a relation: knowing that an individual is somehow mutated can somehow foretell that biological relatives will also be the same. Interrelationship of genetic knowledge provides certain ethics, legal and social concerns, such as the duty that individuals owe to their family members, the equitable provision of health care of genetic health care, and the tension between the national health concern and individual rights. The discussion of such barriers presupposes the expertise of family relationships, principles of cultures, and social expectations and draws attention specifically to the issue of privacy, consent, and justice. Among the essential aspects of genetic medicine is the fact that it may be necessary to make an individual disclose to the family members the dangers that they may inherit. Particularly, when the patient is positive on the basis of BRCA1 mutation, his/her siblings or children might possess this mutation too and they are likely to suffer breast cancer and ovarian cancer. The moral issue is, would the patient be given the consent to disclose the information to the family members, and to what level is it the duty of the medical professionals to disclose the information disclosed? On the one hand, it is the ethical concern of patient confidentiality and autonomy as by the ethical principle medical information people are free to address their issues. Conversely, concealing the risk can lead to a scenario where the affected family of the at-risk would be unable to prevent the risk or even seek early interventions that would make the damage possible. Ethical models will be more inclined to promote voluntary disclosure, which is facilitated by counseling instilling the skills of disclosing sensitive genetic information to the patients. There are cases where the potential harm to the relatives or other persons is a high risk and the harm can be avoided, then a bit of disclosure among the medical staff is ethically acceptable, but the balance between confidentiality, patient rights and potential good to other persons must be considered. Social attitudes, insurance policies and employment are also intervened by genetic data social impacts. One of the issues that are likely to arise is the aspect of genetic discrimination within the health insurance scheme, life insurance or even employment that will result in stigmatization or isolations of people based on their genetic pattern. It has legal and regulatory provisions, including the Genetic information nondiscrimination act (GINA) of the United States that is aimed at preventing misuse of genetic information, but has loopholes in application and coverage. It is more pressing to train and sensitize the society to promote good application of the genetic information and stigma to enable people take good decisions about the testing without fear of being socially and economically stigmatized.

It also makes the issue of autonomy of individuals and social good more complicated because of the issue of the collective health. The use of genetic information can be done in a way that promotes the preventative diseases, screening and resource allocation measures that would be beneficial to the entire population. The fact that the risk groups of some hereditary diseases could be identified can aid in organizing the screening campaigns, early prevention, and prevention which will positively impact the health of the entire population. To make the personal genetic information a societal matter is, nonetheless, ethically strained: a person does not necessarily want his or her genetic information distributed, but such refusal will negatively impact the functioning of the population wide activities. Ethical systems focus on creating a balance between the autonomy respect and the principle of beneficence at the society level. The conflicting priorities can be resolved with the help of such strategies as voluntary participation, aggregation of data with anonymity, and a strong protection strategy towards privacy which will result in the achievement of the objectives of public health. The role of the ethical guidance, counselling, and policy formulation is of high concern due to the distinctiveness of the family responsibility, social exigencies, and the health problems of the population. The medical professionals should assist the patients in recognizing the individual and the overall connotations of the genetic data and instruct them on the complicated choices of disclosure, testing and preventive interventions. Such policies have to be such that ensure the rights of individuals are not neglected, and that equity and elimination of discrimination and, yet, allowing the legitimate use of genetic information in research and to the common good. This is so because cultural competence and cultural sensitivity is required because the ethical requirements are not viewed in the same manner across the societies and the communities. The ethical frameworks must be flexible to the various values but must cover the major tenets of justice, beneficence, non-maleficence and respect of autonomy. Besides these, genetic medicine has social consequences that lead to the problem of intergenerational justice. The current rulings on genetic procedures, whether it is genetic testing, genetic therapy, or genetic editing, can impact the future generations. The ethical factor should be the long-term effects of the taken actions with references to the pros and cons of the possible benefits of the action against the risks of the unthinkable dangers. This is the view which supports the strict regulation, openness in governance and engaging community in coming up with responsible application and use of genetic technologies. Overall, the ethical issues of genetic medicine in general, as it applies to the family and the society, are challenged with complicated ethical dilemmas, which must be deliberated, counselled, and developed with strict policy. People are obliged to their families in terms of the introduction of risks, and the societies will have to struggle with the problem of fairness, availability, and reasonable use of genetic information. Some of the most important ethical considerations would be protecting privacy and the promotion of healthy societies, balancing individual freedom and the overall good, and fair access to the best genetic risk management. To fight these issues, clinicians, ethicists, policymakers, and communities must be involved in order to combine the ethical values with the cultural understanding, social responsibility, and patient-centered care. The health care systems will not only be in a position to reap maximum benefits of the concept of scientific advances, but also minimize the prospects of the potential abuse of the concept in question and protect human dignity, justice, and respect of personal rights.

INEQUALITY AND JUSTICE AND GENETIC MEDICINE

The rapid development of genetic medicine has presented a high potential of enhancement in human health as well as has shown the immense pomposity in provision of genetic services. Although technologies (genome sequencing, predictive tests, treatment according to genes) may be potentially used as an opportunity to diagnose, prevent, and treat diseases in the early stage, not every population utilizes such technology equally. The socioeconomic status, physical location and healthcare infrastructure and systemic inequities may be more likely to limit the access and create serious ethical concerns about justice, fairness, and social responsibility. Genetic medicine should have fair access to prevent the further worsening of the current health disparities besides to make sure that the fruits of scientific advancement are distributed throughout the society. It is expressed in the differences in the access to the genetic service on several levels (Kumar et al., 2025). It is expected that poor neighborhoods or the rural population will create a major obstacle to genetic testing, counseling, and advanced therapy. Such obstacles may be a small number of medical institutions in the area, a lack of trained specialists, treatment and examination costs too much, and they lack insurance. In developed countries, healthcare is developed in such a way that the services are urbanized or delivered to people with more developed socioeconomic background and neglect vulnerable populations. The resulting inequalities are likely to create unequal health outcomes, as only a section of the population, will be in a position to anticipate and treat their health issues, as the rest of the population is left at high risk of acquiring genetic diseases which could have been avoided. To eliminate these inequalities, the policy planning, resources and structural interventions should be availed to offer more genetic services to different population groups.

Another valuable attribute of just genetic healthcare is cultural sensitivity. The former, cultural beliefs, and social norms necessitate ethical inclusiveness that acknowledges that the attitude towards genetic testing, revelation of the findings, and medical treatment is inflicted with the aid of cultural beliefs, social norms, and previous experiences. To take the example of some communities, they can be very structured in the decision-making process regarding family or community and others with individual freedom. The attitudes towards genetic testing or therapeutic interventions, specifically, the germline editing or prenatal screening, can be fostered by religious, ethical, and philosophical ideologies. The medical staff should discover these cultural peculiarities in a respectful and subtle manner and make sure that the patients can be informed and helped in a manner that does not oppose their values (Talukder et al., 2024). The cultural competence of providing genetic counseling and communication and service delivery involves the establishment of trust and the minimization of misunderstandings and empower the patients to make decisions in a way that reflects their own and cultural orientation. Ethical inclusivity is also based on the under-served and marginalized population actively being taken into consideration in the procedure of establishing and delivering genetic services. In the past, people have been divided into parts that have not been addressed in research study hence causing gaps in knowledge on genetic risks, response to treatment, and prevalence among various segments of people. Such exclusion does not only kill the extrapolation of scientific outcomes, but it also claims injustices in healthcare outcomes. This inclusivity can be achieved in the sense that the various populations are enlisted in the studies, the education programs are culturally sensitive and participation barriers non-existent. Moreover, the language barrier and the health literacy and socioeconomic barrier are also to be taken into consideration as all people have to be capable of receiving the discoveries in the field of genetic medicine. The ethical models focus on the importance of justice that connotes the fact that the resources must be distributed equally, the accessibility of the interventions must be equal, and the needs of historically disadvantaged groups must be met.

The intervention policy is the critical role that is played in ensuring equity in genetic medicine. Governments and health agencies may explore the ways of mitigating the financial strains, preparing more skilled employees and assistance in bringing the genetic services in the primary care and community health systems. I think the insurance of the genetic testing, counseling and therapies should be covered in a way that will restrict the out-of-pocket expenditure of the patients or the at high risk or underserved segments of the population. By government funding in the genetic research and infrastructure, the government can make sure that the new developments are benefiting a greater number of the population and not just a small section of the society. The policies are also needed to manage and assess access disparities, gaps in service delivery and service provision correction policies. The two approaches that can be utilized during the promotion of fair access are public engagement and education. The establishment of awareness of the genetic risks, test possibilities and prevention will empower the people to make informed decisions, request them to participate in genetic research and to build trust in the health care structures. The myths can be shattered by the culturally sensitive educational campaigns which can instill genetic services acceptance in the different communities against the myths against genetic conditions as well as inculcating the acceptance of genetic conditions. Besides this, the isolation of the community leaders, patient advocates, and local organizations in the process of designing and outreach of the program will contribute to the relevance, accessibility, and effectiveness. The policies and programs should also be sensitive to the experiences, values and concerns of the people to whom they are addressed so that ethical based inclusion is enhanced.

Technological solutions are also opportunities on improving access. Genetic counseling and education can be used through Genealogy and education on genetic counseling and health Telemedicine; it will be possible to use telemedicine based on the use of mobile health applications and digital counseling systems to provide genetic counseling and education to remote or underserved populations. The implementation of these innovations must be done in a carefully considered manner that would guarantee privacy of the data, their security and equal accessibility. Technology is not an adequate resource to eradicate the disparities but can act as a medium of facilitating structural changes, policy programmes and culture competent care. Fair genetic medicine by itself, along with personal access, should be also concerned with the factors of the societal level. The health systems should make sure that the funds available on the genetic services are distributed in manners that do not encourage the existing inequities. The balancing process of conflicting needs may be carried out using prioritization systems, moral principles and open decision-making system where high-risk populations, vulnerable communities and under-served historically should receive the relevant attention. The international level of cooperation is also very impressive as the unequal distribution of the genetic services on the international level illustrates that there is the necessity of the international assistance and the dissemination of the knowledge and the policy making. Genetic medicine equity is both local and global as an obligation to social justice, human rights and responsible use of the scientific research. Finally, but not the least, genetic medicine must be promoted in terms of equity, which must be achieved by being regularly reviewed and flexible. The access strategies that have been utilized effectively in the past may be not effective with the changes in technologies, and service delivery, patient outcomes, and barriers to care should be assessed in the course of time. Changes in patient feedback, community feedback, and healthcare provider feedback can be made to programs, policies, and educational initiatives (Obaid et al., 2025). In the context of ethical responsibility, some alertness is necessary to ensure that the genetic medicine breakthroughs do not accidentally amplify inequalities or discriminate vulnerable groups. The equitable and inclusive genetic healthcare is based on the combination of ethical reflection, cultural competence, policy making, and community involvement. Lastly, there are equity and access which are the ethical principles of genetic medicine. Inequality in accessing services, cultural sensitivity, ethical inclusivity and policy-making should have significant roles to play in ensuring the gains of the strides achieved by genomic can be distributed equally in the society. The healthcare systems can render genetic medicine beneficial to all populations and not just the privileged and resourceful populations by addressing the structural, cultural and financial barriers and promoting more inclusive and inclusive research and education and designing more just and fair policies. Genetic healthcare equity is an ethical and feasible requirement and the long-term commitment of policymakers, caregivers and researchers and communities is required to reach the full potential genetic medicine in a fair and equal manner.

GENETIC MEDICINE GOVERNANCE, ACCOUNTABILITY AND LEGAL FRAMEWORKS

The need to have right governance, accountability and good legal systems is increasingly becoming requisite in the present circumstances of the genetic medicine that is taking an unprecedented turn at an extremely rapid rate. Genome sequencing, gene therapy, CRISPR-mediated genome editing, and predictive genetic testing presented opportunities of immense potential to improve human health, along with generating complex ethical, social, and legal problems. The possibility of creating and applying sensitive genetic data undermines data privacy, patient protection, monitoring of clinical and research activities, and international coordination. Without clear and binding adjudicating authorities, there will be possibilities of abuse, injustice and lack of trust that the medical and scientific profession can provide. Following this it is important to note that in order to observe that genetic medicine is being practiced in an ethically, safely and reasonably manner, it becomes vital to institute elaborate regulatory guidelines, institutional systems of accountability and best practice standards elsewhere in the world. Among the most significant problems in the given sphere, the presence of loopholes in the current legal and regulation framework can be mentioned. The majority of the existing legislation was developed even earlier than the high-throughput genomics technologies have become available and are thus not adequately sensitive to the complexities of the modern genetic medicine. There is a case in point of the informed consent laws, the privacy of genetic information, the liability should the results of gene therapy be positive, and the use of germline editing is either incomplete, inconsistent, or fragmented across different jurisdictions. Such regulatory delay is puzzling to the healthcare professionals, researchers, and the patients as well because they may not know what their rights, responsibilities or redress will be in case they become victims or suffer any abuse. Moreover, the rapid rate of technological development can slow down the legislative process to leave much of the genetic practice essentially unregulated until suitable policies are developed. The idea to address these gaps ought to be a proactive, progressive legislation program, which is visionary towards the technological advancement, considers the ethical principles, and harmonizes standards in the majority of the areas and in the international context.

Law and ethics the structures are companionate and need ethical control and responsibility on an institutional basis. The systematic consideration and monitoring of research and clinical practice is known as ethical oversight to ensure the adherence to ethical principles, patient safety, and the social standards. The IRBs, ethics committees and specialized genetic oversight committees have a significant role in the evaluation of the ethical implication of their intended intervention and protection of vulnerable groups and risk and benefit analysis. This is because such mechanisms hold the researchers and clinicians liable in that they not only ensure they adhere to the established ethical standards, but also they can monitor adherence. The role of institutions is not directly supervised but also trained health care workers, making sure that clinical and research practices are transparent and using the policy that guarantees patient confidentiality and autonomy is enforced. Institutional supervision will help in preventing exploitation, help instill trust into the community and enhance the ethical nature of genetic medicine. International regulations and norms are an essential indicator of the harmonization of governance in the area where it is extremely globalized. Genetic investigation, clinical trials and treatment practice are prone to transnational collaboration, and this raises the demand of shared ethical principles and regulations harmonies. Some of the organizations that provide information on the way genetic research ought to be conducted responsibly, the ethical implications of germline editing, and the informed consent are the world health organization, international society of stem cell research, and the human genome organizations. In the case of the interventions, be it international or local, such best practices matter in assuring that the practices are carried out in a safe, ethical, and consistent way. Knowledge sharing, capacity building and policy congruency are also facilitated by these guidelines and hence allow the countries with limited resources to practice responsible genetic medicine.

One of the significant areas of governance is patient privacy protection and sensitive genetic information. Genetic information is personal, and may be inclined to forecast the possibility of disease in the subject as well as in the family. The storage, sharing, and access of data should have a clear guideline through legal regulations on how the information can be avoided to be misused by the insurers, employers, or third parties the information stored. An accountability system that has penalties against malpractice, redress systems and compliance monitoring should exist. The confidentiality in the digital era also needs to be guaranteed through the incorporation of technology based security measures such as encryption and safe databases. The privacy of genetic data is not only legal necessity but the ethical need to maintain confidentiality in ensuring that there is trust required by patients to engage in genetic testing and treatments. Accountability and governance are closely related with the equity considerations. Access to genetic services should be a fairly distributed phenomenon and not exclude vulnerable groups of people in the benefits of genetic medicine in a systematic fashion, as legal and institutional arrangements should do. The control agencies can implement control mechanisms that identify the differences, establish whether the equity standards are being met and offer remedial measures. Moreover, it is recommended that the necessity to be inclusive in research enrolment, show different population in clinical trials and offer genetic services in a culturally competent manner should be exemplified using ethical principles. Governance systems that entrench equity within their core values reinforce genetic medicine. Indeed, the rapid advancement of genome editing technology, particularly the one functioning on a germline basis, suggest the need to regulate it strictly. The effects of decision-making on interventions of heritable outcome do not only have an implication to the individual patients but also to the generations to come. The overall recommendation of global community is to take a more conservative approach, and permit clinical use of germline editing only in case of high medical need, high safety information, and morality justification. The regulatory mechanisms ought to provide a no-go criterion of approval, monitoring and follow-up of the long term where the interventions ought to be executed in a responsible and accountable way. Very critical are the ethical oversight committees to review and control the outcomes of the applications, as well as amend policies, related to emerging scientific knowledge. The implication of the people is the other important thing in governance in genetic medicine. An open discussion on the benefits, negative or healthy effects of genetic interventions, promotes informed involvement and confidence in society. The agencies and government should involve the patient groups, communities and advocacy groups in the regulations, ethics and research processes. Public consultation comes in handy to ensure that the systems of governance reflect all the aspects of society, culture and community agendas and not necessarily by scientific or commercial goals. The methods of engagement might also include advisory panels, open forums, educative programs and stakeholder consultation and all this is in support of accountability, transparency and ethical responsiveness.

Situations of liability and accountability in the cases of clinical and research should also be addressed on the legal level. Genetic treatment, genome editing, and proactive testing are laden with risks and clear instructions are required to explain the position of the professionals, entitlement of the patients, and compensations. Conditions on reporting of adverse outcomes, monitoring and high-quality documentation of consent and adherence to procedures need to be mentioned as regulatory standards. The responsibility is validated by the fact that the accountability is reinforced by the routine audit checks, peer review, and enforcement procedures, which enable the adherence to the legal and ethical values. These will protect the patients and the practitioners and enhance the integrity of the genetic medicine business. Finally, genetic medical governance and responsibility ought to be dynamic and persistent. The scientific knowledge and the technological abilities are ever evolving and hence there is necessity to revamp and reformulate the laws, policies and regulation methods. Flexibility gives that the structures of governance are maintained abreast, as effective and ethical as new interventions, research findings and societal problems emerge. The real nature of the governance systems being highly responsive and transparent and being closely related to the ethical and social needs is the key to the existence of the ongoing debate of the scientists, ethicists, policymakers, and the people. The responsible and ethical genetic medicine depends on governance, accountability, and legal systems. Closing loopholes in the current regulations, strengthening institutional responsibility, adherence to the international regulations, patient confidentiality, fairness, and the community are all modifiable elements that are significant in an elaborate governance plan. A mix of the legal, ethical and social aspects can ensure the genetic medicine is safely, responsibly and fairly done and the populace is trusting the system that is in place and at the same time the science invention can do the greatest good. It is through good governance that genetic technologies are provided with a framework through which the potential of altering the health of human beings can be achieved without jeopardizing the ethical standards or social justice.

INCLUSION OF BIOETHICS IN GENETIC MEDICINE

The rapid evolution of genetic medicine is providing the human health with new opportunities in the history of humanity, and, simultaneously, it gives rise to complex ethical, social, and moral issues. Among the predictive genetic testing, the gene therapy, and genome editing, these advances require the organization of the introduction of bioethical principles into the clinical practice, research, and policy-making. Bioethics provides a methodology of how to evaluate the outcomes of genetic interventions, weigh personal rights and interests against the interests of the society, and how to make choices when there is uncertainty, risk, and great personal and social results provided. By offering the ethical rationale onto the practice of genetic medicine, health professionals, scientists, and policymakers will be capable of navigating the dilemmas of the modern genomics safely and ensuring that the advancement of science does not harm the well-being of humanity but rather does not violate any moral and social norms. This is because the core concepts of respecting autonomy, beneficence, non-maleficence, and justice are the primary concepts of bioethics that will be introduced to genetic medicine. The autonomy principle requires that the patients be at a position to make informed decisions on their genetic information, testing and treatment decisions. The genetic information can be so intimate and sentimental such that it can determine the choice of life, family planning and even social interactions. Patient-centered ethical decision-making is one of the most significant aspects of genetic medicine in terms of its application in bioethics. Compared to the majority of other fields of healthcare, genetic interventions often consider very complex, probabilistic data, which can not only affect the individual but also their family members and, in the case of germline editing, their heirs. The patients will be placed in a difficult position regarding the need to test, to disclose the findings to the family members, or to undergo gene therapies or otherwise. Ethical practice, in this respect, implies active involvement of patients in making decisions, providing them with proper explanations of risks and benefits, and taking into account emotional, psychological, and cultural factors that affect preferences of people. This counseling must be one-on-one founded on the values and beliefs among other influences in the life of the patient and interpretation of his or her knowledge regarding the consequences of the genetic information. Support, decision aids, and visual risk communication could be the means of helping patients make informed and independent decisions that rely on their priorities and their decreased anxiety and confusion. The patient-centered ethical practice may be also applied to the recognition of the decisions to decline testing or intervention as autonomy also includes the right not to act on the information available about genetic changes.

Cultural competence is one of the prerequisites of bioethical practice in genetics. The information that is genetic can be interpreted by the patient and families based on cultural, religious, and social experience. The ethical decision making must then take into account the various interpretations in which the term autonomy, family responsibility and acceptable interventions will vary under varying circumstances. What is significant is that genetic counselors and clinicians ought to be trained to navigate through such cultural complexities employing strategies that will not offend the values, but will provide the appropriate information to help in making the appropriate decisions. The practice is not only associated with enhancing ethical inclusivity, but also better patient engagement and compliance with recommendations and content with care.

There is also bioethics integration in the broader view of the society. Policies governing genetic medicine, including access, privacy of information and consent to join a study should be guided by ethical reasoning in order to enhance further fairness, equity and trust in the community. Indicatively, genetic privacy legislation should be struck at the personal privacy and the possible health benefits in society. The research inclusion policies should also be such that they allow diversity in the representation in ways that do not pose a risk to the vulnerable members of the population. Ethical systems are used to shape the decision to practice responsible use of new technology, e.g. genome editing by establishing boundaries to protect human dignity, avoid harm and ensure that any intervention is justifiable and acceptably reasonable to the society. Besides this, bioethical incorporation of genetic medicine is significant in the prediction and reduction of the unintended outcomes of genetic medicine. The availability of the advanced genetic interventions might become the cause of ethical dilemma with respect to improvement, discrimination, or social division. Trying to make inequalities more effective, create an incites to live up to genetic norms or stigmatize people with traits that cannot be altered, unless we meditate on the ethical issues, gene therapies or predictive testing can contribute to the inequalities. Ethical management requires vision, dynamism and continuous assessment of policies and practices following discovery of new issues. It is a proactive solution because the technological innovation would be pursued in a manner that would be ethically sound and in the interests of the society. Genetic medicine has brought a revolution in the medical sphere, offering an opportunity in the healthcare sector that it has never had before, early diagnosis, personalized treatment and prevention of diseases. Recent advances in genome sequencing, predictive testing, gene therapy and genome editing have ensured the vehicle through which the biology of human beings could be studied to a level that was not even thought of several years before and interventions could be formulated to alter the flow of inherited conditions and add to the health outcomes across the whole lifespan. Such scientific progress however comes with the profound moral and ethical concerns that cross the whole worlds of practice, research, and policy. The issues of privacy, informed consent, equal access, family considerations, implications in the society, and limits of medical intervention compel health practitioners, researchers and policy makers to pay special consideration to ethical issues of genetic medicine. All these problems must be argued out to give genetic innovations a positive contribution to the human health in a responsible manner and ensure that human dignity is also secured and in line with the values of the society.

The psychological and social effects of genetic information can also be highlighted as the ethical consideration. Receiving information on genetic risks can be a source of anxiety, stress, or even moral dilemma to the patients and family members and can influence life planning, reproductive choices and family relationships. The medical care providers must anticipate those effects and offer adequate counseling and help and balance out the benefits of early diagnosis and the possibility of psychological harm. Genome editing and predictive testing further introduce a layer of uncertainty and ethical sophistication particularly in cases where there is a generational implication of the act. The use of these technologies should be guided by ethical concerns keeping in mind the principles of beneficence, non-maleficence, justice, and respect towards autonomy and promote the idea of informed and thoughtful decision-making. Equity and access is one of the key problems that are connected with the fair allocation of the benefits of genetic medicine. The access inequality to genetic testing, counseling, and treatment intervention can create a potential of enhancing social and economic disparities within the healthcare environment, benefiting the populations with the resources at the disadvantage of the vulnerable populations (Petersen et al., 2016). Such differences that may result in ethical practices must be addressed proactively, and this approach can be reflected in the policies to reduce the number of financial obstacles, expand the number of healthcare facilities, and provide genetic services more sensitively to different cultures. The inclusion research philosophy, minority inclusion to clinical trials, and involvement in terms of community are also contributing factors to equitable access since all individuals can potentially benefit by using the advancement of genetic medicine.

CONCLUSION

The rapid advancements in the field of genetics and genomics have established solid possibilities of improving healthcare, turning it into more early-diagnosed, therapy-focused on individuals, and preventive medicine. However, this has prompted some grave moral and ethical issues to be posed concerning genetic information, diagnosis and medical intervention. They should pay much attention to the questions connected with the protection of the privacy of the information, the possibility of the informed consent, the likelihood of the genetic discrimination, and the inequalities of the access to the genetic services, and the psychological consequences of the genetic information. To stem such problems, there is an urgent need to establish effective ethical values, explicit policies and effective legal frameworks which could manage to keep abreast with the advances in science. Healthcare professionals, policymakers, and researchers must cooperate to make sure that the application of genetic technologies is implemented in a responsible fashion, in the process of safeguarding the rights and the human dignity of the individuals. It is also essential to spread patient-centered care and educate the population, and offer equal access to genetic services. Lastly, there is the necessity to reconcile the scientific advancement and the ethically accountable to make sure that the advances of genetic medicine prove to be beneficial to the society in general. Genetic innovations can be applied in ethically, socially and morally acceptable way by applying bioethics principles to medicine and social issues and concerns to the best of the present and future generation.

REFERENCES

Andersson, P. L., Petersén, Å., Graff, C., & Edberg, A.-K. (2016). Ethical aspects of a predictive test for Huntington's Disease: A long term perspective. *Nursing Ethics*, *23*(5), 565–575. DOI: 10.1177/0969733015576356 PMID: 25899725

Bergner, A. L., Bollinger, J., Raraigh, K. S., Tichnell, C., Murray, B., Blout, C. L., Telegrafi, A. B., & James, C. A. (2014). Informed consent for exome sequencing research in families with genetic disease: The emerging issue of incidental findings. *American Journal of Medical Genetics. Part A*, *164*(11), 2745–2752. DOI: 10.1002/ajmg.a.36706 PMID: 25251809

Bunnik, E. M., Schermer, M. H., & Jw Janssens, A. C. (2012). The role of disease characteristics in the ethical debate on personal genome testing. *BMC Medical Genomics*, *5*(1), 4. DOI: 10.1186/1755-8794-5-4 PMID: 22260407

Clarke, A. J. (2014). Managing the ethical challenges of next-generation sequencing in genomic medicine. *British Medical Bulletin*, *111*(1), 17–30. DOI: 10.1093/bmb/ldu017 PMID: 25122627

Clayton, E. W., Halverson, C. M., Sathe, N. A., & Malin, B. A. (2018). A systematic literature review of individuals' perspectives on privacy and genetic information in the United States. *PLoS One*, *13*(10), e0204417. DOI: 10.1371/journal.pone.0204417 PMID: 30379944

Cordeiro, J. V. (2014). Ethical and legal challenges of personalized medicine: Paradigmatic examples of research, prevention, diagnosis and treatment. *Revista Portuguesa de Saude Publica*, *32*(2), 164–180. DOI: 10.1016/j.rpsp.2014.10.002

De Groot, N. F. (2023). Commercial genetic information and criminal investigations: The case for social privacy. *Big Data & Society*, *10*(2), 20539517231216957. DOI: 10.1177/20539517231216957

Gainotti, S., Mascalzoni, D., Bros-Facer, V., Petrini, C., Floridia, G., Roos, M., Salvatore, M., & Taruscio, D. (2018). Meeting Patients' Right to the Correct Diagnosis: Ongoing International Initiatives on Undiagnosed Rare Diseases and Ethical and Social Issues. *International Journal of Environmental Research and Public Health*, *15*(10), 2072. DOI: 10.3390/ijerph15102072 PMID: 30248891

Gerke, S., Jacoby, M. B., & Cohen, I. G. (2025). Bankruptcy, Genetic Information, and Privacy—Selling Personal Information. *The New England Journal of Medicine*, *392*(10), 937–939. DOI: 10.1056/NEJMp2415835 PMID: 40029207

Hachmeriyan, M., Levkova, M., Yahya, D., Stoyanova, M., & Dimitrova, E. (2025). Ethical and Psychosocial Issues Associated with Genetic Testing for Hereditary Tumor Predisposition Syndromes. *Health Care, 13*(8), 880. DOI: 10.3390/healthcare13080880 PMID: 40281828

Hays, P. (2021). Moral, Societal, and Ethical Issues: Claims, Consequences, and Caveats. In P. Hays, *Advancing Healthcare Through Personalized Medicine* (pp. 689–726). Springer International Publishing. DOI: 10.1007/978-3-030-80100-7_13

Heath, D., Ardestani, A., & Nemati, H. (2016). Sharing personal genetic information: The impact of privacy concern and awareness of benefit. *Journal of Information. Communication and Ethics in Society, 14*(3), 288–308. DOI: 10.1108/JICES-07-2015-0025

Kaye, D. K. (2023). Addressing ethical issues related to prenatal diagnostic procedures. *Maternal Health, Neonatology and Perinatology, 9*(1), 1. DOI: 10.1186/s40748-023-00146-4 PMID: 36737803

Kothinti, R. R. (2024). Artificial intelligence in healthcare: Revolutionizing precision medicine, predictive analytics, and ethical considerations in autonomous diagnostics. *World Journal of Advanced Research and Reviews, 19*(3), 3395–3406.

Kumar, H. V. K., A., & Kumar, S. (2025). Converging Realms of Social Health, Domestic Workers and Telemedicine Landscape: Challenges and Prospects. In P. Thaichon, P. K. Dutta, A. K. Haghi, & S. Dutta (Eds.), *Digital Disruption in Hospitality, Sustainable Hospitality* (pp. 213–228). Emerald Publishing Limited. DOI: 10.1108/978-1-83662-360-120251010

Kurnat-Thoma, E. (2020). Educational and Ethical Considerations for Genetic Test Implementation Within Health Care Systems. *Network and Systems Medicine, 3*(1), 58–66. DOI: 10.1089/nsm.2019.0010 PMID: 32676590

Li, J. (2016). Genetic Information Privacy in the Age of Data-Driven Medicine. *2016 IEEE International Congress on Big Data (BigData Congress)*, 299–306. DOI: 10.1109/BigDataCongress.2016.45

Lorenzo, D., Esquerda, M., Bofarull, M., Cusi, V., Roig, H., Bertran, J., Carrera, J., Torralba, F., Cambra, F. J., Vila, M., Garriga, M., & Palau, F. (2023). The reuse of genetic information in research and informed consent. *European Journal of Human Genetics : EJHG, 31*(12), 1393–1397. DOI: 10.1038/s41431-023-01457-y PMID: 37699995

O'Neill, O. (2001). Informed Consent and Genetic Information. *Studies in History and Philosophy of Science Part C Studies in History and Philosophy of Biological and Biomedical Sciences, 32*(4), 689–704. DOI: 10.1016/S1369-8486(01)00026-7

Obaid, A. J., Kumar Shukla, V., Dutta, S., Bhattacharya, A., & Chakraborti, S. (Eds.). (2025). *Blockchain Technology for Healthcare Applications: Challenges, Privacy, and Securing of Data*. Nova Science Publishers, Inc., DOI: 10.52305/AUFT8731

Prince, A. E. R., & Roche, M. I. (2014). Genetic Information, Non-Discrimination, and Privacy Protections in Genetic Counseling Practice. *Journal of Genetic Counseling, 23*(6), 891–902. DOI: 10.1007/s10897-014-9743-2 PMID: 25063358

Saulnier, K. M., Cinà, M., Chan, B., Pelletier, S., Dorval, M., & Joly, Y. (2018). Communication of genetic information in the palliative care context: Ethical and legal issues. *Medical Law International, 18*(4), 219–240. DOI: 10.1177/0968533218762239

Talukder, M. B., Kumar, S., & Das, I. R. (2024). Mindfulness of Digital Detoxification: Healthy Lifestyle in Tourism. In Kankaew, K., Chaudhary, S., & Widtayakornbundit, S. (Eds.), (pp. 56–71). Advances in Logistics, Operations, and Management Science. IGI Global., DOI: 10.4018/979-8-3693-1273-5.ch004

Ursin, F., Timmermann, C., & Steger, F. (2021). Ethical Implications of Alzheimer's Disease Prediction in Asymptomatic Individuals through Artificial Intelligence. *Diagnostics (Basel), 11*(3), 440. DOI: 10.3390/diagnostics11030440 PMID: 33806501

Vears, D. F., Borry, P., Savulescu, J., & Koplin, J. J. (2021). Old Challenges or New Issues? Genetic Health Professionals' Experiences Obtaining Informed Consent in Diagnostic Genomic Sequencing. *AJOB Empirical Bioethics, 12*(1), 12–23. DOI: 10.1080/23294515.2020.1823906 PMID: 33017265

Chapter 4
Early Identification, Intervention Models, and Developmental Screening

Atul Kumar
http://orcid.org/0000-0003-3859-0686
Dnyaan Prasad Global University, India

Zairullo Okboyev
Termez University of Economics and Service, Termez, Uzbekistan

Nasiba Jumaniyazova
Mamun University, Khiva, Uzbekistan

Nurjanova Sevara
Mamun University, Khiva, Uzbekistan

Gazibayeva Khadicha
Mamun University, Urgench, Uzbekistan

Tojiyev Rahmatilla
Tashkent State University of Economics, Uzbekistan

Bobanov Xurshid Abdiraxmatovich
Shahrisabz State Pedagogical Institute Teacher of Psychology, Uzbekistan

ABSTRACT

Early identification of genetic syndromes and neurodevelopmental disorders represents a critical window for intervention that can significantly alter developmental trajectories. This chapter examines contemporary approaches to developmental screening, diagnostic protocols, and evidence-based intervention models for children with genetic syndromes. Through systematic analysis of recent advances in screening technologies, including digital phenotyping and genomic workflows, we explore how multidisciplinary teams implement early detection strategies across diverse populations. The chapter synthesizes current evidence on family-centered

DOI: 10.4018/979-8-3373-8485-6.ch004

intervention approaches, naturalistic developmental behavioral interventions, and parent-mediated programs that demonstrate measurable improvements in child outcomes and family quality of life.

1. INTRODUCTION

The landscape of early identification and intervention for children with genetic syndromes has undergone profound transformation over the past decade, driven by technological innovations in genetic testing, refined screening methodologies, and accumulating evidence supporting the efficacy of early intervention programs. The imperative for early detection stems from well-established neurodevelopmental principles demonstrating that brain plasticity is greatest during the earliest years of life, creating optimal conditions for intervention to produce meaningful and lasting changes in developmental outcomes (Sandbank et al., 2023).

1.1 The Critical Importance of Early Detection

Early identification of genetic syndromes and associated neurodevelopmental challenges serves multiple essential functions within the healthcare ecosystem. First, it enables families to access appropriate medical care, therapeutic services, and educational supports during periods of maximal developmental plasticity. Second, early diagnosis facilitates genetic counseling, allowing families to make informed decisions about future family planning. Third, it provides opportunities for participation in research studies and clinical trials that may offer access to emerging treatments and contribute to scientific knowledge (Manickam et al., 2021).

1.1.1 Neurobiological Foundations of Early Intervention

The developing brain exhibits remarkable capacity for adaptation and reorganization during infancy and early childhood, with critical periods for different developmental domains occurring at specific timeframes. Synaptic density reaches peak levels during the first years of life, with subsequent pruning shaped by environmental experiences and learning opportunities. This neurobiological reality creates a compelling rationale for early intervention, as therapeutic experiences introduced during these sensitive periods can harness neuroplasticity to optimize developmental trajectories (Franz et al., 2022).

1.1.2 Shifting Paradigms in Diagnostic Approaches

Traditional diagnostic pathways for genetic syndromes often involved lengthy diagnostic odysseys, with families encountering multiple specialists over extended periods before reaching conclusive diagnoses. Contemporary approaches increasingly emphasize expedited diagnostic processes through advanced genetic testing technologies, including chromosomal microarray analysis, whole exome sequencing, and whole genome sequencing. These methodologies have dramatically reduced time to diagnosis while simultaneously increasing diagnostic yield, particularly for children presenting with congenital anomalies, intellectual disability, or complex neurodevelopmental presentations (Chaves et al., 2024).

1.2 Scope and Organization of This Chapter

This chapter provides a comprehensive examination of current knowledge regarding early identification, screening methodologies, and intervention models for children with genetic syndromes. We organize our discussion around six major themes: developmental screening tools and their psychometric properties, syndrome-specific developmental profiles and identification strategies, genetic testing and diagnostic protocols, evidence-based early intervention models, family-centered care approaches, and emerging technologies in early detection.

1.2.1 Target Audience and Applications

This chapter is designed to serve multiple audiences including pediatricians, geneticists, developmental specialists, early intervention professionals, researchers, and policymakers. Clinical practitioners will find practical guidance on screening tool selection, interpretation of genetic testing results, and implementation of evidence-based interventions. Researchers will benefit from synthesis of recent empirical findings and identification of research gaps requiring further investigation. Policymakers will gain insights into the public health implications of universal developmental screening and the economic benefits of early intervention investments.

2. DEVELOPMENTAL SCREENING: TOOLS, METHODS, AND IMPLEMENTATION

Developmental screening represents the first tier in a multi-stage process of identifying children who may benefit from further evaluation and intervention services. Unlike comprehensive developmental assessments, screening tools are designed for rapid administration, often by non-specialists, to detect children at risk for developmental delays or disabilities within broader populations.

2.1 Psychometric Properties of Screening Instruments

The utility of any screening instrument depends fundamentally on its psychometric characteristics, particularly sensitivity (proportion of children with delays correctly identified) and specificity (proportion of typically developing children correctly identified as not having delays). Optimal screening tools achieve balance between these properties, minimizing both false positives (which create unnecessary anxiety and consume assessment resources) and false negatives (which result in missed opportunities for early intervention).

2.1.1 The Ages and Stages Questionnaire System

The Ages and Stages Questionnaire (ASQ) represents one of the most widely implemented developmental screening tools globally, designed for parent completion across multiple developmental domains including communication, gross motor, fine motor, problem-solving, and personal-social skills. Recent validation studies have examined ASQ performance across diverse populations and cultural contexts, revealing important considerations regarding maternal education level, socioeconomic factors, and cultural interpretations of developmental milestones (Lockhart et al., 2023).

Research by Pitchik et al. (2023) examining concurrent validity between the ASQ and the Bayley Scales of Infant and Toddler Development in rural Bangladesh demonstrated moderate correlations across domains, with variation in performance based on specific developmental areas and age ranges. These findings underscore the importance of understanding screening tool performance characteristics within specific populations and contexts rather than assuming universal applicability of psychometric properties established in different settings.

Figure 1. Multi-tiered framework for early identification and intervention in genetic syndromes

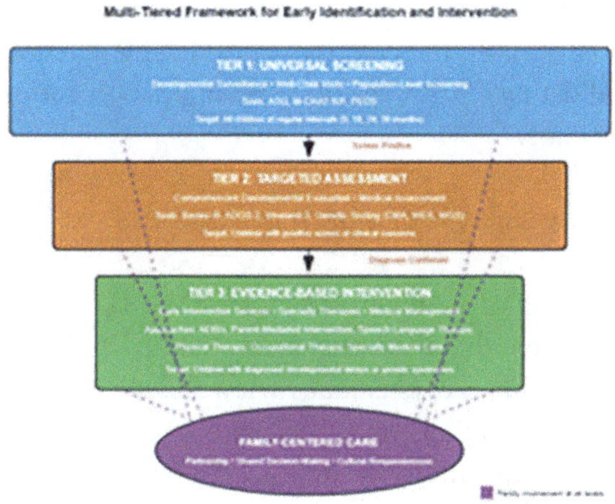

Figure 1. the comprehensive pathway from universal screening through targeted intervention, showing the integration of developmental surveillance, screening tools, diagnostic evaluation, and evidence-based intervention models. The framework emphasizes family-centered care as a central organizing principle across all tiers.

2.1.2 Meta-Analytic Evidence on Screening Accuracy

A comprehensive systematic review and meta-analysis by Rah et al. (2023) evaluated the real-world accuracy of commonly used developmental screening tests, examining data from over 100 studies. The analysis revealed considerable heterogeneity in sensitivity and specificity across different screening instruments, with performance varying based on factors including age at screening, developmental domain assessed, and population characteristics. Notably, screening tools demonstrated generally higher specificity than sensitivity, suggesting greater accuracy in identifying children without delays than in detecting those with delays.

This pattern of findings has important practical implications, indicating that negative screening results should be interpreted with caution and that ongoing developmental surveillance remains essential even when initial screening results fall within typical ranges. The meta-analysis also highlighted the importance of two-stage screening processes, where initial broad screening is followed by more targeted assessment for children with positive results.

2.2 Autism-Specific Screening Instruments

Given the high prevalence of autism spectrum disorder (ASD) and the well-established benefits of early intervention, considerable attention has focused on developing and validating autism-specific screening tools for use in primary care and community settings.

2.2.1 Modified Checklist for Autism in Toddlers

The Modified Checklist for Autism in Toddlers (M-CHAT) and its revised version (M-CHAT-R/F) represent the most extensively studied autism screening tools for toddlers aged 16-30 months. A systematic review and meta-analysis by Wieckowski et al. (2023) examined sensitivity and specificity across 48 studies, finding pooled sensitivity of 0.85 and specificity of 0.84 for the M-CHAT-R/F when using the two-stage process including follow-up interview.

These psychometric properties position the M-CHAT-R/F as an effective population-level screening tool, though the authors note important limitations including lower positive predictive value in lower-risk populations and concerns about equity in screening access and follow-up across diverse socioeconomic and cultural groups.

2.2.2 Comprehensive Review of ASD Screening and Diagnostic Tools

A broader systematic review by dos Santos et al. (2024) evaluated multiple screening and diagnostic instruments for ASD, including the Autism Diagnostic Observation Schedule (ADOS), Autism Diagnostic Interview-Revised (ADI-R), and various parent-report screening measures. The review emphasized the distinction between Level 1 screening tools (designed for universal application in general populations) and Level 2 tools (intended for children already identified as at-risk), with different psychometric expectations and clinical applications for each category.

The authors highlighted emerging approaches to autism screening, including digital technologies and artificial intelligence applications that show promise for enhancing early detection capabilities. These innovations are discussed further in subsequent sections addressing emerging technologies.

2.3 Implementation Challenges and Solutions

Despite strong evidence supporting developmental screening, implementation in real-world clinical practice faces numerous challenges including time constraints in primary care settings, limited reimbursement for screening activities, inadequate follow-up systems for positive screens, and workforce capacity limitations in diagnostic and intervention services.

2.3.1 Telehealth Applications for Developmental Screening

The COVID-19 pandemic accelerated adoption of telehealth approaches across healthcare, including applications for developmental screening and diagnosis. A systematic review by La Valle et al. (2022) evaluated telehealth methods for facilitating diagnosis in children with developmental concerns, finding that remote assessment approaches demonstrated feasibility and validity across various developmental domains and age ranges.

Telehealth screening offers potential advantages including increased access for families in rural or underserved areas, reduced travel burden, and ability to observe children in natural home environments. However, limitations include technology access barriers, concerns about rapport-building and observation quality, and need for caregiver support during assessment procedures.

3. SYNDROME-SPECIFIC DEVELOPMENTAL PROFILES AND EARLY IDENTIFICATION

Different genetic syndromes present characteristic developmental profiles, necessitating syndrome-specific approaches to screening, identification, and intervention planning. Understanding these unique patterns enables more targeted and effective early identification strategies.

3.1 Down Syndrome: Contemporary Developmental Milestones and Health Supervision

Down syndrome, occurring in approximately 1 in 700 live births, represents the most common chromosomal condition associated with intellectual disability. Recent years have seen important advances in understanding developmental trajectories and optimizing health supervision for children with Down syndrome.

3.1.1 Updated Developmental Milestones

Baumer et al. (2024) published landmark research establishing syndrome-specific developmental milestones for children with Down syndrome across multiple domains including gross motor, fine motor, communication, and adaptive skills. This work addressed a critical gap in clinical care, as previous practice relied on comparison to general population norms that did not reflect the unique developmental trajectory of children with Down syndrome.

The new milestone data enable more appropriate developmental surveillance, setting realistic expectations for families while identifying children with Down syndrome who demonstrate delays even relative to syndrome-specific norms and may benefit from additional intervention or evaluation for co-occurring conditions. For example, the median age for walking independently was established at 24 months, compared to 12 months in the general population, providing families and clinicians with appropriate benchmarks for motor development.

3.1.2 Comprehensive Health Supervision Guidelines

The American Academy of Pediatrics published updated health supervision guidelines for children and adolescents with Down syndrome (Bull et al., 2022), providing evidence-based recommendations for screening, monitoring, and management across multiple systems including cardiac, endocrine, orthopedic, sensory, and developmental domains. The guidelines emphasize the importance of anticipatory guidance, regular developmental screening, and early referral to intervention services.

Particularly relevant for early identification, the guidelines recommend hearing assessment within the first month of life, ophthalmologic evaluation by 6 months, thyroid screening at birth and regularly thereafter, and referral to early intervention services immediately upon diagnosis. This proactive approach to health supervision and developmental support reflects current understanding of the benefits of early, comprehensive care.

3.2 Autism Spectrum Disorder: Advances in Early Detection

Autism spectrum disorder presents unique challenges for early identification due to variable age of symptom onset, heterogeneity in presentation, and the behavioral nature of diagnostic criteria. Recent research has focused on identifying early markers and developing novel detection approaches.

3.2.1 Digital Behavioral Phenotyping

A groundbreaking study by Perochon et al. (2023) demonstrated the potential of digital behavioral phenotyping for early autism detection. Using computer vision analysis of video recordings during structured play activities, the researchers developed machine learning algorithms capable of distinguishing children with autism from typically developing children and those with developmental delays with high accuracy.

This approach analyzes multiple behavioral features including attention patterns, motor movements, social engagement, and response to social bids, generating objective behavioral profiles that complement traditional clinical observation. The technology shows particular promise for reducing age at diagnosis and enabling earlier intervention initiation, though questions remain regarding generalizability across diverse populations and settings.

3.2.2 Parent-Mediated Early Intervention Approaches

Recognizing the benefits of early intervention and the central role of parents in young children's learning environments, substantial research has evaluated parent-mediated intervention models for autism. A systematic review and meta-analysis by Conrad et al. (2021) examined outcomes of parent-mediated interventions, finding significant benefits across multiple domains including social communication, language development, and reduction in autism symptom severity.

These findings support the integration of parent coaching and parent-mediated strategies into early intervention programs, empowering families as active intervention agents and potentially extending intervention intensity beyond what would be possible through clinician-delivered services alone.

3.3 Fragile X Syndrome and Rare Genetic Disorders

Fragile X syndrome, the most common inherited cause of intellectual disability, presents unique considerations for early identification and intervention. Similarly, numerous rare genetic syndromes pose challenges related to delayed diagnosis and limited syndrome-specific intervention research.

3.3.1 Advances in Fragile X Screening and Intervention

Tassone et al. (2023) synthesized current understanding of fragile X-associated conditions, highlighting the importance of cascade testing (screening family members of identified individuals), early intervention focusing on language and behavioral support, and emerging pharmacological approaches targeting underlying neurobiological mechanisms. The review emphasized the variable phenotype associated with FMR1 premutation status, with implications for genetic counseling and family planning.

3.3.2 Parent Experiences with Rare Genetic Disorders

A systematic review by von der Lippe et al. (2022) examined parent experiences when children have rare congenital genetic disorders, identifying common themes including prolonged diagnostic odysseys, challenges accessing appropriate care and information, emotional burden, and resilience. The review highlighted the critical importance of support systems, access to specialized expertise, and connection with other families affected by similar conditions.

These findings underscore the need for improved approaches to rare disease diagnosis, including implementation of advanced genetic testing as first-tier evaluation, development of undiagnosed disease programs, and creation of support networks for families navigating rare genetic conditions.

4. GENETIC TESTING AND NEWBORN SCREENING INNOVATIONS

Recent advances in genetic testing technologies have revolutionized diagnostic capabilities for genetic syndromes and neurodevelopmental disorders, enabling earlier identification and more precise characterization of underlying genetic etiologies.

4.1 Clinical Guidelines for Genetic Testing

The American College of Medical Genetics and Genomics (ACMG) published evidence-based guidelines for exome and genome sequencing in pediatric patients with congenital anomalies or intellectual disability (Manickam et al., 2021). The guidelines recommend chromosomal microarray analysis as first-tier testing for patients with multiple congenital anomalies, intellectual disability, or autism spectrum disorder, with exome or genome sequencing considered when microarray results are non-diagnostic.

Figure 2. Timeline of developmental screening and key intervention points for common genetic syndromes

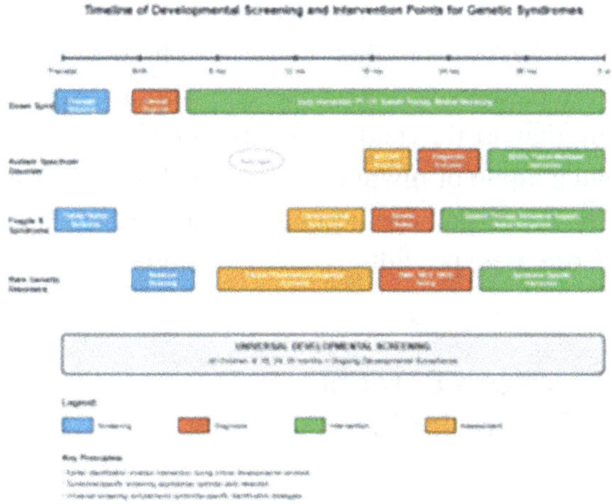

Figure 2. Critical screening timepoints from prenatal diagnosis through early childhood, highlighting syndrome-specific identification opportunities and optimal intervention initiation windows for Down syndrome, autism spectrum disorder, fragile X syndrome, and other genetic conditions

4.1.1 Diagnostic Yield and Clinical Utility

Research examining the performance of genome sequencing as a first-tier test for neurodevelopmental disorders (van der Sanden et al., 2023) demonstrated diagnostic yields ranging from 30-50%, representing substantial improvement over traditional cytogenetic approaches. Genome sequencing offers advantages including detection of sequence variants, copy number variants, and structural variants in a single test, potentially reducing time to diagnosis and eliminating the need for sequential testing approaches.

The clinical utility of genetic diagnosis extends beyond immediate medical management to include recurrence risk counseling, access to condition-specific supports and resources, connection with disease-specific organizations and other affected families, and eligibility for research participation and emerging treatments.

4.1.2 Chromosomal Microarray Analysis for Neurodevelopmental Disorders

A cohort study by Chaves et al. (2024) examined high-resolution chromosomal microarray analysis in patients with neurodevelopmental disorders and congenital anomalies, reporting diagnostic yields and variant classifications. The study emphasized the particular value of microarray analysis for autism spectrum disorder, where pathogenic or likely pathogenic copy number variants were identified in approximately 10% of cases, providing etiologic diagnosis and informing clinical management.

4.2 Expanded Newborn Screening Using Genomic Technologies

Traditional newborn screening programs focus on metabolic and endocrine conditions amenable to early treatment, using biochemical assays to detect elevated or reduced analyte levels indicative of specific disorders. Emerging approaches explore the potential for genomic newborn screening to identify additional conditions, including genetic syndromes, before symptom onset.

4.2.1 Proof-of-Concept Studies in Genomic Newborn Screening

Ziegler et al. (2025) reported results from a study implementing genome sequencing for newborn screening, targeting early actionable conditions including immunodeficiencies, metabolic disorders, and genetic syndromes amenable to preventive intervention. The study demonstrated feasibility of integrating genomic testing into newborn screening workflows, though important questions remain regarding optimal condition inclusion criteria, return of results policies, and long-term outcomes.

4.2.2 Screening for Specific Genetic Syndromes in Newborn Populations

Godler et al. (2022) described a novel genomic workflow for screening newborns for chromosome 15 imprinting disorders, including Prader-Willi syndrome and Angelman syndrome. The study screened over 16,000 newborns, identifying affected individuals before clinical symptom development and enabling early intervention initiation. This approach demonstrates proof-of-concept for expanded newborn screening targeting specific genetic syndromes, though implementation faces challenges related to cost, infrastructure requirements, and ethical considerations regarding early disclosure of diagnoses for conditions with variable presentations.

5. EVIDENCE-BASED EARLY INTERVENTION MODELS

The evidence base supporting early intervention for children with developmental delays and disabilities has expanded substantially, with particular attention to intervention approaches that demonstrate effectiveness across diverse populations and settings while remaining feasible for implementation within real-world service delivery systems.

5.1 Naturalistic Developmental Behavioral Interventions

Naturalistic developmental behavioral interventions (NDBIs) represent a family of intervention approaches that blend principles from developmental psychology and applied behavior analysis, implementing teaching within natural environments and daily routines using child-initiated activities as learning opportunities.

5.1.1 Meta-Analytic Evidence for Autism Interventions

Sandbank et al. (2023) conducted an updated systematic review and meta-analysis of early childhood autism interventions (Project AIM), examining outcomes across developmental domains, intervention types, and moderating factors. The analysis included over 150 studies and found that NDBIs demonstrated significant benefits for social communication outcomes, with effect sizes in the small to medium range.

Notably, the meta-analysis found substantial heterogeneity in outcomes across studies, suggesting that intervention effectiveness varies based on child characteristics, intervention intensity, implementation quality, and other factors. This heterogeneity underscores the need for individualized intervention planning and ongoing progress monitoring to ensure optimal outcomes for individual children.

5.1.2 Impact on Family Quality of Life

Duncan et al. (2024) conducted a systematic review and meta-analysis specifically examining whether NDBIs improve family quality of life, recognizing that intervention success should be evaluated not only through child outcomes but also through family-level impacts. The analysis found small but significant improvements in family quality of life associated with NDBI participation, with particular benefits in domains of parent confidence, family interactions, and access to community resources.

These findings support the value of family-centered intervention approaches that consider family priorities and outcomes as essential components of intervention planning and evaluation.

5.2 Speech and Language Interventions for Genetic Syndromes

Communication challenges represent common features across many genetic syndromes, necessitating targeted speech and language intervention approaches tailored to syndrome-specific profiles.

5.2.1 Interventions for Children with Down Syndrome

Seager et al. (2022) conducted a systematic review of speech, language, and communication interventions for children with Down syndrome from birth to 6 years, examining evidence for various intervention approaches including parent-focused training, direct therapy targeting specific speech and language skills, and augmentative and alternative communication systems.

The review found limited high-quality evidence supporting specific intervention approaches, highlighting a critical research gap in this area. However, available evidence suggested benefits of early intervention focusing on prelinguistic communication skills, parent responsiveness training, and multimodal communication strategies incorporating gestures and visual supports alongside spoken language.

5.2.2 Early Social Communication Interventions

Stojanovik et al. (2024) reported results from a feasibility randomized controlled trial evaluating an early social communication intervention for young children with Down syndrome (ASCEND). The intervention focused on enhancing social communication skills through parent coaching and play-based activities implemented in home settings.

Feasibility outcomes were positive, with high rates of family recruitment, retention, and intervention fidelity. Preliminary child outcomes suggested improvements in joint attention, social engagement, and early communication skills, though definitive efficacy conclusions await larger-scale trials. The study demonstrates the feasibility of implementing manualized early intervention programs for Down syndrome within community settings.

5.3 Family-Centered Care and Tele-Intervention

Contemporary early intervention increasingly emphasizes family-centered care principles, recognizing families as essential partners in intervention planning and implementation. The COVID-19 pandemic accelerated adoption of tele-intervention approaches, prompting evaluation of effectiveness and implementation considerations.

5.3.1 Family-Centered Care Processes and Outcomes

McCarthy and Guerin (2022) conducted a systematic review examining processes and outcomes of family-centered care in early intervention, analyzing factors that facilitate or impede family-centered practice. The review identified key elements of family-centered care including collaborative partnerships between families and professionals, family-directed goal setting, intervention embedded within natural environments and routines, and provision of family support and resources.

Outcomes associated with family-centered care included improved family satisfaction, enhanced family functioning and quality of life, increased parent confidence and competence, and positive child developmental outcomes. However, the review also identified barriers to family-centered implementation including time constraints, professional training limitations, and systemic factors within service delivery organizations.

5.3.2 Evidence for Tele-Intervention Approaches

Jimenez-Arberas et al. (2024) systematically reviewed evidence regarding implementation of family-centered models through tele-intervention platforms in early childhood services. The review found that tele-intervention can effectively deliver family-centered services with comparable outcomes to in-person intervention across various developmental domains and diagnostic categories.

Benefits of tele-intervention included increased access for families facing geographic or transportation barriers, flexibility in scheduling, reduced family stress associated with clinic visits, and opportunities for intervention within natural home environments. Challenges included technology access and literacy barriers, limitations in hands-on guidance and modeling, and reduced opportunities for incidental learning through observation of other children.

Figure 3. Diagnostic yield of genetic testing technologies by indication

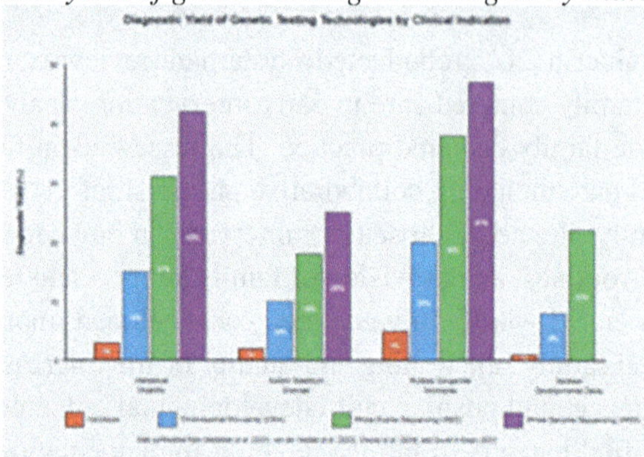

Figure 3. Comparative diagnostic yields for different genetic testing modalities (karyotype, chromosomal microarray, exome sequencing, genome sequencing) across various clinical indications including intellectual disability, autism spectrum disorder, multiple congenital anomalies, and isolated developmental delay.

6. DEVELOPMENTAL TRAJECTORIES AND LONGITUDINAL OUTCOMES

Understanding typical developmental trajectories for children with specific genetic syndromes enables more accurate prognostic counseling, appropriate expectation-setting for families, and identification of children who may benefit from additional evaluation or intervention due to development significantly below syndrome-specific expectations.

6.1 Cohort Studies of Development in Genetic Syndromes

Longitudinal cohort studies tracking development over time provide essential data regarding expected developmental trajectories, factors associated with outcome variability, and effectiveness of intervention approaches.

6.1.1 Down Syndrome Developmental and Service Utilization Patterns

Soccorso et al. (2024) analyzed data from a clinical database tracking children with Down syndrome, examining developmental progress, educational placements, and service utilization patterns. The study documented variability in developmental outcomes across individuals, with factors including early intervention participation, co-occurring medical conditions, and family socioeconomic status associated with outcome differences.

Table 1. Comparative analysis of developmental screening tools: Psychometric properties and clinical applications

Screening Tool	Age Range	Admin Time	Sensitivity	Specificity	Domains Assessed	Completion Method	Clinical Applications	Key Advantages	Limitations
Ages and Stages Questionnaire-3 (ASQ-3)	1-66 months	10-15 min	0.70-0.90	0.76-0.91	Communication, Gross Motor, Fine Motor, Problem Solving, Personal-Social	Parent-completed	Universal screening in primary care, early intervention programs	Low cost, available in 30+ languages, parent-friendly	Influenced by maternal education level, moderate sensitivity
Modified Checklist for Autism in Toddlers-Revised with Follow-Up (M-CHAT-R/F)	16-30 months	5-10 min (screen) + 5-10 min (follow-up)	0.85	0.84	Autism-specific behaviors: social communication, repetitive behaviors	Parent-completed with follow-up interview	Level 1 ASD screening in primary care	Free, well-validated, two-stage process improves accuracy	ASD-specific only, lower PPV in low-risk populations
Parents' Evaluation of Developmental Status (PEDS)	0-8 years	2-5 min	0.74-0.79	0.70-0.80	Global development, parental concerns across all domains	Parent interview	Universal screening, identifies concerns requiring referral	Brief, elicits parental concerns, guides clinical decision-making	Relies on parent awareness, requires clinical interpretation
Bayley Scales of Infant and Toddler Development-III (Bayley-III)	1-42 months	50-90 min	0.80-0.95	0.86-0.93	Cognitive, Language (Receptive/ Expressive), Motor (Fine/ Gross), Social-Emotional, Adaptive	Clinician-administered	Comprehensive diagnostic assessment (Tier 2)	Gold standard assessment, detailed developmental profile	Time-intensive, requires trained administrator, expensive
Autism Diagnostic Observation Schedule-2 (ADOS-2)	12 months-adulthood	40-60 min	0.91-0.97	0.87-0.94	Social communication, restricted/ repetitive behaviors	Clinician-administered structured observation	ASD diagnostic evaluation (Tier 2)	Comprehensive, multiple modules for different ages/ abilities	Requires extensive training, time-intensive, expensive

continued on following page

Table 1. Continued

Screening Tool	Age Range	Admin Time	Sensitivity	Specificity	Domains Assessed	Completion Method	Clinical Applications	Key Advantages	Limitations
Denver Developmental Screening Test-II (DDST-II)	0-6 years	10-20 min	0.56-0.83	0.43-0.80	Personal-Social, Fine Motor-Adaptive, Language, Gross Motor	Clinician-administered	Quick developmental surveillance	Widely known, direct observation	Lower psychometric properties, outdated norms
Vineland Adaptive Behavior Scales-3 (Vineland-3)	0-90 years	20-60 min	0.75-0.88	0.82-0.91	Communication, Daily Living Skills, Socialization, Motor Skills	Parent/caregiver interview or questionnaire	Adaptive functioning assessment for diagnosis and intervention planning	Comprehensive adaptive profile, useful across lifespan	Time-intensive, parent report may be biased
Communication and Symbolic Behavior Scales Developmental Profile (CSBS-DP)	6-24 months	15-25 min	0.88-0.89	0.82-0.84	Social (emotion/eye gaze), Speech, Symbolic (understanding, object use)	Parent questionnaire + behavior sample	Early social-communication screening, ASD risk identification	Identifies subtle communication delays, free screener available	Limited to young age range, requires clinical interpretation

continued on following page

Table 1. Continued

Screening Tool	Age Range	Admin Time	Sensitivity	Specificity	Domains Assessed	Completion Method	Clinical Applications	Key Advantages	Limitations
Screening Tool for Autism in Toddlers and Young Children (STAT)	24-36 months	20 min	0.83-0.95	0.86-0.90	Play, requesting, directing attention, motor imitation	Clinician-administered interactive screening	Level 2 ASD screening for high-risk children	Interactive format, good for follow-up to M-CHAT	Requires training, not for universal screening
Battelle Developmental Inventory-2 (BDI-2)	0-8 years	60-90 min (full); 10-30 min (screener)	0.80-0.92	0.84-0.90	Adaptive, Personal-Social, Communication, Motor, Cognitive	Clinician-administered with parent input	Comprehensive assessment and eligibility determination	Includes screening and diagnostic versions, multiple data sources	Time-intensive for full assessment, requires trained examiner

Notes:

- Sensitivity = proportion of children with delays correctly identified (True Positive Rate)
- Specificity = proportion of typically developing children correctly identified (True Negative Rate)
- Admin Time = Administration time
- PPV = Positive Predictive Value
- Ranges reflect variation across studies, age groups, and populations
- Tool selection should consider: purpose (universal vs. targeted screening), setting, available resources, population characteristics, and psychometric requirements
- Tier 1 tools = universal population screening; Tier 2 tools = comprehensive diagnostic assessment

7. EMERGING TECHNOLOGIES AND FUTURE DIRECTIONS

The field of early identification and intervention continues to evolve rapidly, driven by technological innovations, accumulating research evidence, and changing service delivery models. Several emerging areas show particular promise for enhancing early detection capabilities and intervention effectiveness.

7.1 Artificial Intelligence and Machine Learning Applications

Artificial intelligence and machine learning applications offer potential to enhance both early identification and intervention personalization. Digital behavioral phenotyping, as demonstrated by Perochon et al. (2023), represents one application area, using computer vision and machine learning to identify subtle behavioral patterns indicative of developmental differences. Complementing these approaches, deep learning techniques applied to behavioral surveillance data offer additional promise for anomaly detection in developmental monitoring, enabling automated identification of atypical behavioral patterns that may warrant clinical follow-up (Agrawal et al., 2026).

7.1.1 Predictive Modeling for Developmental Outcomes

Emerging research explores development of predictive models that integrate multiple data sources (genetic testing results, neuroimaging findings, early developmental measures, family factors) to generate individualized outcome predictions and inform intervention planning. Such approaches could enable more precise targeting of intensive intervention to children most likely to benefit while identifying protective factors that could be enhanced through intervention.

7.1.2 Personalized Intervention Approaches

Machine learning approaches also show promise for optimizing intervention selection and intensity for individual children, analyzing patterns in treatment response data to identify child characteristics associated with particular intervention effectiveness. This precision medicine approach to early intervention could improve outcomes while enhancing efficient resource allocation. Notably, the increasing reliance on digital platforms for intervention delivery also raises questions about digital engagement patterns among caregivers and professionals, with emerging research on digital hoboism highlighting how fragmented digital behaviors may affect the consistency and quality of technology-mediated early intervention practices (Gupta, Azizbek et al., 2026).

7.2 Advances in Genetic Diagnostic Technologies

Genetic testing technologies continue advancing rapidly, with emerging approaches including long-read sequencing, optical genome mapping, and multi-omic integration promising to further increase diagnostic yield and reduce time to diagnosis.

7.2.1 Rapid Diagnostic Pathways

Implementation of rapid whole genome sequencing in acute clinical settings has demonstrated feasibility of returning genetic diagnoses within days rather than months, enabling time-sensitive medical management decisions. Extension of rapid diagnostic approaches to outpatient developmental settings could accelerate access to intervention services and family support.

7.2.2 Ethical Considerations in Expanded Genetic Screening

As genetic testing capabilities expand, important ethical considerations emerge regarding which conditions should be included in screening programs, how results should be communicated to families, and how to ensure equitable access to testing and follow-up services. Ongoing stakeholder engagement, including affected individuals and families, remains essential for developing ethically sound policies and practices. Building institutional trust and social license to operate within communities served by genetic screening programs requires sustained investment in moral capital and transparent, values-aligned practice (Gupta, Halaswamy et al., 2026).

7.3 Integration of Screening and Intervention Systems

Despite evidence supporting both developmental screening and early intervention, significant gaps often exist between identification and service initiation. Systematic efforts to integrate screening and intervention systems, including development of streamlined referral processes, enhanced care coordination, and capacity building within intervention service systems, represent critical priorities for translating research evidence into improved outcomes for children and families.

8. IMPLEMENTATION SCIENCE PERSPECTIVES

Translating research evidence into effective real-world practice requires attention to implementation factors including organizational readiness, workforce capacity, financing mechanisms, and family engagement strategies.

8.1 Barriers and Facilitators to Evidence-Based Practice

Multiple factors influence successful implementation of evidence-based screening and intervention practices. Facilitators include leadership support, adequate resources, training and ongoing consultation, alignment with existing workflows, and perceived benefit to children and families. Barriers include time and resource constraints, competing priorities, limited training opportunities, reimbursement challenges, and workforce shortages.

8.1.1 Workforce Development Needs

Effective implementation of early identification and intervention requires a skilled, adequately sized workforce across multiple disciplines including primary care providers, specialists, early intervention professionals, and support staff. Current workforce capacity falls short of need in many regions, with particular shortages in rural areas and for professionals with expertise in specific genetic syndromes or cultural competencies serving diverse populations.

8.2 Policy Implications and System-Level Recommendations

Optimizing early identification and intervention systems requires coordinated action across multiple system levels, from individual practice to state and federal policy.

8.2.1 Financing and Reimbursement

Sustainable financing mechanisms supporting developmental screening, diagnostic evaluation, and evidence-based intervention represent essential infrastructure for effective early identification systems. Current reimbursement structures often create barriers to optimal practice, with inadequate payment for screening and care coordination activities and limitations in intervention service authorization.

Policy reforms could include enhanced reimbursement for preventive developmental services, alternative payment models supporting comprehensive care coordination, and adequate funding for early intervention service systems to meet growing demand.

8.2.2 Quality Measurement and Accountability

Implementation of quality measures related to developmental screening rates, timely follow-up of positive screens, and evidence-based intervention provision could drive system improvement while providing accountability for service quality. Such measures should be developed collaboratively with families, professionals, and policymakers to ensure they capture meaningful outcomes while avoiding unintended consequences.

9. CULTURAL CONSIDERATIONS AND HEALTH EQUITY

Ensuring equitable access to early identification and intervention services across diverse populations represents both an ethical imperative and a practical necessity for maximizing population-level outcomes.

9.1 Disparities in Screening and Diagnosis

Research consistently documents disparities in age of diagnosis for developmental disabilities and genetic syndromes across racial, ethnic, and socioeconomic groups. Wheeler et al. (2023) examined age of diagnosis for children with chromosome 15q syndromes, finding significant delays in diagnosis for children from underrepresented minority backgrounds and those with limited healthcare access.

These disparities result from multiple factors including differential access to healthcare, provider biases in screening and referral practices, cultural differences in symptom interpretation and help-seeking behavior, language barriers, and structural inequities in resource distribution.

9.1.1 Culturally Responsive Screening Practices

Development and validation of screening tools that perform equitably across diverse populations requires attention to cultural factors influencing developmental expectations, language used in screening items, and format of tool administration. Research examining screening tool performance across diverse populations, such as the work by Lockhart et al. (2023) examining maternal education effects on ASQ performance, provides important insights for ensuring equity in screening practices.

9.2 Enhancing Access and Engagement

Strategies for improving equitable access to early identification and intervention include community-based screening initiatives, navigation and care coordination services supporting families through diagnostic and intervention processes, culturally adapted intervention approaches, and workforce diversity enhancement to better reflect communities served.

10. CONCLUSION

Early identification and intervention for children with genetic syndromes represents one of the most dynamic and rapidly evolving domains within pediatric healthcare, developmental science, and medical genetics. The convergence of technological innovation, expanding research evidence, implementation science insights, and growing emphasis on family-centered, equitable practices has fundamentally transformed the landscape of care for children with genetic syndromes and their families. This transformation extends across the entire continuum from initial identification through sustained intervention and long-term support, creating unprecedented opportunities to optimize developmental trajectories and enhance quality of life for affected individuals and families.

10.1 Synthesis of Major Advances and Current Knowledge

The past decade has witnessed remarkable progress across multiple interconnected domains that collectively enhance our capacity to identify and support children with genetic syndromes. Genetic testing capabilities have expanded dramatically, with chromosomal microarray analysis now established as first-tier testing for children presenting with developmental delays, intellectual disability, autism spectrum disorder, or multiple congenital anomalies. The diagnostic yield of genetic testing has increased substantially through implementation of whole exome sequencing and whole genome sequencing, enabling molecular diagnosis in 30-50% of previously undiagnosed cases (Manickam et al., 2021; van der Sanden et al., 2023). These advances have profound implications not only for individual families seeking answers about their children's conditions but also for the broader scientific understanding of genetic contributions to neurodevelopmental disorders.

Developmental screening methodologies have been refined and validated across increasingly diverse populations and settings, with particular attention to psychometric properties, cultural appropriateness, and implementation feasibility. Meta-analytic evidence synthesizing findings across hundreds of studies has clarified the performance characteristics of major screening instruments, enabling more informed tool selection and interpretation (Rah et al., 2023). Emerging technologies including digital behavioral phenotyping demonstrate promise for further enhancing early detection capabilities, potentially enabling identification of developmental differences at younger ages and with greater precision than traditional screening approaches (Perochon et al., 2023).

The intervention evidence base has strengthened considerably, with large-scale systematic reviews and meta-analyses providing increasingly clear guidance regarding effective intervention approaches, optimal timing and intensity parameters, and factors that moderate treatment response. Naturalistic developmental behavioral interventions have emerged as a leading approach for young children with autism spectrum disorder, demonstrating benefits for social communication outcomes while remaining feasible for implementation within community-based service systems (Sandbank et al., 2023). Parent-mediated intervention models have gained prominence, recognizing parents as essential intervention agents and potentially extending intervention intensity beyond what would be achievable through clinician-delivered services alone (Conrad et al., 2021).

Family-centered care principles have moved from aspirational ideals to concrete implementation frameworks, with research documenting both the processes that characterize high-quality family-centered practice and the outcomes associated with this approach. Evidence demonstrates that family-centered care improves not only child developmental outcomes but also family-level outcomes including parent confidence, family functioning, and quality of life (McCarthy & Guerin, 2022). These findings validate the importance of authentic family partnership in intervention planning and delivery, moving beyond token family involvement to genuine collaboration that respects family expertise, priorities, and cultural contexts.

10.2 Persistent Challenges Requiring Sustained Attention

Despite substantial progress, significant challenges persist that constrain our collective capacity to optimize outcomes for all children with genetic syndromes. Implementation gaps between research evidence and routine practice remain substantial, with many children who would benefit from early intervention not receiving timely access to evidence-based services. These implementation challenges reflect multiple factors including workforce capacity limitations, financing and reimbursement barriers, geographic service distribution inequities, and systemic fragmentation between screening, diagnostic, and intervention systems.

Workforce capacity represents a particularly pressing challenge, with shortages of qualified professionals across multiple disciplines including developmental-behavioral pediatrics, genetics, speech-language pathology, occupational therapy, physical therapy, and psychology. These shortages are most acute in rural areas and for professionals with specialized expertise in specific genetic syndromes or cultural competencies serving diverse populations. Addressing workforce challenges requires coordinated action including enhanced training pipeline capacity, retention strategies, alternative service delivery models including telehealth and tiered workforce approaches, and improved compensation and working conditions.

Health equity concerns remain central challenges requiring sustained attention and systemic reform. Research consistently documents disparities in age of diagnosis, access to genetic testing, participation in early intervention services, and intervention quality across racial, ethnic, socioeconomic, and geographic groups (Wheeler et al., 2023). These disparities reflect structural inequities in healthcare access, implicit biases in clinical decision-making, cultural barriers to service engagement, and differential resource allocation. Addressing equity requires multifaceted approaches including bias reduction training for professionals, culturally adapted screening and intervention approaches, community-based service delivery models, navigation and care coordination support, and policy reforms addressing fundamental resource distribution inequities.

Research gaps persist despite the expanding evidence base. Syndrome-specific intervention research remains limited for many genetic conditions, with most intervention studies focusing on Down syndrome and autism spectrum disorder while children with rarer genetic syndromes have limited access to evidence-based, syndrome-tailored interventions. Implementation science research examining effective strategies for translating evidence to practice requires expansion, particularly regarding approaches that prove effective in resource-constrained settings and with diverse populations. Long-term outcome studies tracking developmental trajectories across childhood and into adolescence and adulthood remain insufficient, limiting our understanding of sustained intervention effects and optimal transition planning.

10.3 Future Directions and Transformative Opportunities

Looking forward, multiple promising directions offer potential for substantial advances in early identification and intervention. Continued refinement of screening approaches through integration of artificial intelligence and machine learning may enable earlier detection of developmental differences and more precise characterization of individual profiles. Predictive modeling approaches integrating multiple data sources including genetic testing results, neuroimaging findings, early developmental measures, and environmental factors could generate individualized outcome predictions to inform intervention planning and enable more efficient resource allocation.

Expansion of genetic testing, potentially including genomic newborn screening for early actionable conditions, represents a transformative possibility that could enable identification and preventive intervention before symptom onset for certain conditions (Ziegler et al., 2025). However, implementation of expanded newborn screening raises complex ethical considerations regarding condition selection criteria, return of results policies, psychosocial impacts of early diagnosis disclosure, and equitable access to follow-up services. Addressing these ethical dimensions requires sustained stakeholder engagement including affected individuals, families, professionals, ethicists, and policymakers.

Development of personalized intervention approaches represents an important frontier, moving beyond one-size-fits-all intervention protocols toward precision medicine approaches that match specific intervention strategies to individual child characteristics, developmental profiles, family contexts, and preferences. Machine learning analyses of large intervention response datasets may identify patterns indicating which children respond optimally to which interventions under which conditions, enabling more efficient matching of interventions to individual needs.

System integration efforts addressing fragmentation between screening, diagnostic, and intervention systems represent critical priorities for translating research evidence into improved population-level outcomes. Streamlined referral processes, enhanced care coordination, co-located services, shared data systems, and integrated financing mechanisms could reduce the substantial delays and dropout that currently characterize pathways from screening to intervention access.

10.4 Imperative for Coordinated Action

Realizing the promise of early identification and intervention requires coordinated action across multiple stakeholder groups, each contributing essential elements to the larger ecosystem of support for children with genetic syndromes and their families. Healthcare systems must prioritize developmental screening and timely referral as core components of well-child care, investing in workforce training, decision support tools, and care coordination infrastructure. Policymakers must ensure adequate, sustainable financing for screening, diagnostic evaluation, and intervention services while promoting workforce development, system integration, and quality measurement. Researchers must continue advancing the evidence base while attending to implementation considerations and equity implications, ensuring that research priorities reflect needs of diverse communities and that findings are translated into accessible, actionable guidance for practitioners and families.

Educational systems must partner effectively with early intervention and healthcare systems, ensuring smooth transitions from early intervention to preschool and school-based services while maintaining continuity of evidence-based supports. Community organizations, advocacy groups, and family support networks provide essential peer support, information dissemination, and advocacy functions that complement professional services.

Most fundamentally, all stakeholders must partner authentically with families, recognizing them as experts on their children and essential collaborators in the shared enterprise of supporting optimal development for all children. This partnership requires moving beyond superficial family engagement to genuine shared decision-making, cultural humility, responsiveness to family priorities and values, and commitment to addressing the structural barriers that constrain opportunity and wellbeing for many families.

The convergence of scientific advances, technological capabilities, and growing commitment to equity and family partnership creates unprecedented opportunity to transform outcomes for children with genetic syndromes. Converting this potential into reality requires sustained commitment, coordinated action, adequate resource investment, and unwavering focus on the ultimate goal: ensuring that every child with a genetic syndrome has access to timely identification, comprehensive evaluation, evidence-based intervention, and family-centered support that enables them to reach their fullest potential and experience optimal quality of life.

REFERENCES

Agrawal, A., Bhaskar, R. S., Badhe, S., Thakur, S. K., Bhandari, A., Jain, K., & Gupta, D. (2026). Anomaly detection in behavioral surveillance using deep learning techniques. In Ahmad, S., Jha, S., & Haque, M. (Eds.), *AI-Based Data Mobility and Intelligent Modeling for Smart Cities* (pp. 255–290). IGI Global Scientific Publishing., DOI: 10.4018/979-8-3373-4202-3.ch009

Baumer, N., DePillis, R., Pawlowski, K., Zhang, B., & Mazumdar, M. (2024). Developmental milestones for children with Down syndrome. *Pediatrics*, *154*(4), e2023065402. Advance online publication. DOI: 10.1542/peds.2023-065402 PMID: 39279536

Bull, M. J., Trotter, T., Santoro, S. L., Christensen, C., & Grout, R. W. (2022). Health supervision for children and adolescents with Down syndrome. *Pediatrics*, *149*(5), e2022057010. Advance online publication. DOI: 10.1542/peds.2022-057010 PMID: 35490285

Chaves, T. F., Ocampos, M., Barbato, I. T., de Camargo Pinto, L. L., de Luca, G. R., Barbato Filho, J. H., Bernardi, P., Muniz, Y. C. N., & Maris, A. F. (2024). A cohort study of neurodevelopmental disorders and/or congenital anomalies using high resolution chromosomal microarrays in southern Brazil highlighting the significance of ASD. *Scientific Reports*, *14*(1), 3762. Advance online publication. DOI: 10.1038/s41598-024-54385-2 PMID: 38355898

Conrad, C. E., Rimestad, M. L., Rohde, J. F., Petersen, B. H., Korfitsen, C. B., Tarp, S., Cantio, C., Lauritsen, M. B., & Händel, M. N. (2021). Parent-mediated interventions for children and adolescents with autism spectrum disorders: A systematic review and meta-analysis. *Frontiers in Psychiatry*, *12*, 773604. DOI: 10.3389/fpsyt.2021.773604 PMID: 34867556

dos Santos, C. L., Barreto, I. I., Floriano, I., Tristão, L. S., Silvinato, A., & Bernardo, W. M. (2024). Screening and diagnostic tools for autism spectrum disorder: Systematic review and meta-analysis. *Clinics (São Paulo)*, *79*, 100323. Advance online publication. DOI: 10.1016/j.clinsp.2023.100323 PMID: 38484581

Duncan, A. L., Keene, H., & Shepley, C. (2024). Do naturalistic developmental behavioral interventions improve family quality of life? A systematic review and meta-analysis. *Autism*, *28*(9), 2152–2165. DOI: 10.1177/13623613241227516 PMID: 38318790

Franz, L., Goodwin, C. D., Rieder, A., Matheis, M., & Damiano, D. L. (2022). Early intervention for very young children with or at high likelihood for autism spectrum disorder: An overview of reviews. *Developmental Medicine and Child Neurology*, *64*(9), 1063–1076. DOI: 10.1111/dmcn.15258 PMID: 35582893

Godler, D. E., Ling, L., Gamage, D., Baker, E. K., Bui, M., Field, M. J., Rogers, C., Butler, M. G., Murgia, A., Leonardi, E., Polli, R., Schwartz, C. E., Skinner, C. D., Alliende, A. M., Santa Maria, L., Pitt, J., Greaves, R., Francis, D., Oertel, R., & Amor, D. J. (2022). Feasibility of screening for chromosome 15 imprinting disorders in 16,579 newborns by using a novel genomic workflow. *JAMA Network Open*, *5*(1), e2141911. Advance online publication. DOI: 10.1001/jamanetworkopen.2021.41911 PMID: 34982160

Gupta, D., Azizbek, I., Suxrob, P., & Abdullaeva, I. Ravshan kizi, B. M., Abdukabilovna, T. D., & Jumayev, U. (2026). Digital hoboism. In E. Kaygisiz (Ed.), *Digital Ideologies in the Age of Algorithmic Culture* (pp. 307–338). IGI Global Scientific Publishing. DOI: 10.4018/979-8-3373-4531-4.ch010

Gupta, D., & Halaswamy, D. G., A. M., Srivastava, A., Arya, S., Karthiga, V., & Patil, S. (2026). Moral capital, trust reserve, and social license to operate. In S. Sajib (Ed.), *Investigating Moral Capital in Value Creation* (pp. 111–142). IGI Global Scientific Publishing. DOI: 10.4018/979-8-3373-6043-0.ch004

Jimenez-Arberas, E., Casais-Suarez, Y., Fernandez-Mendez, A., Menendez-Espina, S., Rodriguez-Menendez, S., Llosa, J. A., & Prieto-Saborit, J. A. (2024). Evidence-based implementation of the family-centered model and the use of tele-intervention in early childhood services: A systematic review. *Health Care*, *12*(1), 112. Advance online publication. DOI: 10.3390/healthcare12010112 PMID: 38201017

La Valle, C., Johnston, E., & Tager-Flusberg, H. (2022). A systematic review of the use of telehealth to facilitate a diagnosis for children with developmental concerns. *Research in Developmental Disabilities*, *127*, 104269. Advance online publication. DOI: 10.1016/j.ridd.2022.104269 PMID: 35636261

Lockhart, M., Chaux, R., Chevin, M., Celle, M., Raia-Barjat, T., Patural, H., Chabrier, S., & Giraud, A. (2023). Classification performance of the Ages and Stages Questionnaire: Influence of maternal education level. *Children (Basel, Switzerland)*, *10*(3), 449. Advance online publication. DOI: 10.3390/children10030449 PMID: 36980009

Manickam, K., McClain, M. R., Demmer, L. A., Yu, T. W., & Hisama, F. M. (2021). Exome and genome sequencing for pediatric patients with congenital anomalies or intellectual disability: An evidence-based clinical guideline of the American College of Medical Genetics and Genomics (ACMG). *Genetics in Medicine*, *23*(11), 2029–2037. DOI: 10.1038/s41436-021-01242-6 PMID: 34211152

McCarthy, E., & Guerin, S. (2022). Family-centred care in early intervention: A systematic review of the processes and outcomes of family-centred care and impacting factors. *Child: Care, Health and Development*, *48*(1), 1–32. DOI: 10.1111/cch.12901 PMID: 34324725

Perochon, S., Di Martino, J. M., Carpenter, K. L. H., Compton, S., Davis, N., Eichner, B., Espinosa, S., Franz, L., Krishnappa Babu, P. R., Sapiro, G., & Dawson, G. (2023). Early detection of autism using digital behavioral phenotyping. *Nature Medicine*, *29*(10), 2489–2497. DOI: 10.1038/s41591-023-02574-3 PMID: 37783967

Pitchik, H. O., Tofail, F., Akter, F., Shoab, A. K. M., Sultana, J., Huda, T. M. N., Rahman, M., Winch, P. J., Luby, S. P., & Fernald, L. C. H. (2023). Concurrent validity of the Ages and Stages Questionnaire Inventory and the Bayley Scales of Infant and Toddler Development in rural Bangladesh. *BMC Pediatrics*, *23*(1), 93. Advance online publication. DOI: 10.1186/s12887-022-03800-6 PMID: 36859070

Rah, S. S., Jung, M., Lee, K., Park, J., Yoon, J. Y., & Hong, S. B. (2023). Systematic review and meta-analysis: Real-world accuracy of children's developmental screening tests. *Journal of the American Academy of Child and Adolescent Psychiatry*, *62*(10), 1095–1109. DOI: 10.1016/j.jaac.2022.12.014 PMID: 36592715

Sandbank, M., Bottema-Beutel, K., LaPoint, S. C., Feldman, J. I., Barrett, D. J., Caldwell, N., & Woynaroski, T. (2023). Autism intervention meta-analysis of early childhood studies (Project AIM): Updated systematic review and secondary analysis. *BMJ (Clinical Research Ed.)*, *383*, 383. DOI: 10.1136/bmj-2023-076733 PMID: 37963634

Seager, E., Sampson, S., Sin, J., Pagnamenta, E., & Stojanovik, V. (2022). A systematic review of speech, language and communication interventions for children with Down syndrome from 0 to 6 years. *International Journal of Language & Communication Disorders*, *57*(2), 441–463. DOI: 10.1111/1460-6984.12699 PMID: 35191587

Stojanovik, V., Pagnamenta, E., Sampson, S., Sutton, R., Jones, B., Joffe, V., Harvey, K., Pizzo, E., & Rae, S. (2024). Evaluating an early social communication intervention for young children with Down syndrome (ASCEND): Results from a feasibility randomised control trial. *Pilot and Feasibility Studies*, *10*(1), 127. Advance online publication. DOI: 10.1186/s40814-024-01551-y PMID: 39369246

Tassone, F., Protic, D., Allen, E. G., Archibald, A. D., Baud, A., Brown, T. W., Budimirovic, D. B., Cohen, J., Dufour, B., Eiges, R., Elvassore, N., Gabis, L. V., Grudzien, S. J., Hall, D. A., Hessl, D., Hogan, A., Hunter, J. E., Jin, P., Jiraanont, P., & Hagerman, R. J. (2023). Insight and recommendations for fragile X-premutation-associated conditions from the Fifth International Conference on FMR1 Premutation. *Cells*, *12*(18), 2330. Advance online publication. DOI: 10.3390/cells12182330 PMID: 37759552

van der Sanden, B. P. G. H., Schobers, G., Corominas Galbany, J., Koolen, D. A., Sinnema, M., van Reeuwijk, J., Stumpel, C. T. R. M., Kleefstra, T., de Vries, B. B. A., Ruiterkamp-Versteeg, M., Leijsten, N., Kwint, M., Derks, R., Swinkels, H., den Ouden, A., Pfundt, R., Rinne, T., de Leeuw, N., Stegmann, A. P., & Vissers, L. E. L. M. (2023). The performance of genome sequencing as a first-tier test for neurodevelopmental disorders. *European Journal of Human Genetics : EJHG*, *31*(1), 81–88. DOI: 10.1038/s41431-022-01185-9 PMID: 36114283

von der Lippe, C., Neteland, I., & Feragen, K. B. (2022). Children with a rare congenital genetic disorder: A systematic review of parent experiences. *Orphanet Journal of Rare Diseases*, *17*(1), 375. Advance online publication. DOI: 10.1186/s13023-022-02525-0 PMID: 36253830

Wheeler, A. C., Gantz, M. G., Cope, H., Strong, T. V., Bohonowych, J. E., Moore, A., & Vogel-Farley, V. (2023). Age of diagnosis for children with chromosome 15q syndromes. *Journal of Neurodevelopmental Disorders*, *15*(1), 37. Advance online publication. DOI: 10.1186/s11689-023-09504-x PMID: 37936142

Wieckowski, A. T., Williams, L. N., Rando, J., Lyall, K., & Robins, D. L. (2023). Sensitivity and specificity of the Modified Checklist for Autism in Toddlers (original and revised): A systematic review and meta-analysis. *JAMA Pediatrics*, *177*(4), 373–383. DOI: 10.1001/jamapediatrics.2022.5975 PMID: 36804771

Ziegler, A., Koval-Burt, C., Kay, D. M., Suchy, S. F., Begtrup, A., Langley, K. G., Hernan, R., Amendola, L. M., Boyd, B. M., Bradley, J., Brandt, T., Cohen, L. L., Coffey, A. J., Devaney, J. M., Dygulska, B., Friedman, B., Fuleihan, R. L., Gyimah, A., Hahn, S., & Chung, W. K. (2025). Expanded newborn screening using genome sequencing for early actionable conditions. *Journal of the American Medical Association*, *333*(3), 232–240. DOI: 10.1001/jama.2024.19662 PMID: 39446378

KEY TERMS AND DEFINITIONS

Autism Spectrum Disorder (ASD): A neurodevelopmental disorder characterized by persistent deficits in social communication and social interaction, along with restricted, repetitive patterns of behavior, interests, or activities. Early identification enables timely intervention during critical developmental periods.

Chromosomal Microarray Analysis (CMA): A molecular genetic test that detects submicroscopic deletions and duplications of chromosomal material (copy number variants). CMA is recommended as a first-tier clinical diagnostic test for individuals with developmental disabilities, congenital anomalies, or autism spectrum disorder.

Developmental Screening: A brief assessment process designed to identify children who may be at risk for developmental delays or disabilities and who may benefit from further evaluation. Screening differs from comprehensive developmental assessment in its brevity and use of broad population norms.

Early Intervention: Services and supports provided to infants and young children (typically birth to age 3 years) with developmental delays or disabilities and their families. Early intervention capitalizes on neuroplasticity during critical developmental periods to optimize outcomes.

Family-Centered Care: An approach to planning, delivering, and evaluating healthcare that is grounded in mutually beneficial partnerships among patients, families, and providers. Family-centered care recognizes families as essential participants in treatment decisions and service delivery.

Naturalistic Developmental Behavioral Interventions (NDBIs): A family of intervention approaches for young children with autism that blend developmental and behavioral principles, implementing teaching within natural environments and daily routines using child-initiated activities.

Neurodevelopmental Disorders: A group of conditions with onset in the developmental period, characterized by developmental deficits that produce impairments in personal, social, academic, or occupational functioning. This category includes intellectual disabilities, autism spectrum disorder, attention-deficit/hyperactivity disorder, and specific learning disorders.

Chapter 5
A Family-Centered, Case-Based Approach to Simpson-Golabi-Behmel Syndrome:
Developmental Trajectories and Early Educational Intervention

Assimina Tsibidaki
http://orcid.org/0000-0001-6430-2436
University of the Aegean, Greece

ABSTRACT

This chapter examines how family-mediated early developmental and educational intervention practices support functional participation in a young child diagnosed with Simpson-Golabi-Behmel syndrome type 1 (SGBS1). Adopting a qualitative instrumental case study design, the chapter explores the psychoeducational trajectory of a five-year-old child attending mainstream kindergarten in a semi-urban region of southern Greece. Drawing on clinical documentation, caregiver-reported standardized measures of family quality of life and parental stress, and semi-structured interview data, the chapter investigates how therapeutic goals are integrated into everyday family routines to promote communication, autonomy, and social interaction. Findings highlight the role of parental role reorganization, sibling involvement, and home-based intervention practices in supporting developmental engagement. The chapter further discusses how limited access to specialized services may influence caregiving demands and reliance on family-centered support strategies in early childhood contexts.

DOI: 10.4018/979-8-3373-8485-6.ch005

INTRODUCTION

Rare genetic conditions constitute a diverse group of developmental disorders that, although individually rare, affect a considerable proportion of the global population and are commonly associated with chronic health needs and complex multi-system manifestations. In childhood, these conditions are often accompanied by substantial developmental and neurological implications, while the path to diagnosis may involve a prolonged and complex diagnostic odyssey that delays access to appropriate care and support (Sirchia et al., 2026). Although advances in molecular genetics have significantly improved diagnostic accuracy and early identification, the developmental implications of these conditions extend beyond biomedical management to influence communication, learning, autonomy, and participation in everyday activities (Atkins & Padgett, 2024; Pelentsov et al., 2016). In early childhood, such developmental vulnerabilities may affect access to social interaction, play-based learning opportunities, and adaptive functioning within home and educational environments, thereby shaping the child's developmental trajectory across cognitive, linguistic, and socio-emotional domains (Atkins & Padgett, 2024).

Traditionally, rare genetic syndromes have been approached primarily through a clinical or biomedical framework emphasizing diagnosis, prognosis, and medical surveillance. However, contemporary developmental research increasingly recognizes that the long-term outcomes associated with rare conditions are mediated not only by biological factors but also by environmental influences that shape opportunities for learning and participation (King et al., 2004). Developmental trajectories in children with chronic or rare conditions are understood to emerge through ongoing interactions between the individual and their proximal environments, including family members, peers, and educational practitioners (Bronfenbrenner, 2005). Within this ecological framework, the family microsystem represents a primary context for learning, behavioral regulation, and emotional support during early childhood. Empirical research has further demonstrated that family strengths and parental demographic characteristics may function as protective mechanisms supporting adaptive functioning and developmental participation among children with developmental conditions (Tsibidaki, 2021).

Everyday routines such as play, mealtime interaction, shared caregiving practices, and sibling engagement provide opportunities for repeated practice of communication and adaptive skills in naturalistic contexts. These routine-based interactions may facilitate the generalization of therapeutic gains beyond clinical settings and contribute to functional participation across environments. As a result, intervention models that extend beyond professional-led therapy sessions to include caregiver-mediated strategies within the home environment are increasingly considered essential in supporting developmental progress among children with complex needs (King et al., 2004).

Within caregiving environments, families raising children with rare genetic conditions frequently encounter increased daily demands that may contribute to elevated levels of parental stress and influence perceptions of family quality of life. Capturing caregiver stress alongside family quality of life can therefore provide a more comprehensive understanding of how family-mediated intervention practices are sustained within everyday routines and caregiving contexts (Raina et al., 2005; Whiting et al., 2019).

Children diagnosed with rare genetic syndromes frequently present with global developmental vulnerabilities affecting motor coordination, expressive language, emotional regulation, or social interaction. Hypotonia, sensory processing differences, and communication limitations are among the developmental features commonly reported in rare syndromes, potentially affecting engagement in play-based interaction and early educational experiences (DeBaun et al., 2001; Nisbet et al., 2024). These characteristics may influence autonomy, peer interaction, and participation in structured learning environments during critical periods of early development.

Simpson-Golabi-Behmel syndrome type 1 (SGBS1) is a rare X-linked recessive overgrowth disorder associated with prenatal and postnatal somatic overgrowth, craniofacial anomalies, and multisystem involvement (Behmel et al., 1984; Golabi & Rosen, 1984; Neri et al., 2013). The syndrome is most caused by pathogenic variants in the glypican-3 (GPC3) gene located on chromosome Xq26.2. GPC3 plays a crucial role in cellular growth, embryogenesis, and developmental signaling, including modulation of the canonical Wnt and Hedgehog pathways, while loss of function is regarded as the main pathogenic mechanism underlying SGBS1 (Nisbet et al., 2024; Zhao et al., 2025). In addition to physical manifestations such as macroglossia, organomegaly, and skeletal anomalies, children with SGBS1 may present with delayed motor milestones, expressive language limitations, and reduced endurance related to hypotonia (DeBaun et al., 2001). In addition to physical manifestations such as macroglossia, organomegaly, and skeletal anomalies, children with SGBS1 may present with delayed motor milestones, expressive language limitations, and reduced endurance related to hypotonia (DeBaun et al., 2001). These developmental characteristics may influence functional participation in everyday activities requiring coordination, communication, or sustained attention.

Given the increased risk for associated medical complications, including embryonal tumors such as Wilms tumor, children diagnosed with SGBS1 typically require ongoing clinical surveillance during early childhood (Nisbet et al., 2024). However, the developmental implications of the syndrome extend beyond medical management to include learning, autonomy, and socialization within home and educational environments. Early intervention practices aimed at supporting communication and adaptive functioning are therefore considered essential components of interdisciplinary care for children with rare developmental conditions (Orphanet, 2023).

Contemporary early intervention models increasingly recognize caregivers as active partners in supporting developmental progress. Family-centered approaches emphasize the role of everyday routines as naturalistic learning contexts in which communication, play, and adaptive behaviors may be practiced through meaningful interaction (King et al., 2004). Rather than functioning solely as recipients of professional guidance, parents are positioned as co-facilitators of intervention by embedding therapeutic strategies within shared activities such as play or daily caregiving practices. In families raising children with rare developmental conditions, intervention practices often extend into home environments due to the need for continuous monitoring and limited availability of specialized services (Pelentsov et al., 2016).

In addition to parental involvement, the participation of typically developing siblings in shared routines may further support the generalization of emerging skills across naturalistic contexts. Sibling-mediated interaction has been associated with increased opportunities for imitation, turn-taking, and emotional reciprocity during early childhood (Lummer-Aikey & Goldstein, 2021).

Family resilience theory provides a complementary framework for understanding how families adapt intervention practices over time in response to developmental needs through flexible role organization and collaborative problem-solving (Walsh, 2016).

The Present Study

Despite advances in clinical understanding of SGBS1, limited research has examined how family-mediated early developmental and educational intervention may influence developmental trajectories in children diagnosed with this condition. The present qualitative case study adopts an interdisciplinary and family-centered perspective to explore how therapeutic goals are embedded within everyday family routines to support communication, autonomy, and social participation.

Guided by ecological systems theory (Bronfenbrenner, 2005) and family resilience theory (Walsh, 2016), the study examines the psychoeducational trajectory of a five-year-old child diagnosed with SGBS1 residing in a semi-urban region of Greece. Attention is given to the ways in which caregiver involvement and sibling interaction contribute to the generalization of emerging skills across naturalistic contexts.

Through the integration of caregiver-reported developmental data, standardized family functioning measures, and qualitative interview findings, the chapter aims to provide an in-depth understanding of how family-mediated intervention practices may influence functional participation and developmental engagement in children with rare genetic conditions. By situating early intervention practices within the family microsystem, the study seeks to contribute to interdisciplinary discussions on developmental support, educational inclusion, and family adaptation in the context of rare developmental syndromes.

Based on the family-centered and interdisciplinary framework guiding the present case study, the following research questions were formulated:

1) How does raising a child diagnosed with SGBS1 influence parental role distribution and daily caregiving routines within the family system?
2) What levels of parental stress and perceived family quality of life are reported by caregivers managing long-term developmental needs associated with SGBS1?
3) How does the presence of a chronic developmental condition influence the psychosocial adjustment and involvement of the typically developing sibling?
4) What challenges do families encounter in accessing formal support services within their residential context?

These research questions aim to explore the ways in which family-mediated early developmental and educational intervention practices are embedded within everyday routines and how caregiving environments may function as naturalistic contexts supporting communication, autonomy, and social participation in children diagnosed with rare genetic conditions.

METHOD

Research Design

The present study employed a qualitative instrumental case study design to examine caregiving dynamics and family-mediated early developmental and educational intervention practices associated with raising a child diagnosed with SGBS1. Case study methodology is considered appropriate when the aim is to explore complex developmental phenomena within their real-life context, particularly in situations where contextual variables cannot be easily separated from the phenomenon under investigation (Yin, 2018). Instrumental case studies are commonly used in qualitative research to provide insight into broader theoretical constructs through the in-depth examination of a specific case (Stake, 1995).

Within the context of rare genetic conditions, where clinical heterogeneity and environmental variability are significant, case-based approaches allow for the examination of developmental trajectories and caregiving practices that may not be adequately captured through quantitative methods alone (Creswell & Poth, 2018).

Participants

The participant in this study was a five-year-old boy diagnosed with SGBS1 during infancy following genetic evaluation conducted at a specialized clinical center. The child resides with his biological parents and his typically developing older sibling, aged 9.5 years, in a semi-urban area of southern Greece.

According to available clinical documentation, the child was born with prenatal and postnatal overgrowth features, including a birth weight of 5,900 g, length of 60 cm, and head circumference of 40 cm. Molecular testing confirmed a pathogenic variant in the glypican-3 (*GPC3*) gene located on chromosome Xq26.2, consistent with established clinical descriptions of SGBS1 (Neri et al., 2013; Nisbet et al., 2024). Additional findings during early infancy included hypotonia and organomegaly, necessitating ongoing medical monitoring throughout early childhood, including tumor surveillance protocols for embryonal tumors such as Wilms tumor (DeBaun et al., 2001).

The child's developmental trajectory was characterized by global developmental delay, particularly in motor and communicative domains. Independent walking was achieved after the age of two years, primarily due to reduced muscle tone, while linear growth remained above the 97th percentile throughout early childhood (Behmel et al., 1984). Expressive language limitations prompted the implementation of alternative and augmentative communication strategies, including the Picture Exchange Communication System (PECS) and the use of gestures, to support functional communication within daily family interactions (Orphanet, 2023).

Social interaction difficulties related to imitation, emotion recognition, and emerging autonomy were also reported, in line with previous descriptions of neurodevelopmental variability among individuals with SGBS1 (Nisbet et al., 2024). At the time of data collection, the child was attending a mainstream kindergarten setting with individualized educational support.

Interdisciplinary intervention was coordinated across speech and language therapy, occupational therapy, and physical therapy services, with an emphasis on consistency between clinical sessions and home-based practices. Speech therapy was delivered three times per week, incorporating alternative communication strategies, while motor and sensory integration goals were addressed through individualized therapy programs. Home-based support focused on the integration of therapeutic goals within everyday family routines and sibling interaction to promote autonomy and participation across naturalistic settings (Punnett, 2000).

The father, aged 44 years, is self-employed and maintains full-time professional responsibilities outside the home. The mother, aged 38 years, discontinued paid employment following the child's birth and currently assumes the role of primary caregiver within the home environment. Similar caregiving patterns have been reported in families raising children with rare or chronic developmental conditions, where intensive caregiving demands may lead to adjustments in parental employment and role distribution within the household (Pelentsov et al., 2016; Whiting et al., 2019).

Caregiving responsibilities within the household primarily involve coordination of medical appointments, implementation of therapeutic exercises, and daily supervision of the child's adaptive functioning. The presence of a typically developing sibling introduces additional relational dynamics within the family system that may influence both caregiving routines and opportunities for social interaction (Lummer-Aikey & Goldstein, 2021).

Table 1. Family demographic characteristics

Family Member	Age	Gender	Role in Family	Occupational Status
Father	44	Male	Primary income provider	Self-employed
Mother	38	Female	Primary caregiver	Homemaker
Child with SGBS1	5	Male	Index case	Kindergarten pupil
Typically developing sibling	9.5	Male	Older sibling	Primary school student

Data Collection

Data collection in the present study followed a multi-source case study approach to provide a comprehensive understanding of caregiving dynamics and family-mediated early developmental and educational intervention practices within the naturalistic family environment. In line with qualitative case study methodology, the use of multiple sources of evidence is recommended when examining complex developmental phenomena, as it enhances contextual validity and supports triangulation across data sources (Yin, 2018; Creswell & Poth, 2018).

Accordingly, data were gathered through the integration of clinical and developmental documentation, caregiver-reported standardized family functioning measures, observational information related to daily caregiving routines, and a semi-structured caregiver interview. The inclusion of both structured and open-ended data sources enabled the examination of caregiving practices at descriptive and interpretative levels within the family system. Such multi-method approaches are commonly recommended in research examining family adaptation in the context of rare pediatric conditions, where developmental outcomes are shaped by interactions between medical, environmental, and relational factors (Pelentsov et al., 2016).

Family Quality of Life was examined using the Beach Center Family Quality of Life Scale (FQoL), which assesses perceived well-being across domains including family interaction, parenting, emotional well-being, physical and material well-being, and disability-related support (Hoffman et al., 2006). Parental stress was assessed using the Parental Stress Scale (PSS), a self-report measure designed to evaluate perceived stress associated with parenting roles, including emotional demands and role restriction (Berry & Jones, 1995). The psychosocial adjustment of the typically developing sibling was explored using the Strengths and Difficulties Questionnaire (SDQ), a behavioral screening instrument measuring emotional symptoms, conduct problems, peer relationships, and prosocial behavior (Goodman, 1997).

In addition to standardized measures, qualitative data were collected through a semi-structured interview conducted with the child's primary caregiver to explore caregiving practices, parental role distribution, sibling involvement, emotional adjustment, and access to support services within the home environment. Semi-structured interviews are widely used in qualitative health and developmental research to explore lived experiences and family-mediated adaptation processes within real-life caregiving contexts (Braun & Clarke, 2006; Stake, 1995).

The interview protocol was developed in alignment with the study's research questions, thereby ensuring that thematic domains related to caregiving routines, family functioning, and early developmental and educational intervention practices were systematically addressed during data collection (Creswell & Poth, 2018). Indicative interview questions explored the ways in which the child's diagnosis influenced the distribution of caregiving responsibilities within the family, the extent to which daily family routines had changed following the diagnosis, the management of therapeutic activities within the home environment, and the involvement of the typically developing sibling in daily interaction or caregiving routines. Additional questions focused on emotional challenges associated with managing the child's developmental needs, the impact of the diagnosis on family participation in social or recreational activities, the availability of formal or informal support services, perceived barriers in accessing specialized healthcare or early developmental and educational intervention services, and strategies used to integrate therapeutic goals into everyday family routines.

Examples of verbatim interview questions included the following: *Can you describe how your child's diagnosis has influenced the way caregiving responsibilities are distributed within your family? What changes have occurred in your daily routines since your child began receiving therapeutic or educational support? How is your older child involved in daily interaction or supporting their sibling? What kinds of challenges have you encountered when trying to access specialized health or early educational services?*

An overview of the data collection instruments used in the present study is presented in Table 2.

Table 2. Overview of data collection instruments

Instrument	Target Domain	Informant
FQoL	Family well-being	Primary caregiver
PSS	Parenting-related stress	Primary caregiver
SDQ	Sibling psychosocial adjustment	Primary caregiver
Semi-structured interview	Caregiving practices and routines	Primary caregiver

Procedure

Data collection was conducted over a period of ongoing clinical follow-up and caregiver communication. The procedure involved the systematic organization of developmental information, caregiver-reported outcomes, and contextual observations related to daily family routines and therapeutic engagement within the home environment.

Initially, clinical and developmental documentation related to the child's medical history, intervention planning, and educational support was reviewed to obtain background information regarding developmental trajectory and intervention needs. Subsequently, the primary caregiver completed the FQoL, the PSS, and the SDQ to provide structured information regarding perceived family well-being, caregiving burden, and emotional adjustment.

Following questionnaire completion, a semi-structured interview was conducted with the child's primary caregiver in a private setting within the family home. The interview lasted approximately 45-60 minutes and focused on exploring changes in parental roles, daily caregiving routines, sibling involvement, emotional adjustment, and access to formal or informal support services. Interview responses were documented through written notes and subsequently transcribed for thematic analysis.

Attention was given to the ways in which caregiving responsibilities influenced family routines, employment patterns, participation in social or recreational activities, and the implementation of therapeutic goals within everyday family practices. The inclusion of contextual information related to daily caregiving practices allowed for an in-depth exploration of adaptation processes within the family microsystem (Bronfenbrenner, 2005).

Data Analysis

Data analysis followed a combined measurement-informed qualitative approach to integrate caregiver-reported standardized outcomes with interview-derived thematic data. This analytic strategy enabled the examination of caregiving dynamics at both descriptive and interpretative levels within the family system.

Initially, descriptive statistical analysis was conducted on caregiver responses obtained from the FQoL, the PSS, and the SDQ. Domain-level scores were reviewed to identify patterns related to perceived family well-being, caregiving burden, and sibling psychosocial adjustment. Given the single-case design of the study, these measures were not used for inferential statistical comparison but rather to provide contextualized insight into caregiving demands and family functioning within the household (Raina et al., 2005).

Subsequently, qualitative data derived from the semi-structured caregiver interview were analyzed using thematic analysis procedures as outlined by Braun and Clarke (2006). Thematic analysis is widely used in qualitative developmental and health research to examine lived experiences and meaning-making processes within caregiving environments. Interview responses were initially transcribed and subjected to an inductive coding process in which segments of text were categorized according to recurring caregiving practices, emotional responses, family routines, and role adjustments. Open coding was first applied to identify meaningful units of data related to parental responsibilities, therapeutic routines, sibling involvement, emotional adjustment, and access to support services. Examples of initial codes included parental employment withdrawal, home-based therapeutic implementation, coordination of medical appointments, structured daily routines, sibling participation in interaction, emotional concerns regarding prognosis, shared decision-making, and limited-service accessibility. These codes were subsequently grouped into broader thematic categories reflecting caregiving dynamics within the family system. Through iterative comparison of coded segments and refinement of category boundaries, higher-order themes were developed to represent patterns of family adaptation to the child's developmental needs. The development of themes followed a recursive analytic process involving repeated review of coded interview segments in relation to the study's research questions. Examples of thematic categories included parental role reorganization, integration of therapeutic practices in daily routines, sibling involvement in caregiving contexts, emotional adjustment to developmental uncertainty, and environmental constraints in accessing support services. Credibility of qualitative findings was supported through triangulation between caregiver-reported interview data, clinical documentation, observational information related to daily routines, and standardized family functioning measures (Creswell & Poth, 2018; Yin, 2018). The integration of multiple data sources enabled a more comprehensive understanding of caregiving demands, parental stress, sibling adjustment, and adaptive functioning within the family microsystem. Patterns identified through thematic analysis were interpreted in relation to caregiving burden, family cohesion, sibling participation, and engagement in early developmental and educational intervention practices within the home environment.

An overview of the coding process and thematic categorization derived from interview data is presented in Table 3.

Table 3. Indicative coding framework derived from thematic analysis

Initial Codes	Recoded Categories	Final Themes
Parental employment withdrawal	Parental role redistribution	Parental role reorganization
Coordination of medical appointments	Structured caregiving routines	Integration of therapeutic practices in daily life
Home-based therapy implementation	Daily therapeutic engagement	Integration of therapeutic practices in daily life
Shared decision-making between parents	Collaborative coping strategies	Emotional adjustment to developmental uncertainty
Concerns about developmental prognosis	Future-oriented emotional stress	Emotional adjustment to developmental uncertainty
Sibling participation in play routines	Sibling supportive interaction	Sibling involvement in caregiving contexts
Reduced sibling leisure opportunities	Sibling role adjustment	Sibling involvement in caregiving contexts
Limited availability of services	Service accessibility barriers	Environmental constraints in support access
Transportation challenges	Logistical service constraints	Environmental constraints in support access

Ethical Considerations

Ethical considerations were addressed throughout all stages of the research process in accordance with established qualitative research guidelines for studies involving families of children with developmental or medical conditions (Creswell & Poth, 2018; Yin, 2018). Given the sensitive nature of genetic diagnosis and caregiving experiences, particular emphasis was placed on confidentiality, voluntary participation, and the responsible handling of personal and developmental information.

Prior to data collection, the child's primary caregiver was fully informed about the purpose of the study, the procedures involved, and the intended use of anonymized data for research and publication purposes. Written informed consent was obtained for participation in the completion of standardized questionnaires as well as for involvement in the semi-structured caregiver interview. Participation in all stages of the study was voluntary, and caregivers were informed of their right to withdraw from the research process at any time without consequence.

All identifying information was removed during data transcription and reporting procedures. Pseudonyms were used to ensure participant anonymity and minimize the risk of identification. Developmental, medical, and family-related information was reported only to the extent necessary to address the research aims of the study. Care was taken to avoid the inclusion of contextual details that could indirectly reveal the identity of the participating family, especially given the rarity of SGBS1 within the general population.

Interview data were securely stored in password-protected digital files accessible only to the research team. Questionnaire responses and developmental documentation were handled in accordance with principles of data protection and participant privacy and were retained solely for the purposes of research analysis. No personally identifiable information was included in the final report of findings.

Ethical standards for qualitative case-based research involving vulnerable populations were followed throughout the data collection, analysis, and reporting processes (Creswell & Poth, 2018). The study adhered to internationally recognized ethical principles concerning respect for persons, beneficence, and confidentiality in research involving human participants. The reporting of findings was guided by the aim of contributing to interdisciplinary understanding of family adaptation in rare genetic conditions while safeguarding participant dignity, privacy, and psychosocial well-being.

FINDINGS

The findings of the present case study are presented in relation to both caregiver-reported standardized measures and qualitative data derived from the semi-structured interview. The integration of quantitative descriptive outcomes with thematic interview findings enabled a comprehensive examination of caregiving dynamics, family adaptation processes, and early developmental and educational intervention practices within the home environment.

Outcomes of Standardized Measures

Family Quality of Life

Caregiver responses on the FQoL indicated variability across domains of perceived family functioning. Lower satisfaction levels were reported in relation to time availability for leisure activities and participation in community-based social interactions. The primary caregiver described limited opportunities for family recreation due to the scheduling of therapeutic activities and frequent medical appointments. Moderate levels of satisfaction were reported in domains related to parenting practices and family interaction. Shared involvement in daily caregiving routines, including participation in therapeutic exercises conducted within the home environment, appeared to support communication and collaboration between family members. Emotional well-being was reported as moderately affected by caregiving responsibilities, particularly in relation to uncertainty regarding developmental outcomes and future independence. Perceived availability of disability-related support services was reported as limited. The caregiver noted that access to specialized therapeutic intervention often required travel outside the family's residential area, which influenced both scheduling flexibility and participation in social activities.

Parental Stress

Responses obtained from the PSS suggested elevated levels of stress associated with caregiving responsibilities. Increased stress was reported in relation to role restriction, time demands, and emotional burden associated with managing developmental needs and coordinating intervention services. The distribution of caregiving tasks within the family was primarily centered around the mother, who assumed responsibility for daily supervision and therapeutic engagement following the discontinuation of paid employment. Coordination of medical appointments, implementation of home-based therapy activities, and monitoring of developmental progress were described as contributing to increased daily workload. At the same time, collaborative decision-making between parents regarding treatment planning and intervention strategies was identified as a coping mechanism that supported emotional adjustment within the family system.

Sibling Emotional Adjustment

Scores obtained from the SDQ indicated generally adaptive psychosocial functioning in the typically developing sibling. Elevated scores were observed in the prosocial behavior domain, suggesting supportive involvement in family interactions and positive engagement with the affected child. Mild elevations were noted in domains related to peer relationship difficulties. Caregiver reports indicated that participation in family caregiving routines occasionally influenced the sibling's opportunities for independent social engagement and leisure activities outside the home environment.

Thematic Findings from Semi-Structured Interview

Parental Role Reorganization

Interview data indicated significant changes in parental role distribution within the family system following the child's diagnosis. The mother reported discontinuing paid employment to assume primary caregiving responsibilities within the home environment. Daily caregiving tasks, including supervision of therapeutic activities and coordination of medical appointments, were primarily managed by the mother. The father maintained full-time professional responsibilities to ensure financial stability for the family. This redistribution of roles resulted in a dual-role structure in which caregiving and financial responsibilities were divided between parents.

Integration of Therapeutic Practices in Daily Routines

Caregiving responsibilities associated with the child's developmental needs were integrated into daily family routines and required continuous scheduling of therapeutic and medical activities. Regular visits to healthcare providers, implementation of speech and occupational therapy exercises within the home environment, and coordination of developmental services formed a central component of everyday life. Daily schedules were frequently organized around medical monitoring and therapeutic intervention, which influenced participation in recreational and social activities. Therapeutic goals related to communication, motor development, and autonomy were incorporated into routine family interactions such as play, mealtime, and shared leisure activities.

Sibling Involvement in Caregiving Contexts

The typically developing sibling was reported to participate in daily interactions and occasionally assist with routine caregiving tasks. Interview responses suggested that sibling involvement included participation in therapeutic exercises and engagement in shared daily activities with the affected child. Caregivers described the sibling as actively involved in family routines, particularly in activities involving play and communication. This involvement appeared to support relational bonding within the family system while also reflecting changes in family responsibilities associated with caregiving demands.

Emotional Adjustment to Developmental Uncertainty

Caregivers reported ongoing emotional challenges related to uncertainty regarding developmental outcomes and long-term prognosis. Concerns related to the child's future functioning and access to appropriate support services were identified as sources of stress. Shared decision-making between parents regarding treatment planning and daily caregiving practices was reported as a strategy for managing emotional demands and maintaining balance within the family system.

Environmental Constraints in Accessing Support Services

Interview responses indicated that access to multidisciplinary support services represented an ongoing challenge within the family's residential context. Limited availability of specialized professionals necessitated the continuation of therapeutic exercises within the home environment. Community-based support networks were identified as supplementary resources for managing caregiving responsibilities and coordinating intervention services.

Integrated Synthesis of Findings

The integration of caregiver-reported standardized measures with qualitative interview data provided a comprehensive overview of caregiving dynamics and family adaptation processes within the household. Descriptive outcomes obtained from the FQoL indicated moderate levels of perceived family interaction and emotional functioning, alongside reduced scores in domains related to physical and material well-being. These findings appeared to reflect the ongoing demands associated with coordinating therapeutic activities and accessing multidisciplinary intervention services within a semi-urban context.

Similarly, elevated scores on the PSS suggested increased caregiving burden linked to the implementation of home-based therapeutic practices and the coordination of medical follow-up appointments. Qualitative interview responses further supported these outcomes by illustrating the ways in which caregiving responsibilities influenced parental employment patterns and daily family routines.

Caregiver-reported responses on the SDQ indicated generally adaptive psychosocial functioning for the typically developing sibling, with occasional emotional concerns related to changes in family routines and parental availability. Interview data suggested that sibling involvement in shared play activities and everyday interaction contributed to relational bonding while simultaneously reflecting adjustments in family role distribution.

Across data sources, caregiving practices were consistently integrated into the family's daily routines through structured home-based intervention activities and collaborative parental decision-making. Patterns identified through thematic analysis, including parental role reorganization, integration of therapeutic practices in everyday life, and environmental constraints in accessing support services, appeared to align with descriptive outcomes obtained from standardized family functioning measures.

Taken together, the triangulation of quantitative caregiver-reported measures and qualitative interview data suggests that family-mediated intervention practices may function as adaptive strategies supporting developmental participation and psychosocial adjustment within the caregiving environment.

DISCUSSION

The present study aimed to examine caregiving dynamics and family adaptation processes in a Greek family raising a child diagnosed with SGBS1. Guided by ecological systems theory (Bronfenbrenner, 2005) and family resilience theory (Walsh, 2016), the findings provide insight into the ways in which families respond to long-term developmental needs associated with rare genetic conditions. This broader context is particularly important given that rare genetic conditions in childhood are frequently associated with substantial neurological involvement and often involve a prolonged diagnostic odyssey, which may delay appropriate clinical management and increase psychosocial burden for families (Sirchia et al., 2026). The discussion of results is structured in relation to the research questions guiding the study.

Parental Role Reorganization and Daily Caregiving Practices

The findings of the present study suggest that the child's diagnosis was associated with significant changes in parental role distribution within the family system. Raising a child diagnosed with SGBS1 appears to influence parental role distribution and the organization of daily caregiving routines, as reflected in the discontinuation of paid employment by the mother to assume primary caregiving responsibilities, a pattern commonly observed in families raising children with rare or chronic developmental conditions (Pelentsov et al., 2016; van Niekerk et al., 2026). Recent qualitative evidence further indicates that family caregivers of children with rare diseases often assume multifaceted roles that extend beyond direct daily care to include coordinating healthcare, managing appointments, monitoring symptoms, seeking information, and advocating for their child's needs across services (van Niekerk et al., 2026). Such role reorganization may represent an adaptive response to the increased time demands associated with therapeutic engagement and ongoing medical monitoring.

From the perspective of the family stress and adaptation model, the diagnosis of SGBS1 can be conceptualized as a persistent stressor requiring the mobilization of family resources and adjustment of role expectations (McCubbin & Patterson, 1983). The redistribution of caregiving responsibilities between parents illustrates how families reorganize daily routines to maintain functioning in the presence of long-term developmental challenges. Furthermore, the integration of therapeutic practices into home-based routines reflects an effort to support developmental progress within the family microsystem. Ecological systems theory emphasizes the importance of proximal processes within the family environment in shaping developmental outcomes (Bronfenbrenner, 2005). In this context, daily caregiving practices become embedded within routine family interactions, influencing both the child's developmental experiences and parental availability. In line with previous qualitative findings, caregiving may also involve supporting the child's basic daily functioning and balancing illness-related care with the ordinary demands of parenting, thereby intensifying the need for role flexibility within the family system (van Niekerk et al., 2026).

Parental Stress and Family Quality of Life

The findings of the present study suggest that caregiving demands associated with raising a child diagnosed with SGBS1 may influence levels of parental stress and perceived family quality of life. In the present case, increased caregiving responsibilities were associated with elevated levels of parental stress and moderate levels of perceived family well-being. The time-intensive nature of daily caregiving, including the coordination of therapeutic activities and medical appointments, appeared to affect parental emotional well-being and everyday functioning. In addition, the reorganization of family routines around the child's needs may have contributed to restrictions in employment, leisure, and broader family life. These findings are consistent with previous research showing that parents of children with developmental disabilities often report increased emotional strain and reduced opportunities for employment and leisure activities (Raina et al., 2005). More recent research in the field of rare diseases similarly indicates that caregivers may become overwhelmed by extensive daily care demands, while work disruption, financial pressure, and ongoing caregiving responsibilities can affect family routines, psychological adjustment, and quality of life (Atkins & Padgett, 2024; van Niekerk et al., 2026). Within family quality of life approaches, such caregiving demands may influence multiple domains of family functioning, including emotional well-being, parenting practices, and access to disability-related support (Hoffman et al., 2006; Zuna et al., 2009). At the same time, the findings of the present study suggest that adaptive coping strategies, such as collaborative decision-making between parents and the establishment of structured caregiving routines, may support family cohesion despite increased caregiving demands, a pattern that is broadly consistent with family resilience perspectives (Walsh, 2016).

Sibling Adjustment and Involvement

The findings further indicate that the presence of a chronic developmental condition within the family system may influence the psychosocial adjustment and involvement of the typically developing sibling. In the present case, the sibling was reported to participate in daily interactions and occasionally assist with routine caregiving tasks. Research suggests that siblings of children with chronic developmental conditions may assume supportive roles within the family while simultaneously navigating changes in parental attention and family expectations (Lummer-Aikey & Goldstein, 2021). Sibling involvement in caregiving activities may contribute to the development of empathy and prosocial behavior; however, it may also reflect reduced opportunities for independent social engagement. Previous studies have identified both adaptive and stress-related outcomes among siblings of children with chronic medical conditions, highlighting the importance of examining sibling adjustment within caregiving environments (Atkins & Padgett, 2024). Family resilience theory emphasizes the importance of maintaining balanced relationships within caregiving contexts to support adaptive functioning across all family members (Walsh, 2016). The involvement of the sibling in shared daily routines may therefore represent both relational bonding and the redistribution of family responsibilities associated with caregiving demands, as family life in the context of rare developmental conditions is often reorganized around intensive care needs, emotional demands, and shifting patterns of support within the household (van Niekerk et al., 2026).

Access to Support Services

The findings of the present study suggest that families raising children with SGBS1 may encounter challenges in accessing formal support services within their residential context. In the present case, access to multidisciplinary support services was identified as an ongoing challenge within the family's semi-urban setting. Limited availability of specialized professionals necessitated the continuation of therapeutic exercises within the home environment. Previous research has highlighted the influence of geographical location on access to healthcare and developmental services for families managing rare medical conditions (Pelentsov et al., 2016). Barriers related to transportation, service availability, and coordination of intervention may contribute to increased caregiving burden and reduced flexibility in daily scheduling (Atkins & Padgett, 2024). Community-based support networks may function as supplementary resources in supporting caregiving practices and facilitating continuity of care. The availability of coordinated case management and accessible intervention services has been identified as a key factor influencing family adaptation in the presence of chronic developmental conditions (Atkins & Padgett, 2024).

Implications for Clinical and Educational Practice

The findings of the present case study highlight the importance of adopting family-centered approaches in the clinical and educational support of children diagnosed with rare genetic conditions such as SGBS1. Traditional intervention models frequently focus primarily on the developmental needs of the affected child; however, caregiving environments represent a central context for adaptation, regulation, and learning. The integration of family-centered practices into clinical and educational frameworks may therefore enhance both developmental outcomes and psychosocial adjustment within the family system (Walsh, 2016).

Family-Centered Intervention Planning

Family-centered intervention planning recognizes the interconnected nature of developmental outcomes and caregiving practices. In the present case, parents assumed active roles in implementing therapeutic strategies within the home environment, particularly in contexts where access to specialized services was limited. Such involvement is consistent with contemporary intervention models in developmental disabilities that emphasize the role of caregivers as co-facilitators of learning and adaptive functioning (Pelentsov et al., 2016). Recent qualitative research on rare disease caregiving further suggests that parents often assume multifaceted roles extending beyond direct care to include coordinating healthcare, seeking condition-related information, monitoring symptoms, and advocating for their child across settings (van Niekerk et al., 2026). Providing caregivers with structured guidance and training in communication support strategies, motor development activities, and behavioral regulation techniques may enhance both intervention effectiveness and parental confidence, particularly when professional guidance is communicated in accessible and supportive ways (van Niekerk et al., 2026). Embedding therapeutic goals within daily routines, including play, mealtime interaction, and shared family activities, may further promote generalization of emerging skills across naturalistic contexts. Multidisciplinary collaboration among pediatricians, geneticists, therapists, and educational professionals may support coordinated care that addresses both developmental needs and family functioning. Regular communication between clinical and educational providers may facilitate the alignment of therapeutic and educational goals, thereby promoting continuity of intervention across home and school environments (Bronfenbrenner, 2005).

Supporting Sibling Adjustment

The findings related to sibling involvement underscore the importance of addressing the psychosocial experiences of typically developing sibling within caregiving families. Siblings often participate in daily caregiving routines while simultaneously navigating changes in parental attention and family expectations. Intervention programs that include opportunities for siblings to express concerns and maintain age-appropriate autonomy may contribute to improved emotional adjustment and social participation (Lummer-Aikey & Goldstein, 2021). Family-based support strategies may include structured family counseling sessions, sibling support groups, and psychoeducational resources designed to facilitate open communication regarding caregiving responsibilities. Educational professionals may also contribute to supporting sibling adjustment by recognizing possible changes in peer interaction, emotional functioning, and academic engagement associated with caregiving family environments, as school personnel may be well positioned to identify support needs among siblings of children with chronic conditions (Bortes et al., 2020; Prentice et al., 2026).

Service Accessibility in Semi-Urban Contexts

Families residing in semi-urban or rural areas may encounter logistical barriers in accessing specialized healthcare and developmental services, including repeated travel demands, fragmented service pathways, and limited local availability of specialist care (Atkins & Padgett, 2024; van Niekerk et al., 2026). Flexible service provision, including telehealth-based therapeutic support, may improve access to specialist input and continuity of care for families managing rare genetic conditions (Chen et al., 2024). Supportive policies and services that reduce caregiving burden, including practical assistance and greater flexibility in balancing care and employment demands, may also support family adaptation over time (Pelentsov et al., 2016; van Niekerk et al., 2026). Access to coordinated case management may facilitate communication between healthcare professionals, educators, and family members, thereby reducing the logistical burden associated with scheduling, communication, and service navigation (Walton et al., 2020; Morris et al., 2022).

Implications for Educational Inclusion

Educational professionals play a critical role in supporting children with rare developmental conditions through individualized educational planning and inclusive classroom practices. Collaboration between educators and healthcare providers may facilitate the integration of therapeutic goals into educational environments (Atkins & Padgett, 2024; Bronfenbrenner, 2005). Family-school partnerships may therefore represent an important component of comprehensive intervention planning for children diagnosed with SGBS1. The alignment of clinical intervention goals with educational strategies may support functional participation, communication development, and social interaction within inclusive classroom settings (Atkins & Padgett, 2024).

Implications for Policy and Service Development

The findings of the present case study have important implications not only for clinical and educational practice but also for the design and delivery of support services for families raising children with rare genetic conditions. Rare developmental syndromes such as SGBS1 often require long-term multidisciplinary intervention that extends across medical, educational, and psychosocial domains. As a result, service provision may need to move beyond child-centered intervention models toward more comprehensive family-oriented frameworks of care (Pelentsov et al., 2016; Atkins & Padgett, 2024).

In many healthcare systems, particularly within semi-urban or rural regions, families may encounter challenges in accessing specialized therapeutic services due to geographical distance, repeated travel demands, limited availability of trained professionals, and insufficient coordination between service providers (Atkins & Padgett, 2024; van Niekerk et al., 2026). These barriers may increase reliance on home-based intervention practices, thereby shifting a substantial portion of therapeutic responsibility onto caregivers. In this context, policy initiatives aimed at improving continuity of care may benefit from the implementation of coordinated case management systems that facilitate communication between healthcare professionals, educational practitioners, and family members (Walton et al., 2020; Morris et al., 2022).

National support frameworks for rare diseases may also benefit from the development of integrated service pathways that address both developmental needs and family functioning. The provision of accessible early intervention services, psychological counseling, and caregiver training programs may contribute to more responsive support for families managing chronic developmental conditions (Atkins & Padgett, 2024; Pelentsov et al., 2016). Flexible service delivery models, including telehealth-based therapeutic support and community-based intervention programs, may further help reduce logistical barriers associated with transportation and service availability (Chen et al., 2024).

Supportive employment policies that enable greater flexibility in balancing work and caregiving demands may also facilitate family adaptation over time, particularly in cases where parental role reorganization involves adjustments to employment patterns in response to daily caregiving responsibilities (Pelentsov et al., 2016; van Niekerk et al., 2026). Access to financial assistance, caregiver support services, and respite opportunities may likewise help alleviate some of the emotional and practical strain associated with long-term caregiving demands. Furthermore, the development of sibling support initiatives within community or educational settings may provide additional psychosocial resources for typically developing children living in caregiving environments. Programs designed to promote peer interaction, emotional expression, and age-appropriate understanding of developmental conditions may contribute to improved adjustment outcomes among siblings (Lummer-Aikey & Goldstein, 2021).

Overall, these policy considerations highlight the importance of adopting systemic and family-oriented approaches to service provision for families raising children with rare genetic syndromes. By addressing the needs of caregivers and siblings alongside those of the affected child, service delivery systems may be better positioned to support adaptive family functioning and more sustainable long-term developmental outcomes.

FUTURE RESEARCH DIRECTIONS

Future research examining family adaptation in the context of rare genetic syndromes may benefit from the inclusion of longitudinal study designs to explore changes in caregiving roles and family functioning over time. The cross-sectional nature of the present case study limits the ability to examine developmental transitions across childhood and adolescence, which may influence both caregiving demands and psychosocial adjustment among family members (Atkins & Padgett, 2024).

Further investigation involving multiple families raising children with SGBS1 or related developmental conditions may provide additional insight into patterns of adaptation across diverse caregiving environments. Comparative studies examining families residing in urban versus semi-urban or rural settings may also contribute to a more nuanced understanding of the influence of service accessibility on family functioning and intervention practices (Pelentsov et al., 2016; van Niekerk et al., 2026).

Future research may additionally consider the perspectives of typically developing siblings in order to examine emotional adjustment, coping strategies, and participation in family caregiving routines. The inclusion of sibling-reported measures and qualitative interviews may enhance understanding of family-level adaptation processes in caregiving contexts (Lummer-Aikey & Goldstein, 2021).

In addition, interdisciplinary research integrating clinical, educational, and psychosocial perspectives may contribute to the development of family-centered intervention models that address the complex needs of families managing rare developmental conditions. Such approaches may also inform the design of more coordinated support systems that promote well-being across family members and facilitate continuity of care between home, clinical, and educational settings (Atkins & Padgett, 2024; Walton et al., 2020; Morris et al., 2022).

Additionally, the integration of mixed-methods approaches combining standardized family functioning measures with qualitative case-based analyses may provide a more comprehensive understanding of the mechanisms through which family environments mediate developmental outcomes in children with rare genetic syndromes.

Limitations

The findings of the present study should be interpreted considering several limitations inherent in qualitative case study research. First, the use of a single instrumental case limits the generalizability of the findings to broader populations of families raising children with rare genetic conditions. Case study methodology is intended to provide an in-depth contextualized understanding of complex developmental phenomena rather than to produce statistically generalizable results (Yin, 2018). Consequently, the caregiving dynamics and adaptation processes described in this study may not reflect the experiences of all families managing SGBS1 or other rare developmental disorders.

Second, the reliance on caregiver-reported information may introduce subjective bias related to perceptions of caregiving burden, family routines, and emotional adjustment. While caregiver perspectives are essential for understanding lived experiences within family systems, self-reported data may be influenced by individual coping styles, emotional stress, or recall limitations (Creswell & Poth, 2018). The inclusion of standardized family functioning measures alongside qualitative interview data was intended to enhance contextual understanding; however, the absence of observational data or clinician-reported assessments represents an additional limitation.

Furthermore, the psychosocial adjustment of the typically developing sibling was examined indirectly through caregiver-completed measures rather than through direct self-report or interview-based assessment. Future studies may benefit from incorporating sibling-reported data to obtain a more comprehensive understanding of emotional adjustment and family-level adaptation processes in caregiving environments.

In addition, environmental and contextual factors specific to the family's semi-urban setting may have influenced access to support services and therapeutic resources. Families residing in different geographical or socioeconomic contexts may encounter distinct challenges related to healthcare availability, financial stability, or community-based support systems (Pelentsov et al., 2016). Variability in access to multidisciplinary intervention services may therefore influence caregiving practices and perceptions of family quality of life.

Finally, the cross-sectional nature of the data limits the ability to examine changes in family functioning over time. Caregiving demands associated with rare developmental conditions are likely to evolve across developmental stages, particularly during transitions related to educational placement or adolescence. Longitudinal studies may provide further insight into how caregiving roles, parental stress, and resilience processes develop throughout childhood and adolescence in families managing rare genetic conditions (Atkins & Padgett, 2024).

CONCLUSION

Rare genetic conditions such as SGBS1 present complex developmental challenges that extend beyond clinical management and influence the everyday functioning of the family system. The present case study sought to examine caregiving dynamics and family adaptation processes within a Greek family raising a child diagnosed with SGBS1, with particular emphasis on parental role distribution, caregiving burden, sibling involvement, and access to support services.

The findings indicate that long-term caregiving demands associated with rare developmental conditions may necessitate substantial reorganization of parental roles and daily routines. The integration of therapeutic practices within the home environment, along with collaborative decision-making between parents, reflects adaptive processes that develop over time in response to ongoing medical and developmental needs. These family-mediated practices appear to function as proximal developmental support within the child's everyday environment, shaping opportunities for communication, autonomy, and social participation.

In addition, the involvement of the typically developing siblings in daily interaction and caregiving routines highlights the systemic nature of family adaptation in the presence of chronic developmental conditions. Changes in family routines and parental availability may influence sibling adjustment; however, supportive involvement in shared activities may also contribute to relational bonding and the development of prosocial behaviors within the family context.

Access to multidisciplinary intervention services emerged as an additional factor influencing caregiving practices and family quality of life. Environmental constraints related to service availability within semi-urban settings may increase reliance on home-based intervention strategies, thereby shifting a substantial portion of therapeutic responsibility onto caregivers.

By situating caregiving dynamics within established theoretical frameworks of family stress and resilience, the present study underscores the importance of examining rare genetic conditions through a systemic lens that considers family functioning as a central component of developmental support. The findings suggest that interdisciplinary and family-centered intervention approaches may facilitate improved psychosocial adjustment and functional participation among children with rare developmental disorders.

Future efforts aimed at improving service accessibility, promoting caregiver involvement in early developmental and educational intervention, and supporting sibling adjustment may therefore contribute to more adaptive family functioning and enhanced developmental outcomes in the context of rare genetic syndromes.

REFERENCES

Atkins, J. C., & Padgett, C. R. (2024). Living with a rare disease: Psychosocial impacts for parents and family members – A systematic review. *Journal of Child and Family Studies, 33*(2), 617–636. DOI: 10.1007/s10826-024-02790-6

Behmel, A., Plöchl, E., & Rosenkranz, W. (1984). A new X-linked dysplasia gigantism syndrome: Identical with the Simpson dysplasia syndrome? *Human Genetics, 67*(4), 409–413. DOI: 10.1007/BF00291401 PMID: 6490008

Berry, J. O., & Jones, W. H. (1995). The Parental Stress Scale: Initial psychometric evidence. *Journal of Social and Personal Relationships, 12*(3), 463–472. DOI: 10.1177/0265407595123009

Bortes, C., Strandh, M., & Nilsson, K. (2020). Sibling ill health and children's educational outcomes. *The Journal of School Health, 90*(5), 407–414. DOI: 10.1111/josh.12887 PMID: 32105351

Braun, V., & Clarke, V. (2006). Using thematic analysis in psychology. *Qualitative Research in Psychology, 3*(2), 77–101. DOI: 10.1191/1478088706qp063oa

Bronfenbrenner, U. (Ed.). (2005). *Making human beings human: Bioecological perspectives on human development.* Sage Publications.

Chen, F. H., Hartman, A. L., Letinturier, M. C. V., Antoniadou, V., Baynam, G., Bloom, L., Crimi, M., Della Rocca, M. G., Didato, G., Houge, S. D., Jonker, A., Kawome, M., Mueller, F., O'Brien, J., Puri, R. D., Ryan, N., Thong, M.-K., Tumienė, B., & Parisi, M. A. (2024). Telehealth for rare disease care, research, and education across the globe: A review of the literature by the IRDiRC telehealth task force. *European Journal of Medical Genetics, 72*, 104977. DOI: 10.1016/j.ejmg.2024.104977 PMID: 39374775

Creswell, J. W., & Poth, C. N. (2018). *Qualitative inquiry and research design: Choosing among five approaches* (4th ed.). Sage Publications.

DeBaun, M. R., Ess, J., & Saunders, S. (2001). Simpson-Golabi-Behmel syndrome: Progress toward understanding the molecular basis for overgrowth, malformation, and cancer predisposition. *Molecular Genetics and Metabolism, 72*(4), 279–286. DOI: 10.1006/mgme.2001.3150 PMID: 11286501

Golabi, M., Rosen, L., & Opitz, J. M. (1984). A new X-linked mental retardation-overgrowth syndrome. *American Journal of Medical Genetics, 17*(1), 345–358. DOI: 10.1002/ajmg.1320170128 PMID: 6538755

Goodman, R. (1997). The Strengths and Difficulties Questionnaire: A research note. *Journal of Child Psychology and Psychiatry, and Allied Disciplines*, *38*(5), 581–586. DOI: 10.1111/j.1469-7610.1997.tb01545.x PMID: 9255702

Hoffman, L., Marquis, J. G., Poston, D. J., Summers, J. A., & Turnbull, A. (2006). Assessing family outcomes: Psychometric evaluation of the family quality of life scale. *Journal of Marriage and Family*, *68*(4), 1069–1083. DOI: 10.1111/j.1741-3737.2006.00314.x

King, S., Teplicky, R., King, G., & Rosenbaum, P. (2004). Family-centered service for children with cerebral palsy and their families: A review of the literature. *Seminars in Pediatric Neurology*, *11*(1), 78–86. DOI: 10.1016/j.spen.2004.01.009 PMID: 15132256

Lummer-Aikey, S., & Goldstein, S. (2021). Sibling adjustment to childhood chronic illness: An integrative review. *Journal of Family Nursing*, *27*(2), 136–153. DOI: 10.1177/1074840720977177 PMID: 33305651

McCubbin, H. I., & Patterson, J. M. (1983). The Family Stress Process: The Double ABCX Model of adjustment and adaptation. *Marriage & Family Review*, *6*(1-2), 7–37. DOI: 10.1300/J002v06n01_02

Morris, S., Hudson, E., Bloom, L., Chitty, L. S., Chitty, L., Fulop, N. J., Fulop, N., Hunter, A., Jones, J., Kai, J., Kerecuk, L., Kokocinska, M., Leeson-Beevers, K., Ng, P. L., Ng, P., Parkes, S., Ramsay, A. I., Ramsay, A., Simpson, A., & Walton, H. (2022). Co-ordinated care for people affected by rare diseases: The CONCORD mixed-methods study. *Health and Social Care Delivery Research*, *10*(05), 1–220. DOI: 10.3310/LNZZ5321 PMID: 35312266

Neri, G., Marini, R., Cappa, M., Borrelli, P., & Opitz, J. M. (2013). Simpson-Golabi-Behmel syndrome: An X-linked encephalo-tropho-schisis syndrome. 1988. *American Journal of Medical Genetics. Part A*, *161A*(11), 2697–2703. DOI: 10.1002/ajmg.a.36317 PMID: 24166811

Nisbet, A. F., Hathaway, E. R., & Kalish, J. M. (2024). Simpson-Golabi-Behmel syndrome type 1. In Adam, M. P., Bick, S., & Mirzaa, G. M. (Eds.), *GeneReviews®* [Internet]. University of Washington.

Orphanet. (2023). *Simpson-Golabi-Behmel syndrome*. https://www.orpha.net/en/disease/detail/ 373

Pelentsov, L. J., Fielder, A. L., & Laws, T. A. (2016). The supportive care needs of parents of children with rare diseases: A qualitative descriptive study. *Journal of Pediatric Nursing*, *31*(3), e207–e218. DOI: 10.1016/j.pedn.2015.10.022 PMID: 26651231

Prentice, C. M., Wehrli, S., Zahl, E., Orm, S., Botta, M., Vatne, T. M., Fredriksen, T., Kirchhofer, S., & Fjermestad, K. (2026). Parent-teacher discrepancies about the mental health of siblings of children with chronic disorders: A latent profile analysis. *Journal of Emotional and Behavioral Disorders*, ●●●, 1–11. DOI: 10.1177/10634266261417609

Punnett, H. H. (2000). *Simpson-Golabi-Behmel syndrome. Atlas of Genetics and Cytogenetics in Oncology and Haematology*. https://atlasgeneticsoncology.org/cancer-prone-disease/ 10038/ simpson-golabi-behmel-syndrome

Raina, P., O'Donnell, M., Rosenbaum, P., Brehaut, J., Walter, S. D., Russell, D., Swinton, M., Zhu, B., & Wood, E. (2005). The health and well-being of caregivers of children with cerebral palsy. *Pediatrics*, *115*(6), e626–e636. DOI: 10.1542/peds.2004-1689 PMID: 15930188

Sirchia, F., Kalantari, S., Carli, D., Zadorozhna, M., Bassanese, F., Venti, E. T., Taft, R. J., Kesari, A., Sorasio, L., Antona, V., Guala, A., Feresin, A., Basile, A., Licciardi, F., Garau, J., Gasparini, P., Grosso, E., Mussa, A., Ferrero, G. B., & Giorgio, E. (2026). Advancing Neuropediatric Rare Disease Diagnosis Through Clinical Genome Sequencing. *Pediatric Neurology*, *177*, 28–45. DOI: 10.1016/j.pediatrneurol.2026.01.004 PMID: 41619469

Stake, R. E. (1995). *The art of case study research.* Sage Publications.

Tsibidaki, A. (2021). Children with cerebral palsy: Family and parent demographic characteristics and family strengths in Greece and Italy. *Journal of Health Psychology*, *26*(12), 2071–2083. DOI: 10.1177/1359105319900276 PMID: 31918571

van Niekerk, J., Gush, M., Moosa, S., & Pretorius, C. (2026). Coping with the challenges of caregiving: A qualitative exploration of the experiences of family caregivers of children with rare diseases in South Africa. *Journal of Genetic Counseling*, *35*(2), 1–17. DOI: 10.1002/jgc4.70205 PMID: 41958204

Walsh, F. (2016). *Strengthening family resilience* (3rd ed.). Guilford Press.

Walton, H., Hudson, E., Simpson, A., Ramsay, A. I. G., Kai, J., Morris, S., Sutcliffe, A. G., & Fulop, N. J. (2020). Defining Coordinated Care for People with Rare Conditions: A Scoping Review. *International Journal of Integrated Care*, *20*(2), 14. Advance online publication. DOI: 10.5334/ijic.5464 PMID: 32607101

Whiting, M., Nash, A. S., Kendall, S., & Roberts, S. A. (2019). Enhancing resilience and self-efficacy in the parents of children with disabilities and complex health needs. *Primary Health Care Research and Development, 20*, e33. DOI: 10.1017/S1463423619000112 PMID: 32799971

Yin, R. K. (2018). *Case study research and applications: Design and methods* (6th ed.). Sage Publications.

Zhao, T., Allan, K., Taylor, J., Thorburn, D. R., White, S. M., Tan, T. Y., Christodoulou, J., Tan, N. B., & Stroud, D. A. (2025). Functional characterization of a novel GPC3 missense variant in Simpson-Golabi-Behmel Syndrome. *American Journal of Medical Genetics. Part A, 200*(3), 632–641. DOI: 10.1002/ajmg.a.64287 PMID: 41122961

Zuna, N. I., Turnbull, A., & Summers, J. A. (2009). Family quality of life: Moving from measurement to application. *Journal of Policy and Practice in Intellectual Disabilities, 6*(1), 25–31. DOI: 10.1111/j.1741-1130.2008.00199.x

Chapter 6
Quality of Life in Families of Children With Rare Genetic Syndromes

Christina Krystamtsi
http://orcid.org/0009-0000-1597-3778
University of the Aegean, Greece

Assimina Tsibidaki
http://orcid.org/0000-0001-6430-2436
University of the Aegean, Greece

Dimitra Katsarou
http://orcid.org/0000-0001-8690-0314
University of the Aegean, Greece

ABSTRACT

Families of children with rare genetic syndromes are confronted with complex challenges that extend beyond medical management and substantially affect family functioning, emotional well-being, and everyday life. This chapter presents a systematic review of sixteen recent primary research projects examining the quality of life (QoL) of families of children with rare genetic syndromes, with the aim of synthesizing evidence on QoL dimensions, reported levels, associated factors, and methodological approaches. The findings indicate reduced family QoL, particularly in emotional well-being and family dynamics, with overall levels ranging from low to moderate and varying across dimensions. Family cohesion and access to social and material support emerged as key protective factors. Implications are discussed with a particular focus on family-centered psychosocial interventions that concep-

DOI: 10.4018/979-8-3373-8485-6.ch006

tualize the family as a dynamic and cohesive system, capable, when adequately supported, of constructing meaning, strengthening resilience, and functioning in ways that promote well-being.

INTRODUCTION

Rare genetic disorders affect far more people worldwide than one might assume, with recent estimates suggesting that 450 million individuals are touched by these conditions either directly or as caregivers (Repetto & Rebolledo-Jaramillo, 2020). Although the symptoms and care need often appear from the very first days of life, families frequently endure a long and uncertain "diagnostic Odyssey," sometimes, lasting years (Zurynski et al., 2017). Because most individuals with rare genetic syndromes continue to live within their family environment well into adulthood, families inevitably become the primary source of care something that shapes their daily routines, emotional climate, and overall functioning (Hartmanis et al., 2023; Pelentsov et al., 2016).

Rare Genetic Syndromes and Family Life

Rare genetic syndromes, such as Angelman syndrome, Down syndrome, Fragile X syndrome, and Cri Du Chat syndrome (Katsarou, 2022; Katsarou & Zisi, 2022; Katsarou et al., 2025; Papadopoulou et al., 2024; Walkowiak et al., 2026) are chronic, complex conditions caused by chromosomal abnormalities, gene mutations, or deletions of genetic material (Boycott et al., 2017). They often involve developmental delays, intellectual disability, neurodevelopmental challenges, and multi-system complications (Eiroa-Orosa, 2020). Despite advances in genetic science, diagnosis remains difficult due to the wide range of clinical presentations and the limited specialized knowledge available to many healthcare professionals (McMullan et al., 2020).

Living with a child who has a rare genetic syndrome reshapes the family system in profound ways. From a systemic perspective, any change in one member affects the entire family unit (Giotsa et al., 2015; Watson, 2012). Increased care demands frequently lead to a child-centered family structure, shifts in roles and responsibilities, and reduced opportunities for social participation (Dellve et al., 2006; Tsamparli & Tsibidaki, 2020). Parents, especially mothers, tend to shoulder most daily caregiving tasks, which can be both physically and emotionally demanding (Hartmanis et al., 2023; Kodra et al., 2020).

Family Resilience and Positive Adaptation

Yet, despite these challenges, families often demonstrate remarkable adaptability. Research shows that many develop coping strategies and resilience over time, finding moments of acceptance, pride, hope, and meaning in their experiences (Adams et al., 2018; Horsley & Oliver, 2015; Pelentsov et al., 2016). Perspectives from positive psychology and family resilience theory highlight the capacity of families to mobilize strengths that support cohesion and stability even under demanding circumstances (Beighton & Wills, 2017).

Family Quality of Life: Conceptualization and Research Challenges

Within this context, the concept of Family Quality of Life (FQoL) has emerged as a central analytical framework for capturing the multidimensional experiences of families raising children with disabilities and chronic conditions. FQoL is conceptualized as a multidimensional construct encompassing emotional well-being, family interaction, financial adequacy, social inclusion, and access to supportive services (Zuna et al., 2010). It thus becomes clear that QoL is not a fixed concept, on the contrary, it undergoes changes as the data of society changes (Paxinos, 2022; Verdugo et al., 2005). However, existing research on FQoL varies widely in terms of measurement tools, methodological approaches, and the specific syndromes examined (Lim et al., 2025). This variability highlights the need for more systematic and integrative research.

Study Purpose and Research Questions

The purpose of this study is to highlight the levels of QoL of families of people with rare genetic syndromes through the review and synthesis of international literature, with emphasis on the factors that affect it, the methodological approaches that have been used and the research gaps that are highlighted.

Key Research Question

What are the levels of QoL in families of people with rare genetic syndromes, as reflected in international literature?

Secondary research questions

1. What dimensions of the QoL of families of children with rare genetic syndromes have been studied in international literature?
2. What are the levels of QoL of families, as recorded in quantitative, qualitative, and mixed studies?
3. What factors are associated with higher or lower levels of QoL in families of children with rare genetic syndromes?
4. What methodological approaches and tools are used to assess the QoL of families of children with rare genetic syndromes?

METHODS

The present study is a systematic review of international literature, with the aim of systematically synthesizing research data on the QoL levels of families of children with rare genetic syndromes. The review was conducted in accordance with the PRISMA 2020 guidelines (Preferred Reporting Items for Systematic Reviews and Meta-Analyses) (Page et al., 2021).

Search Strategy

The search was conducted exclusively in the Scopus database, selected for its broad multidisciplinary coverage of peer-reviewed health and social science literature, using a combination of keywords such as rare genetic syndromes, family QoL, parents, and caregivers. The Boolean operators "AND", "OR", and "NOT" were used in combination with the keywords to maximize the sensitivity and specificity of the search (Alharbi & Stevenson, 2020). However, the use of a single database may have limited the inclusion of relevant studies indexed elsewhere. For example, the search string was formulated as follows: ("rare genetic syndrome*" OR "genetic disorder*" OR "hereditary condition*" OR "inherited syndrome*") AND ("family quality of life" OR "family well-being" OR "family functioning" OR "family satisfaction") AND (parent* OR caregiver* OR "family member*" OR "guardian*").

Inclusion and Exclusion Criteria

The identified studies were independently reviewed by three independent reviewers. They then proceeded to select studies, according to the inclusion and exclusion criteria that had been defined (O'Brien et al., 2014). Any disagreements between the reviewers were resolved through discussion.

The study could include primary quantitative, qualitative and mixed studies that examine dimensions of the QoL or/and factors affecting their levels of well-being of families of children with rare genetic syndromes, without limitation as to the type of syndrome. Research articles had to be published in the Scopus database and written in English. The publication date of the articles was chosen to be from 2020 onwards, as it was considered particularly important to highlight modern and, therefore, valid data in relation to the central topic of the research.

Duplicate studies and studies that were not indexed in the Scopus database were excluded from the study. The same goes for studies written in languages other than English. Case studies were also excluded, as it was deemed necessary to contain generalizable research results. Finally, studies that focused solely on the QoL of the person with a rare genetic syndrome and not on the whole family were not included.

In the candidate studies to be included in the final sample of this research, a critical evaluation of the quality of the included studies was carried out, using the Mixed Methods Appraisal Tool (MMAT, Hong et al., 2018), which allows the evaluation of qualitative, quantitative and mixed research designs, as required by the methodology of systematic reviews.

Searching the Scopus database yielded 160 results of published research studies. After reading the titles, the 100 studies were excluded, as they were not related to the research interest of this study.

Of the 60 remaining articles, after evaluation of the abstracts, 44 were excluded. Specifically, 36 articles did not examine the totality of FQoL, but focused on individual family members (e.g., mother, father, siblings) or exclusively on people with genetic syndrome, while 8 articles were systematic reviews or meta-analyses.

Based on the above selection stages, the authors came up with 16 primary research studies, which, after a thorough reading of their full text, were judged to meet all the criteria of validity and suitability for inclusion in the final sample of this research.

In detail, the selection process of the studies is presented through the PRISMA flowchart.

Figure 1. Flowchart PRISMA

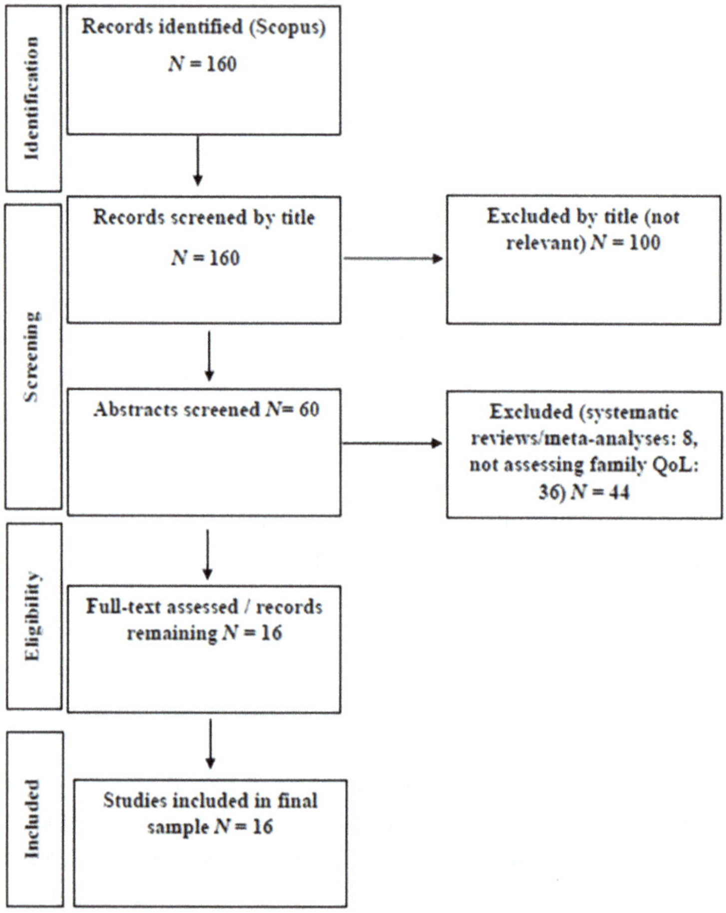

Data Extraction and Analysis

The findings were extracted from the sections of the results of all the studies included in the final sample of this research. After the extraction process, the data were coded and the individual codes were organized into broader conceptual categories, which constituted the so-called descriptive themes. The CK and AT researchers independently proceeded to synthesize the extracted data, before discussion and comparative examination of the emerging issues followed. Subsequently, SK, which had full knowledge of all the included studies, reviewed the proposed topics and the corresponding codes to ensure the coherence and completeness of the thematic grouping. The final agreement on the issues was reached by consensus of all three authors. Interrater reliability was calculated using Cohen's $\kappa = .74$, indicating substantial agreement. The results of the synthesis are presented in analytical topics and sub-themes, as reflected in the section of the results of the present study. Thematic analysis was chosen to synthesize the qualitative data obtained from this systematic review (Saunders et al., 2023).

Following a systematic and thorough examination of the results of the included studies, findings relevant to the review's research questions were extracted. The data were subsequently synthesized and analyzed using thematic analysis, allowing for the coding and organization of findings into conceptually coherent categories.

The thematic synthesis resulted in four central axes encompassing distinct but interrelated quality-of-life dimensions, as summarized in Table 1.

Table 1. Thematic categorization of quality-of-life dimensions in families of children with rare genetic syndromes

Central Thematic Axes	Corresponding QoL Dimensions
Psychosomatic status & resilience	Emotional well-being/functioning, caregiver anxiety/worry, trauma/PTSD, parental resilience, tolerance for uncertainty, cognitive functioning, expression of positive emotions.
Family dynamics & roles	Family interaction & functioning, parental adequacy/role, daily activities/routines, family relationships.
Social & material support	Social functioning & interaction, material/financial well-being, support and resources, disability-related support, leisure, recreation, and outdoor activities.
Child's functioning	Physical functioning, communication, behavioral functioning, autonomy and independence, child HRQoL (Health-Related QoL).

Table 2 presents the codes of factors that positively affect QoL levels in families of children with genetic syndromes.

Table 2. Thematic categorization of factors that positively affect the QoL of families of children with rare genetic syndromes

Central Thematic Axes	Findings included
Social support network & health services	Support from friends, organizations and communities, access to specialized services and resources, accommodation in a care facility, satisfactory support and information in relation to health status, respite care services, diagnosis, and initiation of treatment.
Family cohesion & interaction	Family interaction, strong cohesion, good cooperation between family members, large families, parenting.
Psychological resilience & management	Stress relief interventions, reframing, search for meaning, sense of security, high resilience, religious engagement.
Parental role & empowerment	Positive perception of the parental role.
Socio-economic & educational level	Better financial background, higher income, higher parenting education, satisfactory υλική/φυσική ευεξία.
Child's functionality & condition	Better QoL of the child, high cognitive function, age of the child (older age), disability-related support.
QoL stability	Overall stability of QoL regardless of the existence of the syndrome.

Similarly, Table 3 presents the codes of factors that negatively affect QoL levels in families of children with genetic syndromes.

Table 3. Thematic categorization of factors that negatively affect the QoL of families of children with rare genetic syndromes

Central Thematic Axes	Findings included
Psychological burden	Emotional Charge, High Stress, Anxiety, Post-Traumatic Stress (PTSD), Lack of Emotional Support, Mental Strain of Caregivers.
Care requirements & physical exhaustion	Overload of care, lack of time, high demands of everyday life, sleep problems, effects on work.
Behavioral difficulties & symptom severity	Disease severity, aggravated health condition, heart disease, decreased muscle tone, complexity of the child's symptoms, autistic characteristics, behavioral difficulties, aggressive behavior, low school function.
Social functionality & limitations	Low social participation, difficulty in establishing social relationships for the child, restrictions on autonomy and daily activities, concern for the future.
Deficiencies in the health & support system	Limited access to rehabilitation services, long waits for specialists, insufficient medical knowledge of the syndrome, lack of professional support.
Socioeconomic pressure & family background	Financial burden/difficulty, material constraints, low educational level of parents, dysfunction in family relationships.

The interpretation of QoL levels in the studies included in this systematic review was not based on absolute or theoretical values of the scales used, but on a comparative evaluation in relation to available reference populations, in accordance with the standard interpretation guidelines of the measurement tools and the relevant international literature (Varni et al., 2003). Emphasis was placed on the Pediatric QoL Inventory (PedsQL), which was used in most of the included studies.

In the context of PedsQL, scores on a scale of 0–100 do not reflect a linear continuum from 'low' to 'high' QoL. On the contrary, it is documented that families of children without severe or chronic care needs systematically show high average values, often above 70–90 points (Varni et al., 2003; Varni et al., 2006). Consequently, scores approaching or falling short of 50 points are interpreted as indicative of the frequent and not occasional presence of functional and psychosocial difficulties in the daily life of the family, as they deviate significantly (more than a standard deviation) from the general population (Varni et al., 2003).

Based on this comparative logic, the QoL levels in the individual studies were categorized in an interpretative and proportional way, taking into account: (a) the mean decimal values reported in the results of each study, (b) the comparison with available data of reference populations or control groups (benchmarking), and (c) the internal differentiation of the scores by individual dimension of QoL (Eiser & Morse, 2001).

In particular, scores such as 53.82 were not interpreted as "moderate" based on the theoretical upper limit of the scale (50 is not the "average" of health), but were classified as low or moderate to low, as they deviate substantially from the expected values of healthy populations, approaching the limits that are bibliographically defined as "at risk" for reduced QoL (Varni et al., 2005). The same principle was applied horizontally in all studies, regardless of the tool, to ensure the internal coherence of the narrative composition.

RESULTS

The methodological quality of the included studies was evaluated with MMAT confirming their suitability for thematic synthesis, despite the expected heterogeneity that characterizes investigations in rare genetic syndromes.

The chronological distribution publication of the studies was from 2021 to 2025. Specifically, 5 were published in 2025 (31%), 4 were published in 2022 (25%) and 3 were published in 2023 and 2024 (19% each). 1 study was published in 2021 (6.25%).

The geographical distribution of the studies shows a clear over-representation of European countries, with Poland having the highest percentage (25%), followed by the United States, the United Kingdom and Brazil (12.5% each). Countries such as

Spain, China, Australia, the Netherlands, the Netherlands/Belgium (transnational) are represented with 1 study (6.25% each). One study was also multinational (6.25%).

In the 16 primary research studies included in the systematic review, a total of 1,862 families were evaluated, if each participating parent or caregiver represents one family unit. The sample size varied significantly, ranging from 8 to 462 families, which reflects both the rarity of genetic syndromes and the practical difficulties of assembling large samples in this field of research.

The methodology of most studies, specifically 13 of them (81%) was quantitative. Of the remaining 3, 2 were qualitative methodology (12.5%) and 1 mixed methodology (6.25%).

In terms of QoL assessment tools, the majority of studies used the Pediatric QoL Inventory (PedsQL) in various versions (52.9%), with the most frequent use of the Family Impact Module (41.2%), which indicates an emphasis on the impact of disability on family functionality and well-being. Tools specifically designed for family QoL, such as the Beach Center Family QoL Scale, were used in a smaller percentage of the studies (17.6%). At the same time, tools adapted to populations with disabilities, such as QI-Disability, also appeared in 17.6% of the studies. The use of general QoL tools, such as WHOQOL-BREF and EQ-5D-Y-3L (5.9% respectively), was limited, while three studies (17.6%) adopted qualitative approaches through semi-structured interviews.

The data about basic study information about the country of conduct, genetic syndrome, sample size, type of study, and QoL measurement tools are presented in Table 4.

Table 4. Characteristics of the studies included in the review

Author (Year, Country)	Purpose of study	Sample (*n*=)	Type of study	Assessment tools QoL
Bel-Fenellós et al. (2025), Spain	To examine FQoL in parents of children with WHS.	Parents (34)	Quantitative	BCFQOL
Bolbocean et al. (2022), USA	To evaluate HRQoL in families of children with rare NDDs.	Families (391)	Quantitative	PedsQL
Bos-Roubos et al. (2022), Netherlands	To assess QoL and psychological distress in families of individuals with PWS.	Families (98)	Quantitative	WHOQOL-BREF
Chen et al. (2023), China	To examine associations between child HRQoL and FQoL in WS.	Families (101)	Quantitative	PedsQL GCM, PedsQL-FIM

continued on following page

Table 4. Continued

Author (Year, Country)	Purpose of study	Sample (*n=*)	Type of study	Assessment tools QoL
Dahshi et al. (2024), USA	To assess family impact and QoL in caregivers of individuals with SLC6A1-related NDD.	Caregivers(52)	Quantitative	QI-Disability, PedsQL-FIM
Haseley et al. (2021), Multinational	To explore parental well-being and FQoL in families of children with KS.	Parents (60)	Mixed	PedsQL-FIM, Self-constructed questionnaire
Hoffmann et al. (2025), United Sts. Kingdom	To explore parental experiences and family well-being in rare/ undiagnosed genetic conditions.	Parents (24)	Qualitative	Semi-structured interviews
Jobling et al. (2025), Australia	To examine family functioning in families of children with rare pediatric diseases.	Families (462)	Quantitative	-
Patel et al. (2025), United Sts. Kingdom	To assess QoL and anxiety in parents of children with undiagnosed rare genetic conditions.	Parents (383)	Quantitative	PedsQL-FIM, GAD-7, EQ-5D-Y-3L
Pereira et al. (2023), Brazil	To assess FQoL in families of children with WS.	Families (72)	Quantitative	Beach Center FQoL
Rozensztrauch & Śmigiel (2022), Poland	To evaluate FQoL and family functioning in parents of children with PWS.	Parents (46)	Quantitative	PedsQL- FIM
Rozensztrauch et al. (2023), Poland	To examine associations between child QoL and FQoL in DS.	Parents (52)	Quantitative	PedsQL™ 2.0 PedsQL™ 4.0
Rozensztrauch et al. (2024), Poland	To assess the QoL and the impact of RTS on family functioning.	Caregivers(13)	Quantitative	PedsQL™ 2.0 PedsQL™ 4.0
Telenga et al. (2024), Poland	To evaluate FQoL and family functioning in families of children with PTS.	Families (8)	Quantitative	PedsQL-FIM, QL-Disability
Vale et al. (2022), Brazil	To assess FQoL in families of children with RTS.	Families (51)	Quantitative	Beach Center FQoL
Van Till et al. (2025), Netherlands/Belgium	To explore family-centred outcomes in parents of children with KS.	Parents (15)	Qualitative	Semi-structured interviews

Note. QoL = Quality of Life; FQoL = Family Quality of Life; HRQoL = Health-Related Quality of Life; SLC6A1-related = Solute Carrier Family 6 Member 1 related; NDD = Neurodevelopmental Disorder; WHS = Wolf–Hirschhorn Syndrome; PWS

= Prader–Willi Syndrome; RTS = Rubinstein–Taybi Syndrome; KS = Kleefstra Syndrome; WS = Williams Syndrome; PTHS = Pitt–Hopkins Syndrome; BCFQOL / Beach Center FQoL = Beach Center Family Quality of Life Scale; PedsQL = Pediatric Quality of Life Inventory; GS = genomic sequencing; WHOQOL-BREF = World Health Organization Quality of Life – BREF; PTSD scales = Post-Traumatic Stress Disorder measures; PedsQL GCM = Pediatric Quality of Life Inventory – Generic Core Scales; PedsQL-FIM = Pediatric Quality of Life Inventory Family Impact Module; QI-Disability = Quality of Life with intellectual disabilities; EQ-5D-Y-3L = EuroQol 5 Dimensions – Youth – 3 Levels; IOFS = Impact on Family Scale; GAD-7 = Generalized Anxiety Disorder-7; PedsQL™ 2.0: Pediatric Impact Module; PedsQL™ 4.0: Pediatric Quality of Life.

Regarding the dimensions of the QoL examined by the researchers, the thematic analysis revealed that Family dynamics & roles appeared in fifteen of the sixteen studies (93.75%), which demonstrates that family functionality is the most stable and central axis of FQoL. Psychosomatic status & resilience is found in thirteen studies (81.25%), indicating a strong focus on emotional burden, stress, mental health and family adaptation mechanisms. Social & material support is included in ten studies (62.5%), highlighting the importance of services, social networks, and financial resources, but with a much less systematic nature compared to the intra-family dimensions. Finally, child's functioning is examined in seven studies (43.75%), which shows that, although it is a critical factor in burdening or protecting FQoL, it is not systematically integrated into all studies.

Subsequently, the findings for the central research question of this study reveal that the overall assessment of QoL levels in families of children with rare genetic syndromes shows that the majority of studies report low to moderate QoL levels, with an emphasis on the categories "moderate to low" (43.75%) and "low" (25%). A smaller percentage of studies record clearly moderate levels of QoL (25%), while only one study reports moderate to important levels (6.25%).

Regarding the factors that positively affect the QoL of families, the analysis of the sixteen included studies highlighted the social support network and services as the most frequently cited code, which was identified in nine studies (56.25%). Family cohesion and interaction also recorded a significant presence, a factor highlighted in seven studies (43.75%). Psychological resilience and management, functionality and status of the child, as well as socioeconomic and educational level, follow with equal incidence in four studies (25%). Lower rates were observed in stability of QoL with occurrence in two studies (12.50%), while parental role and empowerment were the least common factor, appearing in only 1 study (6.25%).

Concluding with the results of this research, it is revealed that the dominant factor that negatively affects the QoL levels of families of people with rare genetic syndromes is the psychological burden, which is recorded in ten studies (62.50%).

This is followed by behavioral difficulties & symptom severity, which are found in nine studies (56.25), while socioeconomic pressure and family background seem to weigh on eight studies (50.00%). In smaller percentages, but equally important as findings, follow Care requirements & physical exhaustion are reported in six studies (37.50%) and Deficiencies in the health & support system in the same percentages as social functionality & limitations, which occur equally in four studies (25,00%).

Table 5 presents the main findings that were analyzed through a thematic synthesis and identify key factors that are responsible for the lower or higher levels of QoL experienced by families of people with rare genetic syndromes.

Table 5. Dimensions, levels, and QoL factors

Study	QoL Dimensions Considered	QoL Levels	Positive factors	Negative factors
Bel-Fenellós et al. (2025)	Psychosomatic status & resilience, family dynamics & roles, social & material support	Medium	Social support network & services, family cohesion & interaction, psychological resilience & management, and parental role & empowerment	Psychological burden, care requirements & physical exhaustion social functioning & limitations
Bolbocean et al. (2022)	Family dynamics & roles, psychosomatic status & resilience, social & material support	Medium	Family cohesion & interaction, socio-economic & educational level, QoL stability, social support network & services	Behavioral difficulties & symptom severity psychological burden, socioeconomic pressure & family background
Bos-Roubos et al. (2022)	Psychosomatic status & resilience	Low	Social support network & services	Psychological burden, behavioral difficulties & severity of symptoms
Chen et al. (2023)	Psychosomatic status & resilience, social & material support, child's functioning, family dynamics & roles	Medium–low	Family cohesion & interaction social support network & services, socio-economic & educational level	Socioeconomic pressure & family background care requirements & physical exhaustion, psychological burden, deficiencies in the health & support system
Dahshi et al. (2024)	Psychosomatic status & resilience, social & material support, child's functioning, family dynamics & roles	Medium	Social support network & services	Socioeconomic pressure & family background care requirements & physical exhaustion
Haseley et al. (2021)	Family dynamics & roles, psychosomatic status & resilience, social & material support	Medium–low	Social support network & services	Social functionality & limitations, care requirements & physical exhaustion
Hoffmann et al. (2025)	Psychosomatic status & resilience, child's functioning, family dynamics & roles, social & material support	Low	Psychological resilience & management	Psychological burden
Jobling et al. (2025)	Family dynamics & roles	Low	Child's functionality & condition	Behavioral difficulties & symptom severity, socioeconomic pressure & family background deficiencies in the health & support system

continued on following page

Table 5. Continued

Study	QoL Dimensions Considered	QoL Levels	Positive factors	Negative factors
Patel et al. (2025)	Social & material support, child's functioning, family dynamics & roles. psychosomatic status & resilience	Medium-Low	Psychological resilience & management	Deficiencies in the health & support system, psychological burden, behavioral difficulties & severity of symptoms
Pereira et al. (2023)	Family dynamics & roles, social & material support, psychosomatic status & resilience	Medium–low	Family cohesion & interaction	Psychological burden, socioeconomic pressure & family background behavioral difficulties & severity of symptoms
Rozensztrauch & Śmigiel (2022)	Child's functioning, family dynamics & roles	Medium–low	QoL stability	Social functionality & limitations, care requirements & physical exhaustion
Rozensztrauch et al. (2023)	Child's functioning, family dynamics & roles	Medium	Functionality & status of the child, socioeconomic & educational level	Psychological burden, behavioral difficulties & severity of symptoms
Rozensztrauch et al. (2024)	Family dynamics & roles psychosomatic status & resilience	Medium-Low	Child's functionality & condition, social support network & health services, family cohesion & interaction	Behavioral difficulties & symptom severity social functioning & limitations
Telenga et al. (2024)	Child's functioning, social & material support, family dynamics & roles, psychosomatic status & resilience	Low	Child's functionality & condition social support network & health services	Care requirements & physical exhaustion psychological burden, deficiencies in the health & support system
Vale et al. (2022)	Family dynamics & roles, social & material support, psychosomatic status & resilience	Medium-hight	Family cohesion & interaction, psychological resilience & management	Psychological burden, socioeconomic pressure & family background behavioral difficulties & severity of symptoms
Van Till et al. (2025)	Family dynamics & roles, psychosomatic status & resilience	-	Social support network & services	Behavioral difficulties & symptom severity, socioeconomic pressure & family background

Note. HRQoL = *Health-Related Quality of Life*; PTSD = *Post-traumatic stress disorder.*

DISCUSSION

The present systematic review synthesized evidence from 16 primary studies to examine the QoL of families raising children with rare genetic syndromes. While studies on the QoL of patients with common diseases are readily available, studies that focus on the QoL of patients and their families with rare diseases are much harder to find (Rozensztrauch et al., 2024).

Overall, the findings indicate that FQoL in this population is predominantly reported as low to moderate. The findings confirm the international literature of past years (Fitzgerald & Gallagher, 2022; Gilmore, 2018; Griffith et al., 2011; Jarvis et al., 2025; Pelentsov et al., 2016). It is also characterized by marked variability across dimensions rather than a uniform level of impairment. This pattern confirms that FQoL constitutes a complex, multidimensional construction shaped by the interaction of psychological, relational, social, and child-related factors (Haseley et al., 2021).

A central finding of this review is the overwhelming emphasis placed on family dynamics and psychosomatic well-being. Family dynamics and roles were examined in almost all included studies, while psychosomatic status and resilience emerged as a dominant thematic axis. This suggests that international research conceptualizes FQoL primarily through the lens of emotional burden, stress, and internal family functioning. Such an orientation aligns with systemic and resilience-based frameworks, which view the family as an interdependent unit in which psychological adaptation and relational cohesion play a decisive role in coping with chronic and complex conditions (Bowen, 1978 as cited in Watson, 2012; Patterson, 2002).

At the same time, the comparatively lower frequency with which child functioning and social–material support were examined highlights an important research imbalance. Although child functionality, symptom severity, and communication difficulties were clearly associated with lower FQoL, these factors were not consistently integrated across studies. This gap is noteworthy, given that child-related characteristics often act as proximal stressors that shape daily routines, caregiving demands, and parental mental health (Rozensztrauch et al., 2023).

Similarly, social and material support, despite being repeatedly identified as a strong protective factor, was explored less systematically than intra-family processes. This research imbalance identified in the present review, where intra-family processes outweigh the analysis of systemic factors, is also confirmed by international literature. Researchers such as Anderson et al. (2013) and Jarvis et al. (2025) point out that structural determinants, such as accessibility to coordinated care and financial shielding, often remain on the margins of scientific debate. This suggests that QoL is not only judged within the home, but also in social services and decision-making centers, which often fail to recognize the magnitude of the practical barriers faced by families (Griffith et al., 2011; Walkowiak et al., 2026).

The predominance of low and moderate-to-low QoL levels across studies reinforces the characterization of these families as a population at increased psychosocial risk (Atkins & Padgett, 2024). Importantly, QoL impairment was not uniform across dimensions. Emotional well-being consistently emerged as the most vulnerable domain, while aspects related to physical or material well-being were occasionally reported as relatively preserved. This differentiated profile supports the view that FQoL should not be interpreted as a single global outcome but rather as a constellation of interrelated yet distinct domains, each influenced by different risk and protective mechanisms (Patterson, 2002).

The widespread use of the PedsQL across the included studies reflects the field's need for standardized and comparable measures. However, the limited application of tools specifically designed to capture FQoL, such as the Beach Center FQoL Scale, raises important conceptual considerations. The reliance on instruments that emphasize impact and burden may inadvertently frame families primarily in terms of deficit and dysfunction, rather than as dynamic systems with strengths, adaptive capacities, and evolving meanings. Indeed, the emphasis on negative emotions and burden factors is a fact that has been recorded by other researchers, such as Shrout et al. (2018). That methodological tendency may partially explain why protective factors such as parental empowerment and positive role perception appeared infrequently in the findings (Silibello et al., 2016).

An additional contribution to this review lies in the identification of social support networks and services as the most consistent positive determinant of FQoL. The prominence of this factor underscores the structural dependence of families affected by rare genetic syndromes on organized health, educational, and social care systems. At the same time, the finding that family cohesion was more strongly associated with QoL than child functionality suggests that, through the use of positive coping strategies, families can strengthen their cohesion and overall functioning, thereby buffering the impact of severe clinical presentations and fostering more positive perspectives in the face of daily challenges (Beighton & Wills, 2017). This highlights the importance of family-centered interventions that extend beyond symptom management and explicitly address communication, role negotiation, and emotional connectedness, as evidenced in the findings of Yoonjeong (2023).

Conversely, psychological burden emerged as the most frequently reported negative factor, surpassing even behavioral difficulties and symptom severity. This indicates that chronic stress (Fitzgerald & Gallagher, 2022), uncertainty regarding prognosis, future developments, and emotional exhaustion (Gilmore, 2018) may represent a more universal experience for parents than the specific manifestations of the child's condition. The substantial role of socioeconomic pressure further emphasizes that FQoL is deeply embedded in broader social and economic contexts, reinforcing the need for policies that provide financial relief and practical support alongside medical care (Griffith et al., 2011· Jarvis et al., 2025; Walkowiak et al., 2026).

Taken together, the findings of this systematic review suggest that improving FQoL in rare genetic syndromes requires a shift toward integrated, family-centered models of care. Such models should address emotional well-being, strengthen family relationships, enhance access to social support, and recognize parents not only as caregivers under strain but also as active agents with resilience and adaptive potential.

Contribution to the Field

The present systematic review contributes to the existing literature by offering a contemporary synthesis (2020–2026) of primary research examining FQoL in the context of rare genetic syndromes. Unlike prior reviews that primarily focus on individual caregivers or child-related outcomes, this study adopts a systemic, family-centered perspective, capturing multiple dimensions of family functioning, psychosocial well-being, and living conditions.

By integrating findings from quantitative, qualitative, and mixed-methods studies and applying a consistent interpretative framework for QoL levels, the review advances a more nuanced understanding of how FQoL is shaped not only by clinical severity, but also by relational, emotional, and structural factors. Additionally, the comparative examination of assessment tools highlights both the dominance of generic health-related measures and the underrepresentation of family-specific instruments, thereby identifying critical methodological gaps.

Overall, this review strengthens the conceptualization of FQoL as a multidimensional and context-dependent construction and provides evidence to support the development of family-centered assessment practices, and intervention models within rare disease care.

Implications for Practice

The findings of this systematic review highlight the necessity of adopting family-centered models of care when supporting families of children with rare genetic syndromes. Given the consistently reported low to moderate levels of FQoL, interventions should extend beyond child-focused symptom management and explicitly address parental emotional well-being, family dynamics, and relational functioning.

Health, education, and social care professionals are encouraged to recognize families not only as caregivers under pressure but as active systems with distinct needs, strengths, and adaptive capacities. Enhancing access to coordinated services, psychosocial support, and reliable information may play a crucial role in mitigating caregiver burden and strengthening family resilience.

Furthermore, the prominent role of social and material support identified in the reviewed studies underscores the importance of intersectoral collaboration and policy-level interventions aimed at reducing structural inequalities. Integrating family-specific QoL assessments into routine practice may facilitate early identification of families at risk and inform more personalized and effective support strategies.

Implications for Future Research and Limitations

Future research would benefit from greater methodological diversity. There is a need to collect qualitative data that will allow for the detailed recording and evaluation of the lived experiences of families of people with rare genetic syndromes, examining the factors that influence and shape the profile of their functioning, such as functionality, resilience, cohesion, QoL and stress. At the same time, increased use of family-specific QoL measures is recommended, which will focus on directly intertwined and factors that shape daily family functioning.

The heterogeneity of rare genetic syndromes included in the review represents a limitation, as differences in clinical severity, functional impairment, and care demands may influence FQoL in syndrome-specific ways.

A further limitation concerns the geographical concentration of the included studies, which were predominantly conducted in high-income countries. This limited representation of low- and middle-income countries may affect the generalizability of the findings, particularly with regard to access to services, availability of social support, and structural resources that substantially shape FQoL.

Also, the use of different QoL assessment tools across studies limits direct comparability of findings, despite the application of a structured narrative synthesis.

Despite these limitations, the present systematic review provides a comprehensive and methodologically rigorous synthesis of recent primary research on the QoL of families of children with rare genetic syndromes. By integrating findings across diverse methodological designs and focusing explicitly on the family as a unit of analysis, the review offers valuable insights into common patterns and determinants of FQoL that transcend individual diagnoses. The consistency of key findings across heterogeneous contexts strengthens the credibility of the conclusions and underscores the relevance of family-centered and context-sensitive approaches in both research and practice.

CONCLUSION

Overall, this systematic review demonstrates that families of children with rare genetic syndromes experience persistently reduced QoL across multiple domains, with emotional well-being, family dynamics, and everyday functioning being particularly affected. The findings related to living standards indicate that, despite recent improvements in health and special education services, families within these populations continue to face substantial emotional and practical challenges. Enhancing QoL therefore requires a shift toward integrated models of care that conceptualize parents not merely as caregivers under strain, but as active agents whose well-being is intrinsically linked to equitable access to social, material, and psychosocial resources. By synthesizing evidence across diverse syndromes and methodological approaches, the present review underscores the need for family-centered policies and interventions that address both individual and systemic determinants of FQoL. These findings highlight the need for future research and policy initiatives that systematically integrate family-specific QoL outcomes into rare disease care pathways.

REFERENCES

Adams, D., Clarke, S., Griffith, G., Howlin, P., Moss, J., Petty, J., Tunnicliffe, P., & Oliver, C. (2018). Mental health and well-being in mothers of children with rare genetic syndromes showing chronic challenging behavior: A cross-sectional and longitudinal study. *American Journal on Intellectual and Developmental Disabilities*, *123*(3), 241–253. DOI: 10.1352/1944-7558-123.3.241 PMID: 29671635

Alharbi, A., & Stevenson, M. (2020). Refining Boolean queries to identify relevant studies for systematic review updates. *Journal of the American Medical Informatics Association : JAMIA*, *27*(11), 1658–1666. DOI: 10.1093/jamia/ocaa148 PMID: 33067630

Anderson, M., Elliott, E. J., & Zurynski, Y. A. (2013). Australian families living with rare disease: Experiences of diagnosis, health services use and needs for psychosocial support. *Orphanet Journal of Rare Diseases*, *8*(1), 22. DOI: 10.1186/1750-1172-8-22 PMID: 23398775

Beighton, C., & Wills, J. (2017). Are parents identifying positive aspects to parenting their child with an intellectual disability or are they just coping? A qualitative exploration. *Journal of Intellectual Disabilities*, *21*(4), 325–345. DOI: 10.1177/1744629516656073 PMID: 27352854

Bel-Fenellós, C., Biencinto-López, C., Orio-Aparicio, C., Da Silva-Mori, X., Tenorio-Castaño, J. A., Lapunzina, P., & Nevado, J. (2025). Family well-being in families with children and young people with Wolf-Hirschhorn Syndrome. *Research in Developmental Disabilities*, *160*, 104974. DOI: 10.1016/j.ridd.2025.104974 PMID: 40112494

Bolbocean, C., Andújar, F. N., McCormack, M., Suter, B., & Holder, J. L.Jr. (2022). Health-related quality of life in pediatric patients with syndromic autism and their caregivers. *Journal of Autism and Developmental Disorders*, *52*(3), 1334–1345. DOI: 10.1007/s10803-021-05030-8 PMID: 33937973

Bos-Roubos, A., Wingbermühle, E., Biert, A., Graaff, L. D., & Egger, J. (2022). Family matters: Trauma and quality of life in family members of individuals with Prader-Willi Syndrome. *Frontiers in Psychiatry*, *13*, 897138. DOI: 10.3389/fpsyt.2022.897138 PMID: 35836666

Boycott, K. M., Rath, A., Chong, J. X., Hartley, T., Alkuraya, F. S., Baynam, G., Brookes, A. J., Brudno, M., Carracedo, A., Den Dunnen, J. T., Dyke, S. O. M., Estivill, X., Goldblatt, J., Gonthier, C., Groft, S. C., Gut, I., Hamosh, A., Hieter, P., Höhn, S., & Lochmüller, H. (2017). International cooperation to enable the diagnosis of all rare genetic diseases. *American Journal of Human Genetics, 100*(5), 695–705. DOI: 10.1016/j.ajhg.2017.04.003 PMID: 28475856

Chen, W., Sun, L., He, X., Li, Z., Ji, C., Li, F., Shen, J., Pan, T., Jin, X., Dong, Y., Hu, L., Zou, C., & Bai, G. (2023). Health-related quality of life of children with Williams syndrome and caregivers in China. *Frontiers in Public Health, 11*, 1177317. DOI: 10.3389/fpubh.2023.1177317 PMID: 37361163

Dahshi, H., Kalvakuntla, S., Lee, M., & Goodspeed, K. (2024). Beyond the diagnosis: Evaluation of quality-of-life measures and family functioning in SLC6A1-related neurodevelopmental disorder. *Pediatric Neurology, 155*, 160–166. DOI: 10.1016/j.pediatrneurol.2024.03.030 PMID: 38663152

Dellve, L., Samuelsson, L., Tallborn, A., Fasth, A., & Hallberg, L. R.-M. (2006). Stress and well-being among parents of children with rare diseases: A prospective intervention study. *Journal of Advanced Nursing, 53*(4), 392–402. DOI: 10.1111/j.1365-2648.2006.03736.x PMID: 16448482

Eiroa-Orosa, F. J. (2020). Understanding psychosocial wellbeing in the context of complex and multidimensional problems. *International Journal of Environmental Research and Public Health, 17*(16), 5937. DOI: 10.3390/ijerph17165937 PMID: 32824249

Eiser, C., & Morse, R. (2001). Can parents rate their child's health-related quality of life? Results of a systematic review. *Quality of Life Research: An International Journal of Quality of Life Aspects of Treatment, Care and Rehabilitation, 10*(4), 347–357. DOI: 10.1023/A:1012253723272 PMID: 11763247

Fitzgerald, J., & Gallagher, L. (2022). Parental stress and adjustment in the context of rare genetic syndromes: A scoping review. *Journal of Intellectual Disabilities, 26*(2), 522–544. DOI: 10.1177/1744629521995378 PMID: 33866895

Giotsa, A., Makri, E., Koutelou, S., Stamatelatou, A., & Chavredaki, A. (2015). Systemic family perspective and parent counseling groups. *Scientific Annals of the School of Education University of Ioannina, 4*, 4–35. DOI: 10.12681/jret.8684

Griffith, G. M., Hastings, R. P., Nash, S., Petalas, M., Oliver, C., Howlin, P., Moss, J., Petty, J., & Tunnicliffe, P. (2011). "You have to sit and explain it all, and explain yourself." Mothers' experiences of support services for their offspring with a rare genetic intellectual disability syndrome. *Journal of Genetic Counseling*, *20*(2), 165–177. DOI: 10.1007/s10897-010-9339-4 PMID: 21203808

Hartmanis, S. L., Baker, E. K., Godler, D. E., & Liew, D. (2023). Estimating the impact of Angelman syndrome on parental productivity in Australia using productivity-adjusted life years. *Disability and Health Journal*, *16*(2), 101423. DOI: 10.1016/j.dhjo.2022.101423 PMID: 36639256

Haseley, A., Wallis, K., & DeBrosse, S. (2021). Kleefstra syndrome: Impact on parents. *Disability and Health Journal*, *14*(2), 101018. DOI: 10.1016/j.dhjo.2020.101018 PMID: 33189624

Hoffmann, T. M., Friedrich, B., & Lewis, C. (2025). "I don't grieve as much as I used to": A qualitative study on parents of children with rare and undiagnosed conditions navigating grief in the context of uncertainty. *Journal of Genetic Counseling*, *34*(6), e70149. DOI: 10.1002/jgc4.70149 PMID: 41317142

Hong, Q. N., Fàbregues, S., Bartlett, G., Boardman, F., Cargo, M., Dagenais, P., Gagnon, M.-P., Griffiths, F., Nicolau, B., O'Cathain, A., Rousseau, M.-C., Vedel, I., & Pluye, P. (2018). The mixed methods appraisal Tool (MMAT) version 2018 for information professionals and researchers. *Education for Information*, *34*(4), 285–291. DOI: 10.3233/EFI-180221

Horsley, S., & Oliver, C. (2015). Positive impact and its relationship to well-being in parents of children with intellectual disability: A literature review. *International Journal of Developmental Disabilities*, *61*(1), 1–19. DOI: 10.1179/2047387713Y.0000000026

Jarvis, J., Chertavian, E., Buessing, M., Renteria, T., Tu, L., Hoffer, L., Fischer, R., Moore, A., Cross, M., & Tones, M. (2025). The economic impact of caregiving for individuals with Angelman syndrome in the United States: Results from a caregiver survey. *Orphanet Journal of Rare Diseases*, *20*(1), 82. DOI: 10.1186/s13023-025-03551-4 PMID: 39985061

Jobling, J. M., Teutsch, S. M., Eslick, G. D., & Elliott, E. J. (2025). Impact on the family of a child's rare disease: A large cross-sectional study. *Rare : Open Research in Rare Diseases*, *3*, 100066. DOI: 10.1016/j.rare.2025.100066

Katsarou, D. (2022). Fragile X syndrome and language skills. In Katsarou, D., & Zisi, V. (Eds.), *Disability and mental health* (pp. 133–149). Gutenberg.

Katsarou, D., & Zisi, V. (2022). Down syndrome: Verbal short-term memory from early childhood to old age. *Archives of Hellenic Medicine*, *39*(1), 54–59.

Katsarou, D. V., Theodoratou, M., Sofologi, M., Kougioumtzis, G. A., Efthymiou, E., Argyriadis, A., Patsiaouras, A., Mantsos, E., Argyriadi, A., & Papadopoulou, S. (2025). Angelman Syndrome Neurocognitive and Linguistic Profile, Overlaps, Interventions, and Quality of Life. In Megari, K. (Ed.), *Clinical Applications of Pediatric Neuropsychology from Infancy to Adolescence* (pp. 143–156). IGI Global., DOI: 10.4018/979-8-3693-9689-6.ch007

Kodra, Y., Cavazza, M., De Santis, M., Guala, A., Liverani, M.-E., Armeni, P., Masini, M., & Taruscio, D. (2020). Social economic costs, health-related quality of life and disability in patients with cri du chat syndrome. *International Journal of Environmental Research and Public Health*, *17*(16), 5951. DOI: 10.3390/ijerph17165951 PMID: 32824402

Lim, Y., Hong, I., & Han, A. (2025). Health-related quality of life and family functioning in parents of children with Barth syndrome: An application of the Double ABCX model. *Orphanet Journal of Rare Diseases*, *20*(1), 120. DOI: 10.1186/s13023-025-03636-0 PMID: 40075507

McMullan, J., Crowe, A. L., Bailie, C., Moore, K., McMullan, L. S., Shamandi, N., McAneney, H., & McKnight, A. J. (2020). Improvements needed to support people living and working with a rare disease in Northern Ireland: Current rare disease support perceived as inadequate. *Orphanet Journal of Rare Diseases*, *15*(1), 315. DOI: 10.1186/s13023-020-01559-6 PMID: 33168042

O'Brien, B. C., Harris, I. B., Beckman, T. J., Reed, D. A., & Cook, D. A. (2014). Standards for reporting qualitative research: A synthesis of recommendations. *Academic Medicine*, *89*(9), 1245–1251. DOI: 10.1097/ACM.0000000000000388 PMID: 24979285

Page, M. J., McKenzie, J. E., Bossuyt, P. M., Boutron, I., Hoffmann, T. C., Mulrow, C. D., Shamseer, L., Tetzlaff, J. M., Akl, E. A., Brennan, S. E., Chou, R., Glanville, J., Grimshaw, J. M., Hróbjartsson, A., Lalu, M. M., Li, T., Loder, E. W., Mayo-Wilson, E., McDonald, S., & Moher, D. (2021). The PRISMA 2020 statement: An updated guideline for reporting systematic reviews. *BMJ (Clinical Research Ed.)*, (71), n71. Advance online publication. DOI: 10.1136/bmj.n71 PMID: 33782057

Papadopoulou, S., Anagnostopoulou, A., Katsarou, D. V., Megari, K., Efthymiou, E., Argyriadis, A., Kougioumtzis, G., Theodoratou, M., Sofologi, M., Argyriadi, A., Pavlidou, E., & Toki, E. I. (2024). Enhancing Communication and Swallowing Skills in Children with Cri Du Chat Syndrome: A Comprehensive Speech Therapy Guide. *Children (Basel, Switzerland)*, *11*(12), 1526. DOI: 10.3390/children11121526 PMID: 39767955

Patel, R., Friedrich, B., Sanderson, S. C., Ellard, H., & Lewis, C. (2025). Anxiety and quality-of-life for parents of children with undiagnosed rare conditions: A multi-site quantitative survey study. *Journal of Genetic Counseling*, *34*(4), e70085. DOI: 10.1002/jgc4.70085 PMID: 40767117

Patterson, J. M. (2002). Understanding family resilience. *Journal of Clinical Psychology*, *58*(3), 233–246. DOI: 10.1002/jclp.10019 PMID: 11836706

Paxinos, I. (2022). Is there an "inspiration" of QOL in the field of clinical psychology and psychiatry? *Journal of Biomedical Engineering and Medical Imaging*, *9*(3). Advance online publication. DOI: 10.14738/jbemi.93.12415

Pelentsov, L. J., Fielder, A. L., & Esterman, A. J. (2016). The supportive care needs of parents with a child with a rare disease: A qualitative descriptive study. *Journal of Pediatric Nursing*, *31*(3), e207–e218. DOI: 10.1016/j.pedn.2015.10.022 PMID: 26651231

Pereira, R. C. M., Apis, A., Dos Santos, T. R., De Avó, L. R. D. S., Pilotto, R. F., Germano, C. M. R., & Melo, D. G. (2023). Quality of life of Brazilian families who have children with Williams syndrome. *Journal of Intellectual Disabilities*, *27*(3), 794–807. DOI: 10.1177/17446295221079583 PMID: 35543661

Rozensztrauch, A., Basiak, A., & Twardak, I. (2024). Rubinstein–Taybi Syndrome clinical characteristics from the perspective of quality of life and the impact of the disease on family functioning. *Journal of Clinical Medicine*, *13*(17), 5210. DOI: 10.3390/jcm13175210 PMID: 39274423

Rozensztrauch, A., & Śmigiel, R. (2022). Quality of life in children with Prader–Willi syndrome and the impact of the disease on the functioning of families. *International Journal of Environmental Research and Public Health*, *19*(23), 16330. DOI: 10.3390/ijerph192316330 PMID: 36498413

Rozensztrauch, A., Wieczorek, K., Twardak, I., & Śmigiel, R. (2023). Health-related quality of life and family functioning of primary caregivers of children with down syndrome. *Frontiers in Psychiatry*, *14*, 1267583. DOI: 10.3389/fpsyt.2023.1267583 PMID: 38161724

Saunders, C. H., Sierpe, A., Von Plessen, C., Kennedy, A. M., Leviton, L. C., Bernstein, S. L., Goldwag, J., King, J. R., Marx, C. M., Pogue, J. A., Saunders, R. K., Van Citters, A., Yen, R. W., Elwyn, G., & Leyenaar, J. K. (2023). Practical thematic analysis: A guide for multidisciplinary health services research teams engaging in qualitative analysis. *BMJ (Clinical Research Ed.)*, *074256*, e074256. Advance online publication. DOI: 10.1136/bmj-2022-074256 PMID: 37290778

Shrout, P. E., Stadler, G., Lane, S. P., McClure, M. J., Jackson, G. L., Clavél, F. D., Iida, M., Gleason, M. E. J., Xu, J. H., & Bolger, N. (2018). Initial elevation bias in subjective reports. *Proceedings of the National Academy of Sciences of the United States of America*, *115*(1). Advance online publication. DOI: 10.1073/pnas.1712277115 PMID: 29255039

Silibello, G., Vizziello, P., Gallucci, M., Selicorni, A., Milani, D., Ajmone, P. F., Rigamonti, C., De Stefano, S., Bedeschi, M. F., & Lalatta, F. (2016). Daily life changes and adaptations investigated in 154 families with a child suffering from a rare disability at a public center for rare diseases in Northern Italy. *Italian Journal of Pediatrics*, *42*(1), 76. DOI: 10.1186/s13052-016-0285-0 PMID: 27576488

Telenga, M., Rozensztrauch, A., Giżewska-Kacprzak, K., & Śmigiel, R. (2024). From genotype to phenotype of polish patients with Pitt–Hopkins Syndrome concerning the quality of life and family functioning. *Journal of Clinical Medicine*, *13*(9), 2605. DOI: 10.3390/jcm13092605 PMID: 38731134

Vale, A. R., De Avó, L. R. D. S., Pilotto, R. F., Germano, C. M. R., & Melo, D. G. (2022). Quality of life of Brazilian families who have children with Rubinstein–Taybi syndrome: An exploratory cross-sectional study. *American Journal of Medical Genetics. Part A*, *188*(11), 3294–3305. DOI: 10.1002/ajmg.a.62914 PMID: 35913016

Van Till, S. A. L., Bouman, A., Kleefstra, T., & Bunnik, E. M. (2025). Parental experiences and needs in Kleefstra Syndrome: A semi-structured interview study. *European Journal of Medical Genetics*, *77*, 105037. DOI: 10.1016/j.ejmg.2025.105037 PMID: 40829731

Varni, J. W., Burwinkle, T. M., & Seid, M. (2005). The PedsQL™ as a pediatric patient-reported outcome: Reliability and validity of the PedsQL™ Measurement Model in 25,000 children. *Expert Review of Pharmacoeconomics & Outcomes Research*, *5*(6), 705–719. DOI: 10.1586/14737167.5.6.705 PMID: 19807613

Varni, J. W., Burwinkle, T. M., & Seid, M. (2006). The PedsQLTM 4.0 as a school population health measure: Feasibility, reliability, and validity. *Quality of Life Research: An International Journal of Quality of Life Aspects of Treatment, Care and Rehabilitation*, *15*(2), 203–215. DOI: 10.1007/s11136-005-1388-z PMID: 16468077

Varni, J. W., Burwinkle, T. M., Seid, M., & Skarr, D. (2003). The PedsQL™* 4.0 as a pediatric population health measure: Feasibility, reliability, and validity. *Ambulatory Pediatrics*, *3*(6), 329–341. DOI: 10.1367/1539-4409(2003)003<0329:TPAAP-P>2.0.CO;2 PMID: 14616041

Verdugo, M. A., Schalock, R. L., Keith, K. D., & Stancliffe, R. J. (2005). Quality of life and its measurement: Important principles and guidelines. *Journal of Intellectual Disability Research*, *49*(10), 707–717. DOI: 10.1111/j.1365-2788.2005.00739.x PMID: 16162115

Walkowiak, D., Pospieszyńska-Martysiuk, K., Dianow, H., Węgrzyn, J., & Domaradzki, J. (2026). Measuring economic burden in families of individuals with Angelman Syndrome in Poland: A caregivers' survey. *Orphanet Journal of Rare Diseases*, *21*(1), 24. DOI: 10.1186/s13023-025-04183-4 PMID: 41469742

Watson, W. H. (2012). Family systems. In *Encyclopedia of Human Behavior* (pp. 184–193). Elsevier., DOI: 10.1016/B978-0-12-375000-6.00169-5

Yoonjeong, L. (2023). Impact of raising children with rare diseases on parental quality of life and family functioning. *International Journal of Rare Diseases & Disorders*, *6*(1). Advance online publication. DOI: 10.23937/2643-4571/1710053

Zuna, N., Summers, J. A., Turnbull, A. P., Hu, X., & Xu, S. (2010). Theorizing about family quality of life. In Kober, R. (Ed.), *Enhancing the quality of life of people with intellectual disabilities: From theory to practice* (Vol. 41, pp. 241–278). Springer., DOI: 10.1007/978-90-481-9650-0_15

Zurynski, Y., Deverell, M., Dalkeith, T., Johnson, S., Christodoulou, J., Leonard, H., & Elliott, E. J. (2017). Australian children living with rare diseases: Experiences of diagnosis and perceived consequences of diagnostic delays. *Orphanet Journal of Rare Diseases*, *12*(1), 68. DOI: 10.1186/s13023-017-0622-4 PMID: 28399928

Chapter 7
Assessment of Perceptions of Quality of Life and Stress of Parents of Children With Autism

Krystamtsi Christina
http://orcid.org/0009-0000-1597-3778
University of the Aegean, Greece

Ioannis Paxinos
http://orcid.org/0009-0001-9043-144X
University of the Peloponnese, Greece

Styliani G. Tziaferi
http://orcid.org/0009-0007-2221-9096
University of the Peloponnese, Greece

ABSTRACT

Autism has been recorded as a particularly common coexisting health condition in individuals diagnosed with certain genetic syndromes. Researchers collected data from 114 parents of children with autism aged 4–25 to examine their perceived quality of life and stress levels, as well as the relationship between these variables, while considering selected demographic characteristics. The complexity of care needs in chronic health conditions makes it necessary to systematically study parenting experience. The results showed a strong and statistically significant negative relationship between stress and quality of life, with stress explaining a significant

DOI: 10.4018/979-8-3373-8485-6.ch007

proportion of the variation in quality of life. Differences were found in terms of gender, educational level and marital status. Findings highlight the importance of psychosocial support for parents of children with autism.

INTRODUCTION

Autism has emerged as one of the most widely discussed diagnostic categories within contemporary mental health discourse, not only because of its clinical complexity but also due to its profound impact on family life. Although it is formally classified as a neurodevelopmental condition, its increasing prevalence (Maenner et al., 2023; World Health Organization, 2023) and the broadening of diagnostic criteria (Lord et al., 2020) have intensified scientific and social attention. At the same time, critical perspectives highlight that autism is not merely a biomedical entity, but a construct shaped by sociocultural assumptions and diagnostic frameworks (Boyle, 2002; Timimi et al., 2019). Within this framework, the experience of raising a child with autism extends beyond developmental considerations and enters the domain of family functioning, caregiving demands, and long-term uncertainty. Consequently, parental stress and quality of life emerge as central dimensions for understanding how autism is lived and negotiated within everyday family realities (Hayes & Watson, 2013; Alenazi et al., 2020; Vasilopoulou & Nisbet, 2016).

Concept, diagnosis and basic characteristics of autism

The concept of autism has aroused the interest of the mental health scientific community since the 1940s, when Leo Kanner provided the first description of infantile autism (Neumärker, 2003). It is described by the dominant discourse of psychiatry as a lifelong and highly heterogeneous health condition which is characterized as a neurodevelopmental disorder. The main criteria that place a person in the category of autism are the difficulties in responding and harmonizing with the socially accepted standards of communication and behavior as well as the maintenance of consistently repetitive behaviors. The intensity of symptoms varies in each individual and can range from lower to higher levels of severity, depending on their functional difficulties and support needs (American Psychiatric Association, 2013).

The diagnosis of autism relies primarily on behavioral and developmental assessments rather than on biological markers. Consequently, diagnostic evaluation is based largely on clinical observation, developmental history, and standardized assessment tools. The interview with the child, his developmental history and interaction with the environment are the pre-eminent ways to assess autism (Lord et al., 2020). However, the psychiatric diagnosis cannot explain the person's experiences, as it is constantly moving through a vicious circle of interpretations, the so-called tautology. The question of why the child avoids eye contact, uses literal speech, etc., the answer is that he is on the autism spectrum.

> *"-Why is the child on the autism spectrum?" Precisely because it has literal speech, avoids eye contact, etc. Although diagnostic classification facilitates communication among professionals and access to services, it does not necessarily provide a complete explanation of the underlying developmental processes or eliminate the social stigma that may accompany diagnostic labels. On the contrary, diagnostic classifications decontextualize human problems and then reframe them, inventing concepts such as disorder. Almost all autism diagnosis questionnaires are based on quantitative data (numbering scales), which may create the impression of precise categorical boundaries despite the substantial heterogeneity observed within the autism spectrum (Boyle, 2002:125).*

Epidemiology and prevalence of autism spectrum disorder

In recent decades, there has been a significant increase in the prevalence of autism at international levels, which has caused intense scientific and social concern. According to the World Health Organization, the ratio is estimated at around 1:100 children worldwide (World Health Organization, 2023). Similarly in Greece, a modern national study estimates that the incidence of ASD in children and adolescents aged 2-17 concerns about 1:100 children (Kouznetsov et al., 2023).

Modern epidemiological data show that the prevalence of autism increased from 0.7% in 2000 to 2.3% in 2020, while the incidence was lower in whites compared to other ethnic minorities. Against this background, autism became a cultural disorder, as if we consider that the incidence of the so-called infant autism was only 0.04%, while the incidence of the so-called "autism spectrum disorder" increased to 3% (CDC.gov, 2025).

However, this increase cannot be interpreted in terms of biological etiology, as it has been linked, in part, to the improvement in epidemiological surveillance (Maenner et al., 2023) and the broadening of diagnostic criteria following the introduction of the fifth revised diagnostic and statistical tool for psychiatric disorders (DSM-5) in 2013, which now places autism in a wider range of developmental disorders.

Diagnostic Frameworks and Critical Approaches

In examining this issue, scholars emphasize that autism diagnostic tools are not neutral means of capturing developmental differences, but incorporate theoretical and sociocultural assumptions, which can affect both the diagnostic process and the interpretation of the increasing prevalence of autism diagnoses. This process recognizes each new diagnosis as an achievement and not as a potential therapeutic goal. In this regard, the treatment of autism as a single and strict biomedical diagnostic category has been criticized, as it does not adequately capture the diversity of developmental pathways, causative factors and social influences that make up the autism spectrum (Timimi et al., 2019; Lord et al., 2020).

Idiopathic and syndromic autism

As mentioned earlier, autism includes both people with idiopathic autism and people with syndromic autism, where autistic characteristics coexist with diagnosed genetic or neurodevelopmental syndromes. Relevant meta-analysis shows that coexisting autism occurs more often in people with Rett syndrome, Cohen syndrome, Cornelia de Lange syndrome, nodular sclerosis complex, Angelman syndrome, CHARGE syndrome and fragile X syndrome, especially in men. At lower but clinically significant rates, autism features are also seen in people with neurofibromatosis type 1, Down syndrome, Noonan syndrome, Williams syndrome, and 22q11.2 deletion syndrome (also known as Di George syndrome or velo-cardio-facial syndrome) (Katsarou, 2022; Katsarou & Zisi, 2022; Katsarou et al., 2025; Richards et al., 2015).

This distinction increases the complexity and heterogeneity of autism, as in addition to social communication and behavioral difficulties, particularly important and critical health conditions are added to the syndromic forms of autism (Besag & Vasey, 2020).

Autism and the family system

This highly heterogeneous profile, which a person with autism can present, does not exclusively burden the child's developmental profile but extends to the family system, affecting the way parents give meaning to the diagnosis (Shah et al., 2026), manage care requirements and address expectations for the future. In this light, parental stress and quality of life emerge as critical dimensions of parenting experience, shaped through the interaction of developmental, medical, and social factors (Alenazi et al., 2020; Hayes & Watson, 2013).

Parenthood and Autism

Parenthood represents a complex and demanding life experience that involves a wide range of responsibilities and emotional challenges, while at the same time it can offer feelings of joy and a sense of purpose and meaning in the lives of individuals (Musick et al., 2016). The demands of parenthood are significantly intensified when it comes to raising children who experience complex health conditions such as autism. In these cases, parents are often faced with prolonged care obligations, needs for particular educational and therapeutic situations, as well as uncertainty about their children's future (Stoner et al., 2005; Befkadu & Adamek, 2022). Continued exposure to such living conditions can significantly affect parents' mental health, functioning, and overall well-being (Abolkheirian et al., 2022; Chan et al., 2018).

Stress and Parents of Children with Autism

Stress is often approached unilaterally as an individual state of physical and mental restlessness, cutting it off from the structural elements that produce it (socio-economic conditions, competition, pressure for productivity, precarious working conditions) aiming at a state of bliss, well-being, prosperity. Proper functioning of core activity and appropriate stress system response are critical for a sense of well-being, efficient performance of tasks, and healthy social interactions (Chrousos, 2009).

All people experience stress to some degree, and their reaction to it has a significant effect on their well-being (World Health Organization, 2023). However, in the context of neoliberal ideology, where individuals are identified as inherently vulnerable and inadequately equipped against stressful stimuli, the mental health system shifts the emphasis from social structures to individual skills (Cohen, 2025). The promotion of "resilience" acts as a mechanism for individualizing responsibility for mental pain, while allowing it to be commercialized through a set of variables such as parenthood, childhood, and family relationships (Gill & Orgad, 2018).

From a social constructivist perspective, the emphasis shifts away from internal mental processes, such as individual anxiety, etc., to interactive processes. In this way, all thoughts, perceptions, and therefore stress, are understood as products of communication, rather than of the individual mind. To put it another way, stress is shaped as an experience and perception through communication between dyads, groups, and communities, rather than simply by the individual's internal state (Anderson & Goolishian, 1992:30).

Chronic stress has been identified as one of the most important factors affecting the overall functioning of parents of children with autism. In particular, the parental stress experienced by parents of children with autism is significantly higher compared to the stress experienced by parents of children without developmental disorders or with other disabilities (Warreman et al., 2023). As a factor, it is directly related to the physical and mental health of parents, but also to their overall quality of life, indirectly affecting the developmental course of their children (Musick et al., 2016).

Quality of Life and Parents of Children with Autism

Quality of life as a concept has always been of particular research interest by experts in various scientific fields. It is a multidimensional concept, shaped by both individual and external factors (Paxinos, 2022; Verdugo et al., 2005). However, no single definition representing quality of life has yet prevailed, and as Teoli and Bhardwaj (2025) characteristically dared to point out, if a common quality of life model existed or was universally applied, it would be a mistake.

The complexity of the factors affecting the quality of life from society to society and from person to person is in itself an important factor that hinders its universal definition. It encompasses as a concept various areas such as mental satisfaction, health and social relationships which are evaluated completely differently in each socio-cultural context (Diener & Suh, 1997; Pukeliene & Starkauskiene, 2011).

In the case of parents of children with autism, the quality of life is shaped through a complex interaction between individual, family and social factors (Vasilopoulou & Nisbet, 2016). The international literature shows that parents of children with autism systematically show lower levels of quality of life and higher levels of stress compared to parents of typically developing children.

Demographics and Parental Experience in the Context of Autism

Of particular importance is the investigation of the demographic and social parameters that affect parenting experience, in order to design effective and targeted support interventions. According to a modern study, the demographic characteristics of the two sexes, regarding professional employment or exclusive care of children, seem to affect the two sexes differently, as they tend to use different strategies to deal with the challenges related to the care of children with autism or to be concerned about different areas related to the upbringing and future of their children (Alenazi et al., 2020). Mothers often report higher levels of psychological burden, which is attributed to the unequal distribution of caregiver roles (Turnage & Conner, 2022). In addition, the existence of partner support and socioeconomic stability can act as protective factors (Hsiao, 2018).

Purpose and Contribution of Research

The aim of the research is to assess the perceptions of quality of life and stress levels of parents of children with autism aged 4–25 years, as well as to investigate the relationship between these two variables in relation to the demographic characteristics of the sample. The research focuses on understanding parenting experience, as reflected through subjective assessments of quality of life and psychological burden, with the aim of highlighting factors that affect the overall well-being of parents of children with autism.

Despite the growing body of international literature on parental stress and quality of life in families of children with autism, empirical evidence from the Greek context remains relatively limited. Investigating these dimensions within specific socio-cultural contexts is important, as parental experiences and coping processes may be shaped by variations in social support systems, healthcare structures, and cultural perceptions of disability.

RESEARCH QUESTIONS & HYPOTHESES

Research Questions

RQ1: How do parents of children with autism evaluate their quality of life?
RQ2: What levels of stress do parents report?
RQ3: Do demographic variables influence the relationship between stress and quality of life?
RQ4: Does stress significantly predict quality of life?
Hypotheses
H1: Parents of children with autism will report lower levels of quality of life.
H2: Parents will report elevated levels of stress.
H3: Demographic variables (gender, education, marital status) will moderate the relationship between stress and quality of life.
H4: Higher levels of stress will significantly predict lower levels of quality of life.

METHOD

Research Design

The study follows a quantitative, non-experimental research design, with the aim of investigating the relationship between quality of life and stress levels of parents of children with autism. The quantitative approach enables the systematic measurement and statistical analysis of psychosocial variables (Ishtiaq, 2019).

The design of the research is cross-sectional, as the data were collected at one point in time, without experimental intervention or manipulation of the variables. The choice of this design was considered appropriate, given that the aim of the study is to describe and investigate correlations between variables and not to draw deterministic conclusions.

The study was conducted in accordance with the principles of the Helsinki Declaration and received approval from the Research Ethics Committee of the University of the Peloponnese, (Protocol No. 4225/21-02-25).

The selection of the participants was based on non-probability convenience sampling, through the distribution of the questionnaires to special schools, special education centers, and social groups of parents who have children with autism. Participation in the survey was voluntary, and all participants signed a form of consent to participate in and process the data they provided.

Data Collection Tools

To collect the data, parents were able to fill in either a paper or digital questionnaire which included demographic questions and the two basic psychometric tools. The participants were informed about the purpose of the survey and the process of completing the questionnaire and participated voluntarily. The completion of the questionnaire was anonymous, and the confidentiality of the data was ensured.

The quality of life of the parents was assessed through the WHOQOL-BREF questionnaire, which examines the participants' overall perception of their quality of life, considering multiple dimensions of daily functioning. The Greek version of the tool was used, translated and weighted by Kokkosis and colleagues (Tzinieri-Kokkosi, 2009). The questionnaire has high levels of validity and reliability (Skevington et al., 2004).

Stress levels were assessed with the State-Trait Anxiety Inventory – State (STAI-State) scale (Spielberger et al., 1970), in its Greek edition (Fountoulaki et al., 2002). The scale is widely used to measure transient anxiety and captures the subjective stress experience of participants at the time of completing the questionnaire. The reliability and validity of the tool have been documented in numerous studies (Fountoulakis et al., 2003).

Sample

In total, 550 questionnaires were sent in printed or electronic form to parents of children with autism through special schools, special clinics and social groups throughout the Greek region. 120 parents responded to the survey and participated. However, six questionnaires were not adequately completed and thus were not included in the final set of data processed by the study. The criterion for the inclusion of parents in the study was to have Greek as their mother tongue or to be able to understand it in writing at a fairly satisfactory level and to have at least one child with a diagnosis of autism and the age of the child to be 4 to 25 years old.

Statistical Analysis

The statistical analysis of the data was performed using IBM SPSS software (2024 version). Descriptive statistics (means, standard deviations, minimum and maximum values) were initially calculated for all key variables in the study.

The regularity of the distributions was examined through visual inspection of histograms and normal probability plots (Q–Q plots). Given the satisfactory approach to normal distribution, parametric statistical controls were used.

The internal coherence of the scales was assessed through Cronbach's index α.

The relationship between quality of life and stress levels was investigated with the Pearson correlation coefficient (r), while the determination factor (r^2) was calculated to estimate the effect magnitude.

Differences between two independent groups (gender, marital status after merging categories) were examined with independent sample t-tests. In cases of violation of the homogeneity of fluctuations, the Welch correction was used. The effect magnitude was calculated using Cohen's index d.

For the comparison of more than two groups (educational level, parent's age, child's age) a one-way variation analysis (One-Way ANOVA) was used. The effect magnitude was estimated via eta squared (h^2). When the overall result was statistically significant, post-hoc comparisons were made with Bonferroni correction.

To investigate the predictive relationship between stress and quality of life, a simple linear regression analysis was conducted, with stress levels (STAI_STATE_TOTAL) as the independent variable and quality of life (QOL_TOTAL) as the dependent variable. The level of statistical significance was set at $\alpha = .05$.

RESULTS

Demographic Characteristics of the Sample

The study sample consisted of 114 parents of children with autism spectrum disorder. The majority of participants were women (71.9%), while 28.1% were men. The largest age group was 40–49 years old (57.9%). Most of the parents were married (86.0%) and employed (80.7%). In terms of educational attainment, 44.7% had completed secondary education and 30.7% tertiary education. The detailed demographic data are presented in Table 1.

Table 1. Demographic characteristics of the sample (n = 114)

Variable	Category	*n*	%
Gender of parent	Male	32	28.1
	Woman	82	71.9
Parent's age	30–39 years old	29	25.4
	40–49 years old	66	57.9
	50–59 years old	17	14.9
	60–67 years old	2	1.8
Educational level	Junior High School	6	5.3
	High School	51	44.7
	Higher education	35	30.7
	Postgraduate	22	19.3
Employment status	Employee	92	80.7
	Unemployed	22	19.3
Marital status	Married	98	86.0
	Unmarried	16	14.0
Child's age	4–7	44	38.6
	8–12	31	27.2
	13–17	34	29.8
	18–25	5	4.4

Descriptive Statistics of Key Variables

Descriptive analysis was performed for the key variables of the study, namely quality of life (QOL_TOTAL) and stress levels (STAI_STATE_TOTAL).

Quality of life showed an average value of M = 3.34 (SD = 0.61), with a range of values from 1.69 to 4.58. Stress levels ranged from 20.00 to 75.00, with an average value of M = 43.56 (SD = 13.30). The results are presented in Table 2.

Table 2. Descriptive statistics of quality of life and stress levels (n = 114)

Variable	*n*	Minimum	Maximum	Mean	SD
QOL_TOTAL	114	1.69	4.58	3.34	0.61
STAI_STATE_TOTAL	114	20.00	75.00	43.56	13.30

Regularity check

Visual inspection of histograms and normal probability plots (Q–Q plots) showed that the distributions of the variables approximate the normal distribution, with no obvious outliers. Therefore, the use of parametric statistical controls was considered appropriate.

Scale reliability

The internal coherence of the quality of life scale was assessed through Cronbach's index α and found to be high ($\alpha > .80$), suggesting satisfactory internal consistency of the individual questions.

Similarly, the stress scale (STAI-State) also showed a high internal consistency ($\alpha > .85$), which confirms the reliability of the tool in the present sample.

Correlation of Quality of Life and Stress Levels

The relationship between quality of life and stress levels was investigated through the Pearson correlation coefficient.

The results, as illustrated in Table 3, showed a strong, negative, and statistically significant correlation between the two variables, $r = -.695$, $p < .001$ ($n = 114$). This finding suggests that higher levels of stress are associated with lower perceived quality of life.

The effect size was large ($r^2 = .483$), indicating that stress levels accounted for approximately 48.3% of the variance in quality of life in the present sample.

Table 3. Correlation between quality of life and stress levels (Pearson r)

Variables	QOL_TOTAL	STAI_STATE_TOTAL
QOL_TOTAL	1	–0,695***
STAI_STATE_TOTAL	–0,695***	1

Note. ***p < 0,001, N = 114

Linear Regression

A simple linear regression was performed with quality of life (QOL_TOTAL) as a dependent variable and stress levels as an independent variable (STAI_STATE_TOTAL).

The model was statistically significant, $F(1,112) = 104.7$, $p < .001$, explaining 48.3% of the variation in quality of life ($R^2 = .483$).

Stress levels negatively predicted quality of life ($\beta = -.695$, $p < .001$), indicating that an increase in anxiety is associated with a decrease in perceived quality of life.

Gender Differences

As shown in Table 4, a t-test of independent samples (Welch correction due to unequal variation) was performed.

Women experienced higher levels of stress (M = 45.01, SD = 13.42) compared to men (M = 39.94, SD = 12.47), t(63.91) = 2.41, p = .019, 95% CI [–11.35, –1.07], with a small to moderate effect magnitude (Cohen's d = 0.39).

Similarly, men reported a higher quality of life (M = 3.41, SD = 0.59) than women (M = 3.31, SD = 0.61), t(74.95) = 2.21, p = .030, 95% CI [0.024, 0.463], with a small effect size (Cohen's d = 0.17).

Table 4. Quality of life and stress levels by gender of the parent (t-test) descriptive statistics (Mean ± SD)

Variable	Gender	*n*	M	SD	t	df	p	Cohen's d
Stress	Male	32	39.94	12.47	2.41	63.91	.019	0.39
	Female	82	45.01	13.42				
QOL	Male	32	3.41	0.59	2.21	74.95	.030	0.17
	Female	82	3.31	0.61				

Note. *Cohen's d values indicate effect size magnitude*

Differences in Educational Level

Table 5 presents a One-Way ANOVA analysis was performed to investigate differences in quality of life between educational levels. The analysis showed a statistically significant difference, $F(3,110) = 4.04$, $p = .009$, with a moderate effect size ($h^2 = .10$).

This was followed by post-hoc comparisons with Bonferroni correction, which showed that parents with lower educational attainment reported a significantly higher quality of life compared to parents with higher education ($p < .05$). No statistically significant differences were observed between the other groups.

In terms of stress levels, no statistically significant differences were found between educational levels, $F(3,110) = 0.80$, $p = .497$, with a moderate effect size ($h^2 = .02$).

Table 5. Quality of life and stress levels of parents: descriptive statistics (Mean ± SD) and in relation to educational level (One-Way ANOVA)

Educational level	N	QOL Mean	QOL SD	STAI Mean	STAI SD
Junior High School	6	3.67	0.30	44.00	7.38
High School	51	3.51	0.57	41.45	11.47
Tertiary	35	3.14	0.61	45.17	15.00
Postgraduate	22	3.17	0.62	45.77	15.55
ANOVA Summary					
Variable	**F**	**df**	**p-value**	**h^2**	
QOL_TOTAL	4.04	(3, 110)	.009	.10	
STAI_STATE_TOTAL	0.8	(3, 110)	.497	.02	

Differences in Marital Status

Due to the very small number of participants in certain categories of marital status (e.g., widowed, divorced), the categories were merged into two groups: married and unmarried parents.

Independent sample t-tests were performed to investigate differences in quality of life and stress levels between the two groups.

Married parents ($n = 98$, $M = 3.42$, $SD = 0.54$) reported significantly higher quality of life compared to single parents ($n = 16$, $M = 2.85$, $SD = 0.78$), $t(112) = 3.64$, $p < .001$, 95% CI [0.26, 0.87]. The effect magnitude was large, Cohen's $d = 0.98$ (95% CI [0.44, 1.52]).

Single parents ($n = 16$, $M = 53.38$, $SD = 13.75$) showed significantly higher stress levels compared to married parents ($n = 98$, $M = 41.96$, $SD = 12.59$), $t(112) = -3.32$, $p = .001$, 95% CI [–18.23, –4.60]. The effect magnitude was large, Cohen's $d = 0.90$ (95% CI [0.35, 1.44]). The detailed results are presented in Table 6.

Table 6. Differences in quality of life and stress by marital status

Variable	Marital status	n	M	SD	t	df	p	Cohen's d
Quality of life	Married	98	3.42	0.54	3.64	112	< .001	0.98
	Non-married	16	2.85	0.78				
Stress	Married	98	41.96	12.59	-3.32	112	.001	0.90
	Non-married	16	53.38	13.75				

Note. *Cohen's d values indicate effect size magnitude*

Other Demographic Variables

No statistically significant differences in quality of life or stress levels were found in relation to the parents' work status (quality of life: F(1,112) = 0.001, p = .971; stress: F(1,112) = 0.001, p = .977).

Accordingly, there were no statistically significant differences in the age of the parents (quality of life: F(3,110) = 0.235, p = .872; stress: F(3,110) = 0.407, p = .749), nor in the age of the children (quality of life: F(3,110) = 1,075, p = .363; stress: F(3,110) = 1,665, p = .179).

These results suggest that these demographic variables do not significantly differentiate either the perceived quality of life or the stress levels in the present sample.

Overall, the findings provide strong empirical support for Hypothesis 4, as increased stress levels predict a significantly lower quality of life. In contrast, Hypothesis 3, which concerned the possible moderating role of demographic variables, was not confirmed. Hypotheses 1 and 2 were partly supported at a descriptive level, based on the average values recorded.

DISCUSSION

The present study investigated the perceived quality of life and stress levels of parents of children with autism, as well as the correlation between them. Although the questionnaires were adapted to be available in both paper and digital formats, the response was very limited in relation to the scope of the call, which confirms the documented difficulties in accessing this population group (Bhakta et al., 2022). At the same time, the literature suggests that parents of children with autism seem to be more motivated when it comes to participation in genetic studies, compared to other types of research related to autism. Their involvement in genetic research is often associated with the need to give meaning to the diagnosis, to manage feelings of guilt, as well as to the desire to contribute to the expansion of scientific knowledge and social awareness. In addition, this involvement may be related to family planning issues and to the expectation of future scientific advances in the diagnosis and treatment of autism (Fletcher-Watson et al., 2017).

At the descriptive level, the results showed that parents reported moderate levels of anxiety, with women recording higher values compared to men. Although this finding confirms the literature that highlights an increased psychological burden on parents of children with autism (Hayes & Watson, 2013; Zablotsky et al., 2013), stress levels in the present sample cannot be classified as extreme or clinically high. Therefore, Hypothesis 2 is partially supported, as stress appears to be at moderate rather than particularly high levels.

Accordingly, the quality of life of parents ranged at moderate to satisfactory levels, without a generalized picture of severely reduced well-being. This finding differs in part from studies reporting significantly lower quality of life in parents of children with autism (Alenazi et al., 2020; Vasilopoulou & Nisbet, 2016). This variation may be related to cultural factors, parental adaptation mechanisms, or sample composition. Hypothesis 1 is therefore partially supported, as it does not confirm a generalized low quality of life, but rather a state of moderate well-being that coexists with psychological burden.

However, the coexistence of moderate levels of stress and moderate quality of life should not be interpreted solely as a sign of individual resilience of parents. Rather, it may reflect a process of adaptation shaped by specific social, institutional, and family contexts (Hsiao, 2018; Sim et al., 2019). Thus, the findings of the present study do not simply suggest personal adaptability but highlight the need to understand the parenting experience as a socially integrated process, which is influenced by the available supportive framework and the wider social conditions.

Beyond the empirical associations identified in the present study, the findings may also be interpreted through broader critical and social constructionist perspectives on mental health and diagnosis. Scholars have argued that diagnostic categories and psychological constructs are not purely neutral descriptions of individual functioning but are shaped within specific social and cultural contexts (Boyle, 2002; Timimi et al., 2019). From this perspective, parental stress should not be understood exclusively as an individual psychological response but also as a phenomenon embedded within caregiving demands, institutional structures, and the availability of social support. Thus, the strong association between stress and quality of life observed in this study may reflect not only personal coping processes but also the broader social conditions under which families of children with autism organize and experience everyday life.

The results showed a strong and statistically significant negative correlation between stress and quality of life, with stress explaining almost half of the variance in quality of life. Regression analysis further confirmed that stress significantly predicts quality of life, accounting for a substantial proportion of its variance. This finding highlights the central role of psychological burden in shaping the well-being of parents of children with autism. At the same time, differences were observed in terms of gender, educational level and marital status, while other demographic variables did not appear to have a significant effect.

These findings are consistent with previous research highlighting the negative impact of parental stress on emotional well-being and family functioning (Hayes & Watson, 2013; Norlin & Broberg, 2013; Priego-Ojeda & Rusu, 2023). Parental stress has been associated with symptoms of psychological distress, reduced emotional resilience, and difficulties in interpersonal functioning. Within this framework, the present study reinforces the view that stress constitutes a central mechanism shaping the overall quality of life of parents of children with autism.

In addition, the strong predictive power of stress on quality of life confirms critical literature analysis that points out that a lack of a supportive environment and increased care requirements lead to long-term burden (Picardi et al., 2018; Rezq et al., 2025).

The gender differences recorded are consistent with the international literature, which shows that mothers of children with autism report higher levels of emotional distress and psychological stress compared to fathers (Davis & Carter, 2008; Li et al., 2022). This trend has mainly been attributed to the unequal distribution of caring roles, as mothers often take on the bulk of daily care (Vernhet et al., 2022), while fathers focus more on financial and practical dimensions of family support (García-López et al., 2016). The findings of the present study reinforce the need, highlighted in previous international research, to design interventions that take into account the differing needs and experiences of mothers and fathers (Alodaili et al., 2026).

The significant differentiation observed in terms of marital status is consistent with previous research highlighting the importance of partner and social support (Sim et al., 2019). Married parents may have a larger emotional and practical support network, which can act as a protector against stress and enhance quality of life. This finding is also linked to the reports of Kuhlthau et al. (2014), who found fewer symptoms of psychological distress in married parents.

The differentiation in educational level in quality of life partially confirms previous studies highlighting the importance of socio-economic resources and access to information (Hsiao, 2018). However, the absence of significant differences in stress levels suggests that psychological distress may be a more universal experience, regardless of educational background.

The absence of differences in parents' age, children's age, and employment status may indicate that the experience of stress and reduced quality of life is not limited to specific demographic categories. This finding differs from some studies that support the influence of demographic factors (Hsiao, 2018), which may be due to cultural or sampling factors.

Although no distinction was made between idiopathic and syndromic autism in the present study, this choice does not negate the relevance of the findings in the context of the syndromes. Autism is often a coexisting condition in a variety of genetic and chromosomal syndromes, while autistic traits occur with increased frequency in syndromic populations (Richards et al., 2015). Thus, the findings of this research can provide meaningful information on parental burden in syndromic contexts as well, since psychosocial pressure seems to be mainly associated with functional difficulty and increased care requirements, which are experienced daily by parents with children experiencing complex health conditions, such as those of genetic syndromes (Hayes & Watson, 2013). However, further specialized research is warranted.

Limitations of the Study

Despite the contribution of the present study to understanding the relationship between stress and the quality of life of parents of children with autism, some methodological limitations need to be considered.

First, the cross-sectional design of the research does not allow causal conclusions to be drawn. Although the results demonstrate a strong predictive relationship between stress and quality of life, the direction of the effect cannot be determined with certainty.

Second, the use of self-reported questionnaires may be influenced by subjective assessments and a possible socially desirable response. Incorporating objective indicators or mixed research approaches could enhance the validity of the findings.

Third, the size and geographical concentration of the sample limit the generalizability of the results. The future expansion of the sample to different cultural and socio-economic contexts would allow to draw more generalized conclusions.

In addition, the use of non-probabilistic ease sampling may further limit the possibility of generalizing the findings.

An additional limitation concerns the relatively low response rate of the study. Although 550 questionnaires were distributed, only 120 were returned and 114 were ultimately included in the analysis, corresponding to a response rate of 21.8%. Such a rate is not uncommon in research involving parents of children with autism, a population often characterized by high caregiving demands and limited availability for research participation. Nevertheless, the low response rate raises concerns regarding potential non-response bias and limits the generalizability of the findings. It is possible that parents who chose to participate differ systematically from those who did not respond, for example in terms of stress levels, available support, or engagement with services. Consequently, the findings should be interpreted with caution and cannot be assumed to represent the broader population of parents of children with autism.

Finally, the present study did not explicitly differentiate between idiopathic and syndromic autism. Given the potential increased clinical complexity in syndromic forms, the lack of this distinction limits the possibility of specialized interpretations.

Future Directions

Based on the above, it is proposed to conduct longitudinal studies that will allow the monitoring of the development of parental stress and the quality of life at different stages of the child's development.

Of particular importance is the investigation of the differences between idiopathic and syndromic autism, in order to reflect the specific needs of families facing increased medical and functional burden.

In addition, it is appropriate to integrate factors such as symptom severity, social support, coping strategies and access to services in order to develop more integrated models for predicting quality of life.

Future research could also examine the effectiveness of targeted psychological support and family strengthening interventions, as well as the impact of social policies on alleviating the financial and practical burden of care.

Finally, adopting mixed methodological approaches (quantitative and qualitative) could provide a deeper understanding of the subjective experience of parents.

IMPLICATIONS

Theoretical Implications

The findings of the present study reinforce the theoretical models that place parental stress as a central mechanism of debilitating quality of life in families of children with autism. The strong predictive relationship between stress and quality of life underlines that psychological burden is not just a parallel experience of care, but a determining factor that shapes the perceived well-being of parents as a whole.

At the same time, the limited impact of certain demographic variables suggests that the experience of stress may be intersectional, transcending age or occupational differences. This finding contributes to the theoretical debate on the “universality” of parental burden in environments of increased care demands.

In addition, highlighting gender and marital status differences confirms the need to integrate the sociological dimension into models of understanding parenting experience, taking into account roles, care distribution and support structure.

Clinical and Practical Implications

At the clinical level, the results highlight the need for systematic psychological support for parents of children with autism, with particular emphasis on stress management. The development of empowerment programs, support groups and coping strategies-based interventions can make a significant contribution to improving the quality of life.

Differences between mothers and fathers suggest that interventions should be gender-sensitive, acknowledging the different experiences and needs of both parents. At the same time, the importance of marital status shows that strengthening marital and family cohesion can have a protective effect.

Particular attention is required in families facing increased clinical complexity, such as in cases of syndromic autism, where medical and functional needs are often more intense.

Policy Implications

At the level of social policy, the findings highlight the need to develop integrated support structures that will reduce the psychological and financial burden of care. Enhancing accessible mental health services, providing financial facilities, and expanding specialized educational and therapeutic interventions are critical priorities.

Especially in the context of syndromic forms of autism, where additional medical needs often coexist, the state is called upon to formulate policies that take into account the increased complexity of care and the long-term effects on family well-being.

Recognizing parental stress as a public health issue can help shape interventions that do not focus solely on the child but adopt a family-centered approach.

CONCLUSION

The present study highlighted the close and strong relationship between parental stress and perceived quality of life in parents of children with autism, confirming that psychological burden is a determining factor in shaping their overall well-being. The findings demonstrate that stress does not just function as an accompanying feature of care, but as a central mechanism that fundamentally influences quality of life.

At the same time, differences in gender, educational level and marital status highlight the importance of social and demographic parameters in shaping parenting experience. However, the absence of variations in other variables suggests that the experience of stress crosses broader societal boundaries.

In the context of a volume dedicated to syndromes, the results are of particular importance, as they underline the need to further investigate the particular challenges faced by families of children with syndromic forms of autism, where clinical complexity may exacerbate the psychological and practical burden.

The relationship between stress and quality of life among parents of children with autism carries implications that extend beyond research, into the domain of social policy and professional practice. Strengthening families through psychological, social and institutional support is a key prerequisite for improving the well-being of both parents and children.

A family-centered and socially informed approach remains essential for the development of effective and sustainable support for families raising children with autism.

REFERENCES

Abolkheirian, S., Sadeghi, R., & Shojaeizadeh, D. (2022). What do parents of children with autism spectrum disorder think about their quality of life? A qualitative study. *Journal of Education and Health Promotion, 11*(1), 169. DOI: 10.4103/jehp.jehp_887_21 PMID: 35847126

Alenazi, D., Hammad, S., & Mohamed, A. (2020). Effect of autism on parental quality of life in Arar city, Saudi Arabia. *Journal of Family & Community Medicine, 27*(1), 15. DOI: 10.4103/jfcm.JFCM_157_19 PMID: 32030074

Alodaili, M. S. M., Cornejo, L. T. O., Saleh, K. A., Alrashedi, H., Alrubaiee, G. G., Almoliky, M. A., Alqalah, T. A. H., & Alkubati, S. A. (2026). Quality of life of caregivers of children with autism spectrum disorder in Saudi Arabia. *Journal of Pediatric Nursing, 86*, 709–716. DOI: 10.1016/j.pedn.2025.12.010 PMID: 41468833

American Psychiatric Association. (2013). *Diagnostic and statistical manual of mental disorders* (5th ed.). American Psychiatric Association., DOI: 10.1176/appi.books.9780890425596

Anderson, H., & Goolishian, H. (1992). The client is the expert: A not-knowing approach to therapy. In McNamee, S., & Gergen, K. J. (Eds.), *Therapy as social construction* (pp. 25–39). Sage.

Befkadu, B., & Adamek, M. E. (2022). The financial challenges of parents of a child with autism in addis ababa, ethiopia: A Qualitative study. *Integrated Journal for Research in Arts and Humanities, 2*(1), 5–10. DOI: 10.55544/ijrasb.2.1.7

Besag, F. M. C., & Vasey, M. J. (2020). Seizures and epilepsy in autism spectrum disorder. *Child and Adolescent Psychiatric Clinics of North America, 29*(3), 483–500. DOI: 10.1016/j.chc.2020.02.002 PMID: 32471597

Bhakta, B. B., Coleman, K. J., & Choi, K. R. (2022). Randomized study of survey recruitment strategies for parents of autistic children. *Journal of Pediatric Health Care, 36*(5), 470–473. DOI: 10.1016/j.pedhc.2022.05.008 PMID: 35705390

Boyle, M. (2002). *Schizophrenia: A scientific delusion?* (2nd ed.). Routledge.

CDC. gov. (2025). Data and statistics on autism spectrum disorder. Available at: https://www.cdc.gov/autism/data-research/index.html

Chan, K. K. S., Lam, C. B., Law, N. C. W., & Cheung, R. Y. M. (2018). From child autistic symptoms to parental affective symptoms: A family process model. *Research in Developmental Disabilities*, *75*, 22–31. DOI: 10.1016/j.ridd.2018.02.005 PMID: 29455076

Chrousos, G. P. (2009). Stress and disorders of the stress system. *Nature Reviews. Endocrinology*, *5*(7), 374–381. DOI: 10.1038/nrendo.2009.106 PMID: 19488073

Cohen, C. I. (2025). Neorecovery: A Critical Analysis of the Relationship between Neoliberalism and the Recovery Movement. *Community Mental Health Journal*, *61*(2), 248–253. DOI: 10.1007/s10597-024-01275-6 PMID: 38874799

Davis, N. O., & Carter, A. S. (2008). Parenting stress in mothers and fathers of toddlers with autism spectrum disorders: Associations with child characteristics. *Journal of Autism and Developmental Disorders*, *38*(7), 1278–1291. DOI: 10.1007/s10803-007-0512-z PMID: 18240012

Diener, E., & Suh, E. (1997). Measuring quality of life: Economic, social, and subjective indicators. *Social Indicators Research*, *40*(1/2), 189–216. DOI: 10.1023/A:1006859511756

Fletcher-Watson, S., Apicella, F., Auyeung, B., Beranova, S., Bonnet-Brilhault, F., Canal-Bedia, R., Charman, T., Chericoni, N., Conceição, I. C., Davies, K., Farroni, T., Gomot, M., Jones, E., Kaale, A., Kapica, K., Kawa, R., Kylliäinen, A., Larsen, K., Lefort-Besnard, J., & Yirmiya, N. (2017). Attitudes of the autism community to early autism research. *Autism*, *21*(1), 61–74. DOI: 10.1177/1362361315626577 PMID: 26975669

Fountoulakis, K., Papadopoulou, M., Kleanthous, S., Papadopoulou, A., Bizeli, V., Agorastos, G., Nimatoudis, I., Iacovides, A., & Kaprinis, G. S. (2003). Reliability and psychometric properties of the Greek translation of the State–Trait Anxiety Inventory Form Y: Preliminary data. *Annals of General Hospital Psychiatry*, *2*(S1, Suppl 1), S80. DOI: 10.1186/1475-2832-2-S1-S80

García-López, C., Sarriá, E., & Pozo, P. (2016). Multilevel approach to gender differences in adaptation in father-mother dyads parenting individuals with autism spectrum disorder. *Research in Autism Spectrum Disorders*, *28*, 7–16. DOI: 10.1016/j.rasd.2016.04.003

Gill, R., & Orgad, S. (2018). The amazing bounce-backable woman: Resilience and the psychological turn in neoliberalism. *Sociological Research Online*, *23*(2), 477–495. DOI: 10.1177/1360780418769673

Hayes, S. A., & Watson, S. L. (2013). The impact of parenting stress: A meta-analysis of studies comparing the experience of parenting stress in parents of children with and without autism spectrum disorder. *Journal of Autism and Developmental Disorders, 43*(3), 629–642. DOI: 10.1007/s10803-012-1604-y PMID: 22790429

Hsiao, Y. (2018). Autism spectrum disorders: Family demographics, parental stress, and family quality of life. *Journal of Policy and Practice in Intellectual Disabilities, 15*(1), 70–79. DOI: 10.1111/jppi.12232

Ishtiaq, M. (2019). Book Review Creswell, J. W. (2014). Research design: Qualitative, quantitative and mixed methods approaches (4th ed.). Thousand Oaks, CA: Sage. *English Language Teaching, 12*(5), 40. https://doi.org/DOI: 10.5539/elt.v12n5p40

Katsarou, D. (2022). Fragile X syndrome and language skills. In Katsarou, D., & Zisi, V. (Eds.), *Disability and mental health* (pp. 133–149). Gutenberg.

Katsarou, D., & Zisi, V. (2022). Down syndrome: Verbal short-term memory from early childhood to old age. *Archives of Hellenic Medicine, 39*(1), 54–59.

Katsarou, D. V., Theodoratou, M., Sofologi, M., Kougioumtzis, G. A., Efthymiou, E., Argyriadis, A., Patsiaouras, A., Mantsos, E., Argyriadi, A., & Papadopoulou, S. (2025). Angelman Syndrome Neurocognitive and Linguistic Profile, Overlaps, Interventions, and Quality of Life. In Megari, K. (Ed.), *Clinical Applications of Pediatric Neuropsychology from Infancy to Adolescence* (pp. 143–156). IGI Global., DOI: 10.4018/979-8-3693-9689-6.ch007

Kouznetsov, R., Angelopoulos, P., Moulinos, S., Dimakos, I., Gourzis, P., & Jelastopulu, E. (2023). Epidemiological study of autism spectrum disorders in greece for 2021: Nationwide prevalence in 2–17-year-old children and regional disparities. *Journal of Clinical Medicine, 12*(7), 2510. DOI: 10.3390/jcm12072510 PMID: 37048594

Kuhlthau, K., Payakachat, N., Delahaye, J., Hurson, J., Pyne, J. M., Kovacs, E., & Tilford, J. M. (2014). Quality of life for parents of children with autism spectrum disorders. *Research in Autism Spectrum Disorders, 8*(10), 1339–1350. DOI: 10.1016/j.rasd.2014.07.002

Li, F., Tang, Y., Li, F., Fang, S., Liu, X., Tao, M., Wu, D., & Jiang, L. (2022). Psychological distress in parents of children with autism spectrum disorder: A cross-sectional study based on 683 mother-father dyads. *Journal of Pediatric Nursing, 65*, e49–e55. DOI: 10.1016/j.pedn.2022.02.006 PMID: 35249769

Lord, C., Brugha, T. S., Charman, T., Cusack, J., Dumas, G., Frazier, T., Jones, E. J. H., Jones, R. M., Pickles, A., State, M. W., Taylor, J. L., & Veenstra-VanderWeele, J. (2020). Autism spectrum disorder. *Nature Reviews. Disease Primers*, *6*(1), 5. DOI: 10.1038/s41572-019-0138-4 PMID: 31949163

Maenner, M. J., Warren, Z., Williams, A. R., Amoakohene, E., Bakian, A. V., Bilder, D. A., Durkin, M. S., Fitzgerald, R. T., Furnier, S. M., Hughes, M. M., Ladd-Acosta, C. M., McArthur, D., Pas, E. T., Salinas, A., Vehorn, A., Williams, S., Esler, A., Grzybowski, A., Hall-Lande, J., & Shaw, K. A. (2023). Prevalence and characteristics of autism spectrum disorder among children aged 8 years—Autism and developmental disabilities monitoring network, 11 Sites, United States, 2020. *MMWR. Surveillance Summaries*, *72*(2), 1–14. DOI: 10.15585/mmwr.ss7202a1 PMID: 36952288

Musick, K., Meier, A., & Flood, S. (2016). How parents fare: Mothers' and fathers' subjective well-being in time with children. *American Sociological Review*, *81*(5), 1069–1095. DOI: 10.1177/0003122416663917

Neumärker, K.-J. (2003). Leo Kanner: His Years in Berlin, 1906-24. The roots of autistic disorder. *History of Psychiatry*, *14*(2), 205–218. DOI: 10.1177/0957154X030142005 PMID: 14518490

Norlin, D., & Broberg, M. (2013). Parents of children with and without intellectual disability: Couple relationship and individual well-being. *Journal of Intellectual Disability Research*, *57*(6), 552–566. DOI: 10.1111/j.1365-2788.2012.01564.x PMID: 22533701

Paxinos, I. (2022). Is there an "inspiration" of QOL in the field of clinical psychology and psychiatry? *Journal of Biomedical Engineering and Medical Imaging*, *9*(3). Advance online publication. DOI: 10.14738/jbemi.93.12415

Picardi, A., Gigantesco, A., Tarolla, E., Stoppioni, V., Cerbo, R., Cremonte, M., Alessandri, G., Lega, I., & Nardocci, F. (2018). Parental burden and its correlates in families of children with autism spectrum disorder: A multicentre study with two comparison groups. *Clinical Practice and Epidemiology in Mental Health*, *14*(1), 143–176. DOI: 10.2174/1745017901814010143 PMID: 30158998

Priego Ojeda, M., & Rusu, P. P. (2023). Emotion regulation, parental stress and family functioning: Families of children with disabilities vs normative families. *Research in Developmental Disabilities*, *139*, 104548. DOI: 10.1016/j.ridd.2023.104548 PMID: 37320995

Pukeliene, V., & Starkauskiene, V. (2011). Quality of life: Factors determining its measurement complexity. *The Engineering Economist*, *22*(2), 147–156. DOI: 10.5755/j01.ee.22.2.311

Rezq, K. A., Albalawi, H. M. H., & Alharbi, H. F. (2025). Exploring social support and quality of life among mothers of children with autism spectrum disorders: A Cross-sectional study. *Health Care*, *13*(2), 95. DOI: 10.3390/healthcare13020095 PMID: 39857122

Richards, C., Jones, C., Groves, L., Moss, J., & Oliver, C. (2015). Prevalence of autism spectrum disorder phenomenology in genetic disorders: A systematic review and meta-analysis. *The Lancet. Psychiatry*, *2*(10), 909–916. DOI: 10.1016/S2215-0366(15)00376-4 PMID: 26341300

Shah, S. M., Madhavan, S. P., Bowden, N., & Nedgungadi, P. (2026). Caregivers' experiences with autism from pre- to postdiagnosis: Multi-country perspectives using ecological systems theory. *Research in Autism*, *132*, 202836. DOI: 10.1016/j.reia.2026.202836

Sim, A., Cordier, R., Vaz, S., & Falkmer, T. (2019). "We are in this together": Experiences of relationship satisfaction in couples raising a child with autism spectrum disorder. *Research in Autism Spectrum Disorders*, *58*, 39–51. DOI: 10.1016/j.rasd.2018.11.011

Skevington, S. M., Lotfy, M., & O'Connell, K. A. (2004). The World Health Organization's WHOQOL-BREF quality of life assessment: Psychometric properties and results of the international field trial. A Report from the WHOQOL Group. *Quality of Life Research: An International Journal of Quality of Life Aspects of Treatment, Care and Rehabilitation*, *13*(2), 299–310. DOI: 10.1023/B:QURE.0000018486.91360.00 PMID: 15085902

Spielberger, C. D., Gorsuch, R. L., & Lushene, R. E. (1970). *Manual for the State-Trait Anxiety Inventory (STAI)*. Consulting Psychologists Press.

Stoner, J. B., Bock, S. J., Thompson, J. R., Angell, M. E., Heyl, B. S., & Crowley, E. P. (2005). Welcome to our world: Parent perceptions of interactions between parents of young children with ASD and education professionals. *Focus on Autism and Other Developmental Disabilities*, *20*(1), 39–51. DOI: 10.1177/10883576050200010401

Teoli, D., & Bhardwaj, A. (2025 Jan). Quality of life. [Updated 2023 Mar 27] In *StatPearls* [Internet]. StatPearls Publishing., Available from https://www.ncbi.nlm.nih.gov/books/NBK536962/

Timimi, S., Milton, D., Bovell, V., Kapp, S., & Russell, G. (2019). Deconstructing diagnosis: Four commentaries on a diagnostic tool to assess individuals for autism spectrum disorders. *Autonomy (Birmingham, England)*, *1*(6), AR26. PMID: 31396391

Turnage, D., & Conner, N. (2022). Quality of life of parents of children with autism spectrum disorder: An integrative literature review. *Journal for Specialists in Pediatric Nursing*, *27*(4), e12391. DOI: 10.1111/jspn.12391 PMID: 35986656

Tzinieri-Kokkosi, M. (2009). *Quality of life manual with the WHOQOL-100 questionnaire as its axis: Sections and content of topics* (Improved version.). *BETA Bulletin of Experimental Treatments for AIDS.*

Vasilopoulou, E., & Nisbet, J. (2016). The quality of life of parents of children with autism spectrum disorder: A systematic review. *Research in Autism Spectrum Disorders*, *23*, 36–49. DOI: 10.1016/j.rasd.2015.11.008

Verdugo, M. A., Schalock, R. L., Keith, K. D., & Stancliffe, R. J. (2005). Quality of life and its measurement: Important principles and guidelines. *Journal of Intellectual Disability Research*, *49*(10), 707–717. DOI: 10.1111/j.1365-2788.2005.00739.x PMID: 16162115

Vernhet, C., Michelon, C., Dellapiazza, F., Rattaz, C., Geoffray, M.-M., Roeyers, H., Picot, M.-C., Baghdadli, A., Baghdadli, A., Chabaux, C., Chatel, C., Cohen, D., Damville, E., Geoffray, M.-M., Gicquel, L., Jardri, R., Maffre, T., Novo, A., Roxane, R., & Vespérini, S.ELENA study group. (2022). Perceptions of parents of the impact of autism spectrum disorder on their quality of life and correlates: Comparison between mothers and fathers. *Quality of Life Research: An International Journal of Quality of Life Aspects of Treatment, Care and Rehabilitation*, *31*(5), 1499–1508. DOI: 10.1007/s11136-021-03045-3 PMID: 34822048

Warreman, E. B., Lloyd, S. E., Nooteboom, L. A., Leenen, P. J. M., Terry, M. B., Hoek, H. W., Van Rossum, E. F. C., Vermeiren, R. R. J. M., & Ester, W. A. (2023). Psychological, behavioural, and physical aspects of caregiver strain in autism-caregivers: A cohort study. *EClinicalMedicine*, *64*, 102211. DOI: 10.1016/j.eclinm.2023.102211 PMID: 37767192

World Health Organization. (2023). *Stress*. https://www.who.int/news-room/questions-and-answers/item/stress

Zablotsky, B., Bradshaw, C. P., & Stuart, E. A. (2013). The association between mental health, stress, and coping supports in mothers of children with autism spectrum disorders. *Journal of Autism and Developmental Disorders*, *43*(6), 1380–1393. DOI: 10.1007/s10803-012-1693-7 PMID: 23100053

Chapter 8

Occupational, Physical, and Recreational Therapy Interventions for Individuals With Genetic Syndromes:

An Interdisciplinary and Lifespan Perspective

Evangelos Mantsos
http://orcid.org/0009-0002-8490-2660
University of Western Macedonia, Greece

ABSTRACT

This chapter provides an integrative overview of occupational therapy, physical therapy, and recreational therapy interventions for individuals with selected genetic syndromes, including Down syndrome, Williams syndrome, Prader–Willi syndrome, Fragile X syndrome, and Rett syndrome. Emphasising person-centred and participation-oriented approaches, it explores how interdisciplinary interventions support daily functioning, motor development, health, leisure, and social inclusion across the lifespan, while highlighting the importance of family involvement, environmental adaptations, and inclusive community practices.

DOI: 10.4018/979-8-3373-8485-6.ch008

INTRODUCTION

Genetic syndromes associated with intellectual and developmental disability—such as Down syndrome, Williams syndrome, Prader–Willi syndrome, Fragile X syndrome, and Rett syndrome—often involve complex profiles of motor, cognitive, communication, sensory, behavioral, and health-related needs that evolve across the lifespan (Bull et al., 2022). These needs commonly affect daily functioning (e.g., self-care, learning, mobility, communication), participation in typical life contexts (home, school, work, community), and long-term health trajectories (e.g., fitness, secondary conditions, mental health, aging-related risks) (World Health Organization, 2007).

This report expands the chapter-style text you provided into a deeper, therapy-focused synthesis that integrates occupational therapy (OT), physical therapy (PT), and recreational therapy (RT) as complementary components of interdisciplinary support. It emphasizes participation-oriented and person-centred practice: (a) defining outcomes as meaningful engagement in everyday activities and life roles, (b) valuing autonomy and preferences (including family preferences for children), and (c) treating environments, routines, and social opportunity structures as legitimate therapeutic "targets," not just impairments (World Health Organization, 2007).

A recurring theme across syndromes is that *single-domain interventions are rarely sufficient*. Functional gains in "body functions" (e.g., strength, balance) are most likely to translate into real-world independence and well-being when programs are designed to (1) generalize skills into daily routines and community settings, and (2) reduce environmental barriers and participation restrictions (World Health Organization, 2007).

CONCEPTUAL FRAMEWORKS FOR PARTICIPATION-FOCUSED INTERVENTION

A widely used foundation for modern rehabilitation thinking is the biopsychosocial model embedded in the World Health Organization's International Classification of Functioning, Disability and Health (ICF). The ICF conceptualizes disability as an interaction among health conditions, body functions/structures, activities, participation, and contextual factors (environmental and personal), shifting clinical reasoning away from a purely medical "deficit" model and toward modifiable participation determinants (Barnes, 2019).

Figure 1. Work related disease/disorder

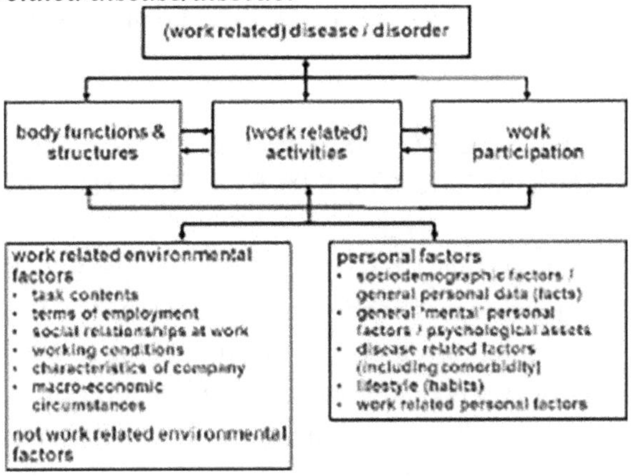

Figure 2. Health condition

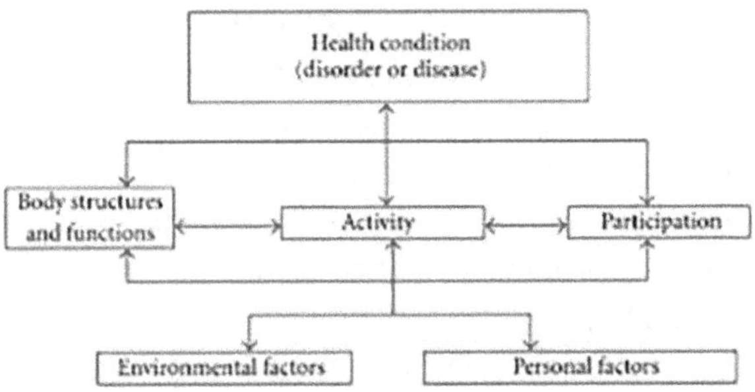

Two complementary traditions deepen the ICF's relevance for genetic syndromes. First, disability studies critiques overly reductionist medical framings and highlights how barriers, stigma, and exclusion shape lived disability—especially in education, employment, and community life (Barnes, 2019). Second, developmental systems theory—often summarized through bioecological approaches associated with Urie Bronfenbrenner—emphasizes that development emerges from dynamic interactions between a person and multiple environmental layers (family routines, school systems, community resources, social policy, and time). This makes "context engineering" (supports, scaffolding, inclusive opportunities) a core mechanism of change, not a secondary add-on (Bronfenbrenner & Morris, 2007).

From these perspectives, rehabilitation outcomes can be reframed as *capabilities for living*: the ability to participate in self-care, learning, friendships, play/leisure, work, and community membership with appropriate supports. This aligns with rights-based views that treat participation in recreation, leisure, and sport as a legitimate social entitlement—not merely a therapeutic luxury (Bantekas et al., 2018).

FUNCTIONAL PROFILES OF SELECTED GENETIC SYNDROMES AND IMPLICATIONS FOR THERAPY PLANNING

Although each syndrome has a distinct genetic etiology and phenotype, several functional challenges recur across conditions relevant to OT, PT, and RT planning: hypotonia and delayed motor development; motor coordination and balance limitations; differences in sensory processing and arousal regulation; executive functioning and cognitive flexibility challenges; communication limitations (often severe in Rett syndrome); and vulnerability to secondary health conditions (e.g., obesity, low fitness, musculoskeletal complications) (Paleg et al., 2025).

Down syndrome is frequently characterized by generalized hypotonia, ligamentous laxity, delayed motor milestones, and increased risk of musculoskeletal issues (e.g., joint instability, scoliosis, hip and patellar instability), which can influence gait efficiency, endurance, and skill acquisition (Foley & Killeen, 2019). These physical features have practical implications for PT dosage and for OT task adaptation (e.g., seating/positioning, fine motor endurance, joint protection (Shields, 2021)). In adulthood, Down syndrome is also strongly associated with early-onset Alzheimer-type neuropathology and elevated dementia risk, making long-term participation planning, environmental supports, and health promotion particularly salient (Fortea et al., 2021).

Williams syndrome often includes a distinctive cognitive profile with relative strengths in sociability and certain language skills but notable weaknesses in visuospatial construction and motor performance; anxiety is commonly reported, which can influence participation and tolerance for novelty in therapy and community settings (Martens et al., 2008). GeneReviews specifically notes that physical therapy is recommended to maximize mobility and reduce later orthopedic complications, and it highlights interventions such as hippotherapy as considerations in management—illustrating the importance of combining traditional therapeutic exercise principles with motivating participation contexts (Kozel et al., 2021).

Prader–Willi syndrome typically involves early hypotonia and later emergence of hyperphagia with high obesity risk, plus behavioral and emotional regulation difficulties (e.g., rigidity with routines, temper outbursts, compulsive behaviors, skin picking (Shaikh et al., 2024). Because food-related drive can dominate daily decision-making, participation outcomes are often tightly coupled to environmental design ("food security"), structured routines, and safe opportunities for enjoyable physical activity—areas where OT (routine design), PT (fitness and functional mobility), and RT (inclusive, motivating activity participation) can be mutually reinforcing (Ho & Dimitropoulos, 2010).

Fragile X syndrome is commonly associated with sensory sensitivities and hyperarousal, along with anxiety and social-communication challenges that can interfere with learning, daily living participation, and community inclusion (Lachiewicz et al., 2024). Large-scale registry work has examined sensory symptoms and hyperarousal across development, supporting the clinical emphasis on arousal regulation, environmental predictability, and individualized sensory supports—while also underscoring variability by age and sex (Lachiewicz et al., 2024). This argues for intervention plans that are "syndrome-informed" but individualized, targeting participation barriers rather than assuming a one-size-fits-all protocol (World Health Organization, 2007).

Rett syndrome involves profound motor and communication challenges for many individuals, including loss of functional hand use, movement disorders, and severe limitations in natural speech, making alternative communication modalities and sustained support for mobility and posture central (Fonzo et al., 2020). Evidence syntheses describe physical therapy as a key aspect of management and highlight that, despite rarity-related research constraints, individuals can improve or maintain aspects of function with rehabilitation (Fonzo et al., 2020).

Across all five syndromes, the practical implication is that *therapeutic targets should be mapped to participation goals* (e.g., mealtime independence, classroom access, friendships, community mobility) and jointly "owned" by the person and family—using body function interventions as means rather than ends (World Health Organization, 2007).

OCCUPATIONAL THERAPY INTERVENTIONS ACROSS THE LIFESPAN

Occupational therapy is distinctive in its explicit focus on enabling engagement in meaningful activities (occupations) and roles through a blend of skill development, task adaptation, environmental modification, and caregiver/partner coaching. In genetic syndromes, OT is often central for translating gains in motor or cognitive capacity into real-world performance in self-care, play, learning routines, social participation, and (later) vocational and community living tasks (World Health Organization, 2007).

A strong participation-oriented trend in pediatric OT is the growing emphasis on caregiver coaching and consultation models, where clinicians build caregiver capacity to embed therapeutic strategies into natural routines and environments. Scoping reviews of coaching in early intervention and across OT populations describe coaching as viable and increasingly used, while also noting variability in definitions and calling for stronger outcome evidence and training standards for implementation fidelity (Seruya et al., 2022). Recent reviews focused on family-centered OT consultation similarly report benefits related to children's participation and caregiver competence, supporting consultation as a complement (or alternative) to exclusively therapist-delivered sessions (Shahbazi et al., 2026).

In syndrome populations, caregiver coaching is particularly relevant because (1) many functional problems emerge in routines that caregivers manage (sleep, dressing, feeding, transitions), and (2) generalization across contexts is often a primary barrier. For example, in Prader–Willi syndrome, occupational performance and emotional regulation are deeply entangled with environmental routines and food access; OT-informed structuring of daily schedules, predictable transitions, and "choice architecture" can reduce conflicts and support participation (Ho & Dimitropoulos, 2010).

OT intervention commonly includes *task and environmental adaptation*. This can involve: assistive technology and communication supports; seating/positioning for attention and hand use; simplified visual supports for routines; motor planning scaffolds; and sensory-environment modifications (lighting, noise, movement breaks) to reduce dysregulation and support learning participation. In Williams syndrome—where visuospatial and motor challenges can limit handwriting, dressing, and classroom tool use—OT often targets fine motor skill acquisition while also adapting tasks and environments to reduce frustration and anxiety-related avoidance (Cure Science Institute, 2024).

Sensory processing and regulation are frequently addressed in OT for neurodevelopmental conditions, including Fragile X syndrome and Down syndrome, where sensory sensitivities or modulation differences may affect attention, behavior, and participation. However, it is essential to treat sensory-based interventions as part of a comprehensive plan with clear functional goals and measurable outcomes (Lachiewicz et al., 2024). The American Academy of Pediatrics policy statement on sensory integration therapies emphasizes that the evidence base is limited and that families should be informed about uncertainty; it recommends that sensory-based strategies be used within a broader treatment plan with monitoring of effectiveness (Lachiewicz et al., 2024). Practically, this supports an OT approach that prioritizes *function-linked sensory supports* (e.g., noise reduction to enable participation in class, or movement breaks to support mealtime sitting) rather than sensory activities as stand-alone outcomes (Section On Complementary And Integrative Medicine et al., 2012).

Across the lifespan, OT is often pivotal during *transitions*: early intervention to school entry; primary to secondary school; adolescence to adulthood; and adult aging-related change. These transitions can destabilize routines and participation, particularly for people with executive function challenges, anxiety, or rigidity (commonly described in Prader–Willi syndrome) and for individuals whose physical needs change over time (e.g., musculoskeletal issues in Down syndrome, evolving motor function in Rett syndrome) (Ho & Dimitropoulos, 2010). OT contributions here often include environmental redesign (home/community accessibility), self-advocacy supports, assistive technology updates, and role participation planning (education, employment, community living) (Moran et al., 2025).

PHYSICAL THERAPY INTERVENTIONS FOR MOTOR FUNCTION AND LONG-TERM HEALTH

Physical therapy for individuals with genetic syndromes typically targets motor development, posture, gait, balance, strength, endurance, and movement efficiency—while also emphasizing long-term health behaviors such as sustained physical activity and safe participation in community mobility (Shields, 2021). This dual focus matters because people with developmental disabilities experience disproportionate health risks linked to inactivity and obesity-related secondary conditions, which can further restrict participation (Rimmer et al., 2010).

For *Down syndrome*, the PT evidence base includes multiple systematic reviews and topical reviews describing benefits from exercise-based and task-specific interventions for strength, balance, and functional skills (Shields, 2021). Meta-analytic work on exercise and balance in children with Down syndrome reports improvements associated with structured exercise programs, although the intervention types and dosing vary widely (Lei et al., 2025). A key conceptual point from physiotherapy reviews is that *task-specific training* (learning real motor skills in contexts that resemble the target activity) appears beneficial for building motor proficiency—supporting PT programs that resemble meaningful participation tasks (walking in the community, cycling, stairs, playground mobility) rather than only isolated impairment drills (Shields, 2021).

Clinical PT planning for Down syndrome also needs to account for syndrome-associated medical considerations such as joint instability and musculoskeletal anomalies (Foley, & Killeen, 2019). Cohort evidence highlights the role of ligamentous laxity and hypotonia in musculoskeletal complications and delayed motor milestone acquisition. Exercise program development papers note that major professional fitness guidelines recommend medical evaluation with attention to joint instability and cardiovascular considerations prior to exercise testing/training—reinforcing the need for individualized screening and interprofessional coordination (Mann et al., 2023).

For *Prader–Willi syndrome*, PT has a prominent role in building physical capacity, preserving lean mass, and supporting weight management strategies in synergy with environmental and nutritional approaches (Shaikh et al., 2024). Recent clinical guidance emphasizes multi-disciplinary care and highlights the life-course pattern of early hypotonia followed by later hyperphagia and rapid weight gain risk, which shapes PT goals from early motor development to long-term activity adherence. Systematic review evidence suggests that physical exercise is generally safe and can improve physical fitness phenotypes in Prader–Willi syndrome, although research remains limited by small samples and heterogeneity—common constraints in rare conditions (Morales et al., 2019).

For *Rett syndrome*, a systematic review focused on evidence-based PT describes a range of interventions, reflecting the reality that high-quality trials are difficult in rare, complex conditions. Still, the synthesis supports PT as integral for maintaining or improving function, with typical PT emphases including mobility maintenance, postural management, scoliosis prevention/management support, and prevention of secondary complications (Fonzo et al., 2020). Importantly, because participation is often constrained by severe motor limitations, PT outcomes in Rett syndrome should be framed not only as motor scores but as *access to participation opportunities* (e.g., supported walking, safe seating to enable communication and leisure) (World Health Organization, 2007).

A participation-oriented PT approach also requires explicit attention to environmental barriers and facilitators. Research on barriers to physical activity participation in youth with intellectual and developmental disabilities highlights structural and contextual obstacles (access, supports, resources), which are often as limiting as impairments themselves (Clemente, 2017). This evidence supports PT practice that includes advocacy and "systems work," such as liaising with schools, designing accessible home activity programs, and partnering with community sports providers (Giummarra et al., 2022).

Finally, PT should be aligned with public health guidance: global recommendations on physical activity explicitly apply to people living with disability and emphasize that any activity is better than none, with age-specific targets for aerobic, strengthening, and (for older adults) balance activity (World Health Organization, 2020). For genetic syndromes that elevate long-term health risks (e.g., obesity risk in Prader–Willi syndrome and broader IDD populations; dementia risk in Down syndrome), the "fitness for participation" framing becomes a central lifespan intervention logic rather than a supplemental wellness add-on (World Health Organization, 2020).

RECREATIONAL THERAPY AND LEISURE PARTICIPATION AS HEALTH AND INCLUSION INTERVENTIONS

Recreational therapy (also called therapeutic recreation or recreation therapy) is designed to use activity-based interventions to restore, remediate, or rehabilitate functioning and to reduce participation restrictions—often serving as the bridge between clinic-based goals and real-world community participation (World Health Organization, 2020). Professional standards describe RT as an evidence-informed process involving assessment, planning, implementation, and evaluation within an interdisciplinary plan of care (Bethel et al., 2024).

A participation-based framing of RT is strongly supported by human rights instruments. United Nations materials on Article 30 of the Convention on the Rights of Persons with Disabilities emphasize the right of persons with disabilities to participate in cultural life, recreation, leisure, and sport, with state responsibilities that include enabling access and equal participation opportunities. In practice, this supports an ethical argument that leisure and sport participation are not merely optional "extras," but legitimate life domains in which disability-related exclusion should be addressed through inclusive design and appropriate supports (Moran et al., 2025).

Empirical work across disability populations consistently links leisure participation to well-being, inclusion, and participation breadth. Systematic reviews on determinants of leisure participation in youth with disabilities highlight that participation is shaped by a combination of individual factors (motivation, functional capacity) and environmental factors (family support, resources, accessibility), reinforcing RT's ecological focus (Shikako-Thomas et al., 2008). Broader evidence syntheses on interventions for social and community participation in adults with intellectual disability also emphasize the importance of context, supports, and implementation facilitators—pointing to the need for community-partnered programs rather than clinic-only approaches (Giummarra et al., 2022).

Within sport and structured activity, systematic reviews report perceived benefits of sport participation for people with disabilities—including improvements in function and psychosocial outcomes such as reduced anxiety—while also noting that many remain inactive due to access barriers (Aitchison et al., 2022). Controlled intervention studies in inclusive sport contexts report improvements in fitness outcomes for athletes with intellectual disability, supporting the plausibility of sport as a health promotion and participation intervention when appropriately adapted (Gallotta et al., 2024).

In genetic syndromes specifically, RT often becomes especially important when clinical therapies alone cannot deliver social inclusion. For individuals with Prader–Willi syndrome, structured, enjoyable physical activities can serve dual functions: improving fitness while providing routine-based engagement that may reduce behavior escalations tied to rigidity and stress (Ho & Dimitropoulos, 2010). For Rett syndrome, participation may depend on accessible environments, supportive technology, and partner training; leisure contexts can be key opportunities for communication through alternative modalities and for social interaction with peers (Wandin et al., 2023).

A practical pathway to inclusion is *universal design and accessible community infrastructure*, especially play and recreation spaces. Guidance documents on inclusive playgrounds explicitly apply universal design principles to reduce physical, sensory, and social barriers, aligning closely with the ICF's environmental factors domain. UNICEF guidance on building inclusive playgrounds, for example, frames universal design as a route to non-stigmatizing access and participation, illustrating how design choices can function as population-level therapeutic supports (UNICEF, 2021).

Finally, RT's professional identity is partly defined by standards and credentialing structures. The American Therapeutic Recreation Association publishes standards of practice that position RT as goal-directed, evidence-based, and individualized, which aligns with the need for outcome tracking and accountability in interdisciplinary care. The National Council for Therapeutic Recreation Certification scope of practice explicitly frames the ultimate goal as facilitating optimal involvement in community life, reinforcing RT's role as a participation bridge (UNICEF, 2021).

INTERDISCIPLINARY INTEGRATION, IMPLEMENTATION CONTEXTS, AND EVIDENCE GAPS

Interdisciplinary care for genetic syndromes is not simply "multiple therapies delivered in parallel," but a coordinated process of (1) shared participation goals, (2) consistent environmental strategies across settings, and (3) reinforcement of skills across routines and community life. This need is particularly salient in syndromes where participation barriers span domains—such as Prader–Willi syndrome (food environment + behavior + activity), Rett syndrome (mobility + posture + communication access), and Down syndrome (motor development + musculoskeletal risk + long-term aging) (Shaikh et al., 2024).

A practical integrative template is to use the ICF (or ICF-aligned participation frameworks) to link discipline-specific interventions to shared outcomes. For example: PT may target strength and balance to enable community mobility; OT may adapt tasks and environments to enable independent self-care and school/work participation; RT may provide inclusive contexts where these skills produce actual social membership, friendships, and identity-building roles. In the intellectual and developmental disability field, quality-of-life supports models emphasize that supports should be conceptualized as coordinated resources and strategies that mitigate disability effects and enhance well-being—an approach compatible with ICF reasoning and interdisciplinary goal alignment (Moran et al., 2025).

Evidence gaps and research design challenges remain substantial. Rare disorders often yield small samples, heterogeneous phenotypes, and practical/ethical constraints on randomized trials, which contributes to dispersed evidence and variable intervention reporting. This pattern is visible in rehabilitation syntheses for Rett syndrome, which catalog diverse interventions but are limited by study designs and inconsistent outcome measures (Fonzo et al., 2020). It is also evident in coaching and consultation literatures in OT, where scoping reviews describe growth in use but persistent inconsistency in definitions, outcome selection, and fidelity reporting (Seruya et al., 2022).

Two methodological priorities emerge from the literature. First, outcomes must better reflect participation and lived experience, not only impairment-level change; this aligns with disability-rights rationales and with ICF participation domains. Second, interventions should be evaluated in real-world contexts with attention to facilitators and barriers (implementation science), because access, transport, inclusive program availability, and caregiver demands often determine whether interventions result in sustained participation (Clemente, 2017).

Ethically, the modern participation-oriented approach requires avoiding ableist assumptions that equate "normalization" with success. Instead, it prioritizes dignity, autonomy, and meaningful life participation with supports—consistent with rights-based commitments to inclusion in recreation, leisure, and community life. As a concrete example of inclusion-oriented systems practice, large-scale inclusive sport initiatives such as Special Olympics are frequently discussed in the literature as mechanisms for social inclusion and opportunity creation for people with intellectual disabilities, illustrating how participation outcomes can be pursued via community institutions, not only clinical services (Harada et al., 2013). In sum, the strongest integrative logic across OT, PT, and RT for genetic syndromes is: *build capacity, adapt context, and expand opportunity*—with success defined by participation, belonging, and quality of life across the lifespan.

DISCUSSION

The present chapter synthesizes evidence on occupational therapy, physical therapy, and recreational therapy interventions for individuals with selected genetic syndromes and situates these practices within contemporary participation-oriented frameworks. Across the literature, a consistent finding is that individuals with genetic syndromes experience complex and evolving functional profiles that require coordinated, interdisciplinary interventions throughout the lifespan. Motor impairments, sensory processing differences, executive functioning challenges, and health-related vulnerabilities are common across conditions such as Down syndrome, Williams syndrome, Prader–Willi syndrome, Fragile X syndrome, and Rett syndrome, although their presentation and severity vary considerably (Paleg et al., 2025). These characteristics affect not only body functions but also daily participation in education, social life, and community activities, reinforcing the importance of interventions that address functional outcomes rather than isolated impairments.

A key theoretical implication of the findings relates to the application of the biopsychosocial perspective articulated in the International Classification of Functioning, Disability and Health (ICF). The ICF conceptualizes disability as a dynamic interaction between health conditions and contextual factors rather than as a fixed individual deficit (World Health Organization [WHO], 2007). From this perspective, the goal of rehabilitation is not simply remediation of impairments but the facilitation of meaningful participation across life domains. The synthesis of occupational, physical, and recreational therapy approaches supports this framework by demonstrating how each discipline contributes uniquely to activity performance and participation outcomes.

From a *clinical perspective*, the evidence highlights the importance of early, individualized, and context-sensitive intervention planning. Occupational therapy plays a critical role in supporting participation in daily occupations, including self-care, play, learning, and social interaction. In young children with genetic syndromes, caregiver coaching and family-centered practice models have gained increasing recognition as effective approaches for embedding therapeutic strategies within natural routines (Seruya et al., 2022; Shahbazi et al., 2026). These approaches acknowledge that families are primary facilitators of children's participation and that intervention effectiveness depends on integration within everyday contexts. For example, structured routines and environmental supports are particularly important for individuals with Prader–Willi syndrome, where behavioral regulation and food-related routines significantly influence participation (Ho & Dimitropoulos, 2010).

Physical therapy contributes primarily to the development and maintenance of motor abilities, postural control, and physical fitness. The literature consistently reports that individuals with genetic syndromes are at increased risk for sedentary lifestyles and associated health conditions, including obesity and reduced cardiovascular fitness (Rimmer et al., 2010). Exercise-based and task-specific training programs have demonstrated benefits for improving balance, strength, and functional mobility, particularly among individuals with Down syndrome (Lei et al., 2025; Shields, 2021). Importantly, effective physical therapy interventions are those that incorporate meaningful functional tasks and encourage long-term engagement in physical activity rather than focusing exclusively on isolated motor exercises. This approach supports sustainable health outcomes and aligns rehabilitation goals with everyday life activities.

Recreational therapy represents an essential component of interdisciplinary intervention because it facilitates participation in leisure, sport, and community activities. Leisure participation has been associated with improved physical health, social competence, and psychological well-being among individuals with intellectual and developmental disabilities (Aitchison et al., 2022; Gallotta et al., 2024). Recreational therapy therefore extends the goals of clinical intervention beyond rehabilitation settings and into inclusive community contexts. Participation in inclusive sport programs, community recreation initiatives, and accessible play environments can provide opportunities for social inclusion and identity development. These contexts are particularly important for individuals whose functional limitations might otherwise restrict opportunities for peer interaction and community engagement.

Beyond clinical practice, the findings also have important *educational implications*. In school settings, interdisciplinary collaboration among therapists, educators, and families is essential to support inclusive participation in learning environments. Occupational therapists often assist with classroom adaptations, assistive technologies, and strategies that facilitate engagement in academic tasks. For students with genetic syndromes who experience motor or sensory processing differences, these supports can significantly enhance access to educational activities. Physical therapists may contribute to mobility planning within school environments, enabling safe navigation of classrooms, playgrounds, and community spaces. Meanwhile, recreational therapists and adapted physical activity specialists can promote inclusive participation in school-based sport and leisure programs.

Educational inclusion also requires attention to environmental and social factors that influence participation. Research has consistently demonstrated that barriers such as inaccessible facilities, limited support resources, and social stigma can restrict participation opportunities for individuals with disabilities (Clemente, 2017). Consequently, educational institutions must adopt inclusive design principles and collaborative support systems to create environments that enable participation for all students. Universal design approaches, particularly in play and recreational spaces, have been identified as effective strategies for reducing barriers and promoting inclusive engagement (UNICEF, 2021).

Another important consideration concerns *lifespan transitions*, including transitions from early childhood services to school settings and from adolescence to adulthood. These periods often involve significant changes in service systems and participation opportunities, which may disrupt established support structures. Occupational therapy has been identified as particularly important during these transitions, supporting individuals in developing adaptive skills, accessing assistive technologies, and navigating new environments (Moran et al., 2025). Similarly, physical activity and recreational engagement can support health and social participation during adulthood and aging, particularly for individuals with conditions such as Down syndrome who may experience early-onset neurodegenerative changes (Fortea et al., 2021).

Despite growing evidence supporting interdisciplinary interventions, significant research gaps remain. Many studies examining therapeutic interventions in rare genetic syndromes involve small sample sizes and heterogeneous methodologies, limiting generalizability and the ability to conduct rigorous randomized controlled trials (Fonzo et al., 2020). Additionally, outcomes in rehabilitation research often focus on impairment-level changes rather than broader participation outcomes. Future research should prioritize longitudinal designs, standardized outcome measures, and participatory research approaches that include individuals with disabilities and their families as active collaborators.

Ethical considerations also emerge from the literature. Contemporary disability scholarship emphasizes the importance of avoiding ableist assumptions that equate success with normalization of functioning. Instead, interventions should prioritize autonomy, dignity, and meaningful participation according to the preferences and goals of individuals and their families (Barnes, 2019). This perspective aligns with rights-based frameworks such as the Convention on the Rights of Persons with Disabilities, which recognizes participation in recreation, leisure, and cultural life as fundamental human rights (Bantekas et al., 2018). Within this context, occupational, physical, and recreational therapy should be viewed not only as clinical services but also as mechanisms for promoting social inclusion and equity.

CONCLUSION

This chapter examined the contributions of occupational therapy, physical therapy, and recreational therapy to the support of individuals with genetic syndromes across the lifespan. The synthesis demonstrates that effective intervention requires a participation-oriented, interdisciplinary approach that integrates motor development, functional skill acquisition, environmental adaptation, and opportunities for social inclusion. Grounded in the ICF framework, contemporary rehabilitation practice emphasizes the interaction between individual capacities and contextual factors, highlighting the importance of family involvement, inclusive environments, and coordinated support systems.

Occupational therapy facilitates engagement in daily occupations and supports adaptive functioning within home, school, and community contexts. Physical therapy contributes to motor development, mobility, and long-term physical health, while recreational therapy provides pathways for social participation and inclusive engagement in leisure and sport. When integrated within interdisciplinary frameworks, these therapeutic approaches can significantly enhance participation, autonomy, and quality of life for individuals with genetic syndromes.

Future research should continue to strengthen the evidence base for interdisciplinary interventions by prioritizing participation-focused outcomes, longitudinal evaluation, and inclusive research methodologies. At the same time, clinical and educational systems must work collaboratively to create environments that enable individuals with genetic syndromes to participate fully in community life. Ultimately, the goal of therapeutic intervention should not be limited to functional improvement but should extend to supporting meaningful lives characterized by inclusion, opportunity, and well-being.

REFERENCES

Aitchison, B., Rushton, A. B., Martin, P., Barr, M., Soundy, A., & Heneghan, N. R. (2022). The experiences and perceived health benefits of individuals with a disability participating in sport: A systematic review and narrative synthesis. *Disability and Health Journal, 15*(1), 101164. DOI: 10.1016/j.dhjo.2021.101164 PMID: 34238729

Bantekas, I., Stephenson, C. P. Y., Karapapa, S., Polymenopoulou, E., Stein, M. A., & Anastasiou, D. (2018). Article 30 Participation in Cultural Life, Recreation, Leisure, and Sport. [1]. *Paragraph, 100*(882), 883.

Barnes, C. (2019). Understanding the social model of disability: Past, present and future. In *Routledge handbook of disability studies* (pp. 14–31). Routledge. DOI: 10.4324/9780429430817-2

Bethel, K. A., Fuhrman, N. E., Kelsey, K. D., & Borron, A. (2024). Recreational therapists and the duty of care. *Journal of Experiential Education, 47*(3), 536–554. DOI: 10.1177/10538259231190844

Bronfenbrenner, U., & Morris, P. A. (2007). Handbook of child psychology: Vol. 1. *The bioecological model of human development.*

Bull, M. J., Trotter, T., Santoro, S. L., Christensen, C., & Grout, R. W. (2022). Health supervision for children and adolescents with Down syndrome. *Pediatrics, 149*(5), e2022057010. DOI: 10.1542/peds.2022-057010 PMID: 35490285

Clemente, I. (2017). Barriers and facilitators to participation in physical activity for children with disabilities. *A systematic literature review.*

CureScience Institute. (2024). Williams Syndrome. *Disease Review*, 1-13.

Foley, C., & Killeen, O. G. (2019). Musculoskeletal anomalies in children with Down syndrome: An observational study. *Archives of Disease in Childhood, 104*(5), 482–487. DOI: 10.1136/archdischild-2018-315751 PMID: 30472668

Fonzo, M., Sirico, F., & Corrado, B. (2020). Evidence-based physical therapy for individuals with Rett syndrome: A systematic review. *Brain Sciences, 10*(7), 410. DOI: 10.3390/brainsci10070410 PMID: 32630125

Fortea, J., Zaman, S. H., Hartley, S., Rafii, M. S., Head, E., & Carmona-Iragui, M. (2021). Down syndrome-associated Alzheimer's disease: A genetic form of dementia. *Lancet Neurology, 20*(11), 930. DOI: 10.1016/S1474-4422(21)00245-3 PMID: 34687637

Gallotta, M. C., Franciosi, E., Giorgi, M., Guidetti, L., Cerbara, E., Pes, G., Silvestri, F., & Curzi, D. (2024). Benefits of inclusive sport training on fitness and health of athletes with and without intellectual disability. *Scientific Reports, 14*(1), 21203. DOI: 10.1038/s41598-024-69334-2 PMID: 39261519

Giummarra, M. J., Randjelovic, I., & O'Brien, L. (2022). Interventions for social and community participation for adults with intellectual disability, psychosocial disability or on the autism spectrum: An umbrella systematic review. *Frontiers in Rehabilitation Sciences, 3*, 935473. DOI: 10.3389/fresc.2022.935473 PMID: 36189003

Harada, C. M., Siperstein, G. N., Parker, R. C., & Lenox, D. (2013). Promoting social inclusion for people with intellectual disabilities through sport: Special Olympics International, global sport initiatives and strategies. In *Disability in the global sport arena* (pp. 63–80). Routledge.

Ho, A. Y., & Dimitropoulos, A. (2010). Clinical management of behavioral characteristics of Prader–Willi syndrome. *Neuropsychiatric Disease and Treatment*, •••, 107–118. PMID: 20505842

Kozel, B. A., Barak, B., Kim, C. A., Mervis, C. B., Osborne, L. R., Porter, M., & Pober, B. R. (2021). Williams syndrome. *Nature Reviews. Disease Primers, 7*(1), 42. DOI: 10.1038/s41572-021-00276-z PMID: 34140529

Lachiewicz, A. M., Stackhouse, T. M., Burgess, K., Burgess, D., Andrews, H. F., Choo, T. H., Kaufmann, W. E., & Kidd, S. A. (2024). Sensory symptoms and signs of hyperarousal in individuals with fragile X syndrome: Findings from the FORWARD registry and database multisite study. *Journal of Autism and Developmental Disorders, 54*(11), 4259–4277. DOI: 10.1007/s10803-023-06135-y PMID: 37840096

Lei, Z., Yuan, K., Xu, J., Miao, Y., Dai, Y., Wang, J., & Chang, J. (2025). Effects of physical exercises on balance in children with down syndrome: A systematic review and meta-analysis. *BMC Sports Science, Medicine and Rehabilitation, 17*(1), 165. DOI: 10.1186/s13102-025-01222-2 PMID: 40604949

Mann, S., Spiric, J., Mitchell, C., & Hilgenkamp, T. I. M. (2023). Development of a physical therapy-based exercise program for adults with Down syndrome. *International Journal of Environmental Research and Public Health, 20*(4), 3667. DOI: 10.3390/ijerph20043667 PMID: 36834362

Martens, M. A., Wilson, S. J., & Reutens, D. C. (2008). Research Review: Williams syndrome: a critical review of the cognitive, behavioral, and neuroanatomical phenotype. *Journal of Child Psychology and Psychiatry, and Allied Disciplines, 49*(6), 576–608. DOI: 10.1111/j.1469-7610.2008.01887.x PMID: 18489677

Morales, J. S., Valenzuela, P. L., Pareja-Galeano, H., Rincón-Castanedo, C., Rubin, D. A., & Lucia, A. (2019). Physical exercise and Prader-Willi syndrome: A systematic review. *Horumon To Rinsho*, *90*(5), 649–661. DOI: 10.1111/cen.13953 PMID: 30788853

Moran, G., Seymour, H., Walsh, N., O'Leary, N., & Gallagher, A. L. (2025). The Optimal Service for Children and Young People With Complex Neurodevelopmental Disabilities: Findings From an Integrative Literature Review. *Advances in Communication and Swallowing*, *28*(2), 87–101. DOI: 10.1177/27725383251339604

Paleg, G. S., Hidalgo Robles, Á., Govender, P., & Livingstone, R. W. (2025). Occupational and Physical Therapy Interventions for Young Children with Developmental Central Hypotonia: An Overview of Systematic Reviews. *Disabilities*, *5*(1), 14. DOI: 10.3390/disabilities5010014

Rimmer, J. H., Yamaki, K., Lowry, B. D., Wang, E., & Vogel, L. C. (2010). Obesity and obesity-related secondary conditions in adolescents with intellectual/developmental disabilities. *Journal of Intellectual Disability Research*, *54*(9), 787–794. DOI: 10.1111/j.1365-2788.2010.01305.x PMID: 20630017

Seruya, F. M., Feit, E., Tirado, A., Ottomanelli, D., & Celio, M. (2022). Caregiver coaching in early intervention: A scoping review. *The American Journal of Occupational Therapy*, *76*(4), 7604205070. DOI: 10.5014/ajot.2022.049143 PMID: 35727822

Shahbazi, M., Abed, E. H., & Esmaili, S. K. (2026). Family-Centered Occupational Therapy Consultation for Children Under 18 Years Old: A Scoping Review. *Occupational Therapy International*, *2026*(1), 1184326. DOI: 10.1155/oti/1184326 PMID: 41522633

Shaikh, M. G., Barrett, T. G., Bridges, N., Chung, R., Gevers, E. F., Goldstone, A. P., Holland, A., Kanumakala, S., Krone, R., Kyriakou, A., Livesey, E. A., Lucas-Herald, A. K., Meade, C., Passmore, S., Roche, E., Smith, C., & Soni, S. (2024). Prader–Willi syndrome: Guidance for children and transition into adulthood. *Endocrine Connections*, *13*(8). Advance online publication. DOI: 10.1530/EC-24-0091 PMID: 38838713

Shields, N. (2021). Physiotherapy management of Down syndrome. *Journal of Physiotherapy*, *67*(4), 243–251. DOI: 10.1016/j.jphys.2021.08.016 PMID: 34511385

Shikako-Thomas, K., Majnemer, A., Law, M., & Lach, L. (2008). Determinants of participation in leisure activities in children and youth with cerebral palsy: Systematic review. *Physical & Occupational Therapy in Pediatrics*, *28*(2), 155–169. DOI: 10.1080/01942630802031834 PMID: 18846895

UNICEF. (2021). *Good practice guide on building an inclusive playground*. UNICEF.

Wandin, H., Lindberg, P., & Sonnander, K. (2023). Aided language modelling, responsive communication and eye-gaze technology as communication intervention for adults with Rett syndrome: Three experimental single case studies. *Disability and Rehabilitation. Assistive Technology*, *18*(7), 1011–1025. DOI: 10.1080/17483107.2021.1967469 PMID: 34455895

World Health Organization. (2007). *International classification of functioning, disability, and health: Children & youth version: ICF-CY*. World Health Organization.

World Health Organization. (2020). *WHO guidelines on physical activity and sedentary behaviour*. World Health Organization.

Zimmer, M., Desch, L., Rosen, L. D., Bailey, M. L., Becker, D., Culbert, T. P., McClafferty, H., Sahler, O. J. Z., Vohra, S., Liptak, G. S., Adams, R. C., Burke, R. T., Friedman, S. L., Houtrow, A. J., Kalichman, M. A., Kuo, D. Z., Levy, S. E., Norwood, K. W.Jr, Turchi, R. M., & Wiley, S. E.Section On Complementary And Integrative Medicine. (2012). Sensory integration therapies for children with developmental and behavioral disorders. *Pediatrics*, *129*(6), 1186–1189. DOI: 10.1542/peds.2012-0876 PMID: 22641765

Chapter 9

Deep Learning Approach Leveraging Optimized Residual Neural Networks for Robust and Early-Stage Alzheimer's Disease Clarification

K. Ramalakshmi
http://orcid.org/0000-0002-3038-643X
P.S.R. Engineering College, India

M. Uvaneshwari
Vel Tech Rangarajan Dr. Sagunthala R&D Institute of Science and Technology, India

L. Krishna Kumari
Ramco Institute of Technology, India

B. Mohan
P.S.R. Engineering College, India

N. Ismayil Kani
AMET University, Chennai, India

M. Ashok Kumar
http://orcid.org/0000-0002-4541-8465
KPR Institute of Engineering and Technology, India & INTI International University, Nilai, Malaysia

R. Santhana Krishnan
http://orcid.org/0000-0001-7930-8072
SCAD College of Engineering and Technology, India

ABSTRACT

This study presents a deep learning-based framework using the ResNet18 architecture for automatic classification of Alzheimer's disease stages from Magnetic Resonance Imaging (MRI) scans. The datasetcomprises Non Demented, Very Mild Demented,

DOI: 10.4018/979-8-3373-8485-6.ch009

Mild Demented, and Moderate Demented—with both original and augmented images to ensure data diversity and balance. The methodology involves several key stages. First, all MRI images were resized to a uniform resolution, normalized, and augmented. The ResNet18 model, a deep residual convolutional neural network pre-trained on ImageNet, was utilized through transfer learning, where the initial layers were frozen to retain low-level feature extraction, and the final fully connected layers were fine-tuned to adapt to the Alzheimer's dataset. The trained model achieved an outstanding test accuracy of 98.18%, indicating strong generalization and discriminative capability. The classification report demonstrates high reliability with F1-scores of 0.99 (Mild Demented), 1.00 (Moderate Demented), 0.98 (Non Demented), and 0.97 (Very Mild Demented).

INTRODUCTION

Alzheimer's disease (AD) is one of the most common neurodegenerative disorders affecting millions of elderly people around the world. It gradually damages brain cells, leading to memory loss, confusion, and difficulty in thinking or performing daily activities. The disease not only impacts patients but also places a heavy emotional and financial burden on families and healthcare systems. Early and accurate diagnosis of Alzheimer's disease is crucial for timely medical treatment, better management, and improved quality of life.

In the last decade, deep learning techniques have become powerful tools for analyzing medical images, helping healthcare professionals detect diseases automatically and with higher accuracy. These methods can learn and recognize complex structures in medical scans without the need for manual feature extraction. This project focuses on developing a deep learning-based classification system using the ResNet18 architecture to identify and classify MRI brain images into different stages of Alzheimer's disease. The system aims to assist radiologists in achieving faster, more reliable, and objective diagnoses.

1.1 Background of Alzheimer's Disease

Alzheimer's disease is a progressive and irreversible brain disorder that causes the gradual deterioration of neurons (nerve cells) in the brain. It is the most common cause of dementia, responsible for about 60–80% of all dementia cases worldwide. The exact cause of Alzheimer's is not fully understood, but it is believed to involve a combination of genetic, environmental, and lifestyle factors.

Patients with Alzheimer's experience symptoms that worsen over time, including memory loss, language problems, confusion, disorientation, and behavioral changes. The disease typically progresses through several stages: Very Mild Demented, Mild Demented, Moderate Demented, and Severe Demented. In the early stages, symptoms are subtle, often mistaken for normal aging. However, as the disease advances, it severely affects a person's ability to perform daily tasks independently.

At the biological level, Alzheimer's is associated with the accumulation of amyloid-beta plaques and tau protein tangles in the brain, which disrupt neural communication and lead to cell death. Modern brain imaging techniques, especially Magnetic Resonance Imaging (MRI), provide detailed structural information that helps identify brain shrinkage and tissue loss in specific regions such as the hippocampus and cerebral cortex — both of which are key indicators of Alzheimer's progression. These MRI-based observations make the disease suitable for analysis using image classification techniques powered by artificial intelligence.

1.2 Importance of Early Detection

Early detection of Alzheimer's disease is one of the most critical challenges in modern neuroscience and healthcare. Identifying the disease at an early stage can significantly slow its progression, allowing patients to benefit from available treatments and lifestyle interventions. Early diagnosis helps patients preserve cognitive function for a longer period, plan for future care, and participate in clinical trials for emerging therapies.

However, manual diagnosis using MRI scans requires expert radiologists to examine numerous brain slices, which is both time-consuming and prone to human error. Subtle structural differences between early-stage Alzheimer's and normal aging are difficult to detect visually. Consequently, there is a growing demand for automated diagnostic systems that can analyze large volumes of MRI data quickly, objectively, and accurately.

Artificial Intelligence (AI), particularly deep learning, can bridge this gap. By learning from large image datasets, AI systems can detect patterns and anomalies that are often invisible to the human eye. Such systems can provide decision support to clinicians, improving diagnostic confidence and ensuring consistent evaluations across healthcare institutions. Ultimately, automated deep learning models can complement medical expertise rather than replace it, making diagnosis faster, more accessible, and less expensive.

1.3 Role of Deep Learning in Medical Imaging

Deep learning is a branch of artificial intelligence inspired by the structure of the human brain, designed to recognize patterns in data through layers of interconnected neurons. In medical imaging, deep learning models, especially Convolutional Neural

Networks (CNNs), have demonstrated exceptional ability in tasks like classification, segmentation, and detection across modalities such as MRI, CT, PET, and X-ray.

Unlike traditional machine learning models that rely on hand-crafted features, CNNs automatically learn hierarchical features directly from raw image data. The early layers detect simple patterns like edges and textures, while deeper layers capture more complex features such as anatomical structures and disease-specific patterns. This automatic feature extraction makes CNNs highly effective for medical diagnosis, where precise image interpretation is vital.

In the case of Alzheimer's detection, deep learning models can identify subtle structural changes in the brain—such as cortical thinning or hippocampal shrinkage—that might not be easily visible in manual analysis. Several CNN-based architectures, including VGG16, Inception, and ResNet, have been successfully used for brain image classification. Among them, ResNet18 (Residual Network 18) has gained attention due to its residual learning mechanism, which allows the network to be deeper and more accurate without facing problems like vanishing gradients.

Figure 1. Image classification process

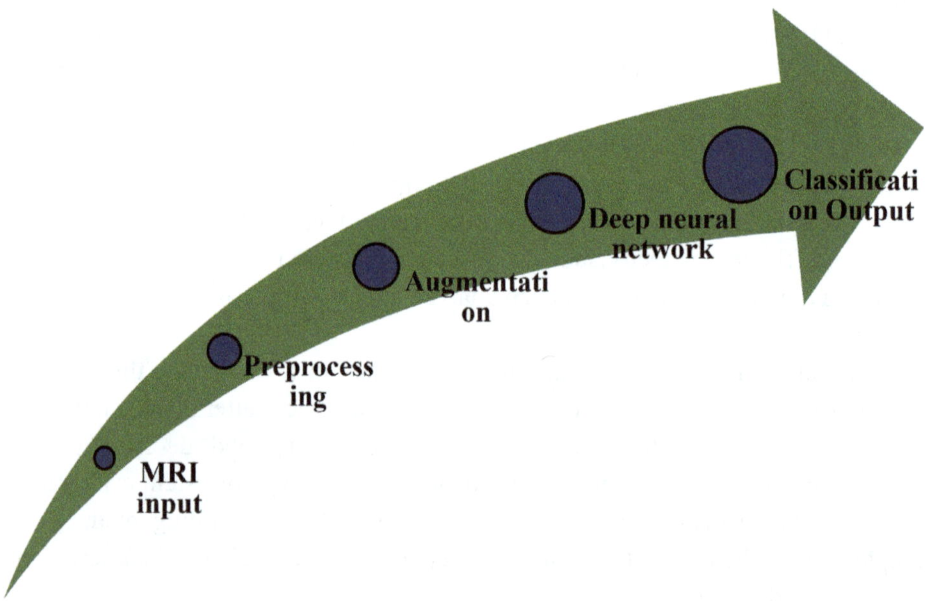

ResNet18 uses skip connections (or residual connections) that help the model retain important information across layers and accelerate convergence during training. This makes it well-suited for complex medical imaging tasks, where maintaining fine details is crucial. Additionally, transfer learning is applied by using a ResNet18 model pre-trained on the ImageNet dataset — a large collection of natural images — and then fine-tuning it with MRI scans. This approach allows the model to leverage previously learned visual features and adapt them to medical contexts, even when the dataset size is limited.

By combining transfer learning with medical imaging, the proposed ResNet18-based framework aims to deliver a high-performing, robust, and efficient system for Alzheimer's disease classification. This methodology not only improves diagnostic accuracy but also demonstrates the potential of deep learning in assisting clinicians with reliable, early, and automated detection of neurodegenerative diseases.

1.4 Objectives of the Project

The main goal of this project is to develop an efficient deep learning model for classifying MRI brain images into different stages of Alzheimer's disease. The specific objectives are:

- To analyze MRI images and identify structural patterns related to Alzheimer's progression.
- To apply ResNet18 architecture with transfer learning for multi-class classification.
- To improve model accuracy and generalization using image preprocessing and augmentation techniques.
- To evaluate the performance of the model using metrics such as accuracy, precision, recall, and F1-score.
- To demonstrate that deep learning can be an effective tool for early and automated Alzheimer's disease detection.

2.LITERATURE REVIEW

2.1 Overview of Previous Research on Alzheimer's Detection

The global prevalence of Alzheimer's disease (AD) continues to increase with ageing populations, creating an urgent need for accurate, early-stage detection strategies. Traditional diagnostic workflows rely on clinical evaluation, cognitive tests, cerebrospinal-fluid biomarkers, and neuroimaging; however, these approaches often detect disease only after significant neuronal loss. Consequently, researchers have focused on automated methods using neuroimaging, particularly structural MRI and PET scans, for quantitative assessment of disease progression. BrainAge models, which estimate the biological age of the brain using neuroimaging and clinical data, have emerged as promising tools for understanding neurodegenerative diseases such as Alzheimer's disease (Garcia Condado et al., 2025). However, their reliance on neuroimaging features like grey matter volume and hippocampal atrophy introduces potential biases, since these biomarkers are affected by both normal aging and Alzheimer's pathology. This overlap can confound the ability of BrainAge models to accurately distinguish between aging-related and disease-specific changes. To address this, Garcia Condado et al. (2025) analyzed how feature selection influences the trade-off between optimizing models for age prediction versus disease classification. Using mutual information to rank neuroimaging and neuropsychological features, they found that neuroimaging variables correlated more strongly with aging, whereas neuropsychological features were more effective in discriminating Alzheimer's stages. Models optimized for age prediction yielded poorer Alzheimer's classification accuracy, and vice versa, revealing an inherent trade-off. Although logistic regression models trained directly on selected features sometimes outperformed BrainAge deltas in classification, BrainAge models still offered a valuable continuous biomarker capable of capturing progression across cognitive stages (Garcia Condado et al., 2025).

The early and accurate detection of Alzheimer's Disease (AD) remains a major clinical challenge due to subtle brain structure changes and overlapping symptoms between disease stages (Almansour et al., 2025). To address this, recent advances in deep learning have focused on transformer-based architectures for medical imaging. The proposed Deformable Attention Vision Transformer (DA-ViT) integrates deformable Multi-Head Self-Attention (MHSA) with a Multi-Layer Perceptron (MLP) block for efficient MRI-based AD classification. Unlike traditional vision transformers, DA-ViT employs learned offset predictions to focus on spatially relevant patches, improving local feature extraction. The model is computationally lightweight, containing only 0.93 million parameters, making it practical for deployment in limited-resource environments. Using an imbalanced dataset of 6,400 MRI images across four AD categories, DA-ViT achieved 80.31% accuracy and a macro F1-score of 0.80. It also reported an exceptional AUC of 1.00 for the Mild Demented class, highlighting its sensitivity to early disease stages. Ablation studies confirmed optimal architectural settings for performance and efficiency. Comparative analysis demonstrated that DA-ViT outperforms several state-of-the-art CNN models. Overall, the study underscores the potential of deformable attention mechanisms for improving AD diagnosis through MRI analysis (Almansour et al., 2025).

Early detection of Alzheimer's disease (AD) is vital for delaying its progression since no effective cure currently exists (Author, Year). Deep learning, particularly convolutional neural networks (CNNs), has shown strong potential for automatic AD diagnosis and stage classification. This study proposes an end-to-end CNN-based framework to classify AD across four stages using 2D and 3D MRI scans from the ADNI dataset. Two methods are explored: simple CNN architectures and transfer learning with pre-trained models such as VGG19. The simple CNNs offer computational efficiency and reduced overfitting, achieving accuracies of 93.61% (2D) and 95.17% (3D), while the fine-tuned VGG19 model reaches 97% accuracy. Additionally, a remote Alzheimer's checking web application is developed to support clinical monitoring during restricted healthcare access (Helaly et. al, 2022).

The rapid advancement of computational power has enabled the development of Artificial Intelligence (AI) models for medical diagnosis, including Alzheimer's disease (AD) detection (Author, Year). Despite their success, many Computer-Aided Diagnosis (CAD) systems face limited clinical adoption due to the opaque, black-box nature of AI models. To address this, the field of Explainable AI (XAI) focuses on enhancing the interpretability and trustworthiness of AI predictions. This systematic review categorizes XAI methods for AD detection into conceptual approaches—such as post-hoc, ante-hoc, model-agnostic, and model-specific—and frameworks like LIME, SHAP, Grad-CAM, and LRP. These methods bridge local and global interpretability, offering meaningful clinical insights. The study also identifies current limitations and outlines future directions for integrating XAI-driven models into practical AD diagnostic workflows (Viswan et. al, 2024).

Recent advances in healthcare technologies have enabled significant progress in diagnosing neurodegenerative diseases such as Alzheimer's disease (AD), the most prevalent cause of dementia (Yousry AbdulAzeem et. al, 2021). The rising economic burden of AD care underscores the importance of early and accurate computer-aided diagnosis. Deep learning, particularly convolutional neural networks (CNNs), has emerged as a superior approach over traditional machine learning for AD classification using brain MRI scans. Numerous studies have demonstrated CNNs' effectiveness in identifying structural brain abnormalities associated with AD. Building on this foundation, the proposed CNN-based end-to-end framework offers high diagnostic performance using MRI data from the Alzheimer's Disease Neuroimaging Initiative (ADNI). The model achieved 99.6% and 99.8% accuracy for binary AD versus cognitively normal (CN) classification, and 97.5% for multi-class classification. These results highlight CNNs' potential for reliable, automated AD detection in clinical settings.

Machine learning (ML) methods, particularly convolutional neural networks (CNNs), have been widely explored for automatic classification of Alzheimer's disease (AD) from brain imaging data (Wen et al., 2020). However, comparing performance across studies is challenging due to differences in participant selection, image pre-processing, and validation procedures. Many studies also suffer from reproducibility issues, as frameworks are often not publicly available and implementation details are insufficient. Some reported results may be biased due to inadequate validation or model selection. Wen et al. (2020) conducted a systematic review and categorized

CNN-based AD classification into four approaches: 2D slice-level, 3D patch-level, ROI-based, and 3D subject-level. They found that over half of surveyed studies might have experienced data leakage, leading to inflated performance. To address these limitations, they developed an open-source framework for AD classification using T1-weighted MRI, including modular preprocessing, classification architectures, and evaluation tools. Using rigorous training, validation, and test splits, they compared different CNN architectures while preventing overfitting. Their results showed that 3D approaches (subject, ROI, patch) performed similarly, whereas 2D slice-level models underperformed. Surprisingly, CNNs did not outperform SVMs with voxel-based features. The framework generalized well to similar populations but less so to datasets with different demographics, emphasizing the need for standardized evaluation in AD research (Wen et al., 2020).

Recent systematic reviews highlight a paradigm shift from handcrafted feature extraction to deep-learning-based feature representation (Malik et al., 2024). These approaches can automatically identify subtle structural and metabolic alterations in the brain associated with AD. Large-scale public datasets such as ADNI, OASIS-3, and AIBL have facilitated this research by providing standardized, multi-modal data that enable reproducible model benchmarking (Mohsen et al., 2025). Studies using these datasets have achieved strong results in differentiating between cognitively normal (CN), mild cognitive impairment (MCI), and AD subjects, yet the majority of models remain limited to single-time-point classification rather than progression prediction (Hafeez et al., 2025).

Moreover, reviews comparing different imaging modalities indicate that multimodal combinations (e.g., MRI + PET + clinical variables) consistently outperform single-modality pipelines (Zia-ur-Rehman et al., 2024). Despite this, MRI remains the modality of choice for early diagnosis because of its wide availability and ability to capture cortical-thickness and hippocampal-volume alterations (European Journal of Medical Research, 2024). Collectively, these studies illustrate that deep learning has transformed AD research but also reveal methodological and interpretability limitations that motivate further innovation.

2.2 Deep Learning Approaches in Medical Image Classification

Convolutional neural networks (CNNs) dominate medical image analysis owing to their capacity to learn hierarchical spatial features directly from images. Early CNN-based frameworks demonstrated substantial gains in AD detection accuracy by leveraging 2D MRI slices or 3D volumes (Khan et al., 2023). More recent work, however, expands beyond conventional CNNs toward architectures such as Vision

Transformers (ViTs) and hybrid CNN–Transformer models that incorporate attention mechanisms to capture long-range dependencies (Saoud and AlMarzouqi, 2024).

For instance, Saoud and AlMarzouqi (2024) developed an explainable ensemble of 138 3D ViTs focused on specific regions of interest (ROIs) and reported both improved interpretability and higher accuracy compared with baseline CNNs. Similarly, the "AlzheimerViT" framework proposed by Akan et al. (2024) achieved over 98% accuracy on the OASIS-3 dataset by applying lightweight self-attention layers. These results underscore how attention-based mechanisms can enhance discriminative performance while offering regional interpretability.

Parallel reviews—such as Malik et al. (2024) and Hafeez et al. (2025) emphasize that reproducibility and transparent evaluation remain critical. They recommend multi-fold cross-validation, independent testing, and external-site validation to counteract overfitting and dataset bias. Turrisi et al. (2024) similarly highlight the importance of standardized preprocessing and augmentation pipelines, noting that inconsistent experimental setups can yield inflated accuracy estimates. Thus, while deep CNNs and transformers exhibit strong potential, methodological rigor continues to be a major concern across studies.

2.3 Transfer Learning and CNN Architectures

Transfer learning has become essential for medical imaging tasks, enabling models pretrained on large natural-image datasets (e.g., ImageNet) to be fine-tuned on smaller, domain-specific datasets. Khan et al. (2023) demonstrated that a VGG-based transfer-learning approach improved multi-class AD classification across ADNI subgroups, outperforming models trained from scratch. Likewise, Pandey et al. (2024) implemented deep transfer learning using ResNet-101 and achieved enhanced sensitivity and specificity for AD versus MCI detection.

Recent studies extend these methods to 3D architectures and transformer frameworks. Gu et al. (2024) showed that pretraining on real-world image features substantially boosts downstream performance in MRI-based AD classification, while Aghdam et al. (2024) proposed the PVTAD architecture—an adaptation of the Pyramid Vision Transformer—for AD diagnosis, demonstrating improved efficiency and robustness. These advances illustrate how transfer learning and attention mechanisms together contribute to both accuracy and model generalizability.

Architectural innovations continue with hybrid CNN–Transformer and CNN–LSTM pipelines. Such hybrids exploit CNNs for local spatial feature extraction and recurrent or attention layers for capturing inter-regional relationships or temporal progression (Akan et al., 2024). MobileNet and EfficientNet variants have also been explored for lightweight deployment in clinical environments (Mohammed, 2024).

Nonetheless, few comparative studies systematically evaluate how different fine-tuning strategies and network depths influence diagnostic performance.

2.4 Research Gap Identification

Despite notable achievements, several key research gaps persist in the literature:

1. Reproducibility and cross-site robustness.

Reviews by Malik et al. (2024) and Hafeez et al. (2025) emphasize that many reported accuracies depend heavily on pre-processing, data partitioning, and scanner characteristics. Models often fail to generalize across independent cohorts, highlighting the need for standardized evaluation and transparent reporting (Zhou et al., 2025).

2. Explainability and clinical interpretability.

Although explainable AI (XAI) approaches—such as Grad-CAM and attention heatmaps are becoming common, clinical interpretability remains limited. Saoud and AlMarzouqi (2024) demonstrated region-specific attention visualization, but similar studies that correlate model attention with neuropathological biomarkers are still scarce.

3. Temporal and longitudinal modelling.

Most deep-learning models treat imaging data as independent samples, ignoring disease progression over time. Akan et al. (2024) and Hafeez et al. (2025) note that longitudinal modelling—using recurrent or transformer-based temporal modules—could provide predictive insight into MCI-to-AD conversion but remains underexplored.

4. Hybrid architectures and attention mechanisms.

While hybrid CNN–Transformer pipelines have shown promise, there is a lack of systematic ablation studies assessing the individual contributions of spatial versus channel attention components. Mohsen et al. (2025) identifies the integration of attention-enhanced CNN–LSTM frameworks as an open area capable of improving interpretability without sacrificing accuracy.

5. Domain shift and generalizability.

Transfer-learning studies (Gu et al., 2024; Pandey et al., 2024) reveal that models trained on ADNI or OASIS often lose performance when tested on unseen datasets, underscoring the necessity of cross-domain adaptation and federated-learning paradigms.

6. Data efficiency and limited annotated data.

ViT-based methods require large training datasets. Aghdam et al. (2024) report that without adequate pretraining or augmentation, transformer models overfit quickly. Few studies have addressed semi-supervised or self-supervised pretraining for AD detection, representing a further opportunity.

These gaps suggest several directions for advancement. Future AD-classification frameworks should (i) combine 3D spatial representation via CNNs with attention-based interpretability; (ii) incorporate temporal or sequence modelling for longitudinal progression analysis; (iii) employ robust cross-site validation to ensure reproducibility; and (iv) address data scarcity through transfer, semi-supervised, or federated learning. The present study builds on this analysis by proposing an attention-enhanced CNN–LSTM architecture designed to capture both spatial and temporal features, thereby directly targeting the limitations identified in recent literature (Malik et al., 2024; Mohsen et al., 2025; Saoud and AlMarzouqi, 2024).

3. PROPOSED METHODOLOGY

3.1 System Architecture Overview

The proposed deep learning framework for Alzheimer's disease (AD) classification consists of a four-stage pipeline: data preprocessing, data augmentation, feature extraction using ResNet18, and classification using a softmax output layer (Figure 5.1). The architecture is designed to process structural MRI scans and automatically classify them into one of four AD stages: Non Demented, Very Mild Demented, Mild Demented, and Moderate Demented.

Figure 2. Proposed system architecture for ResNet18-based Alzheimer's classification

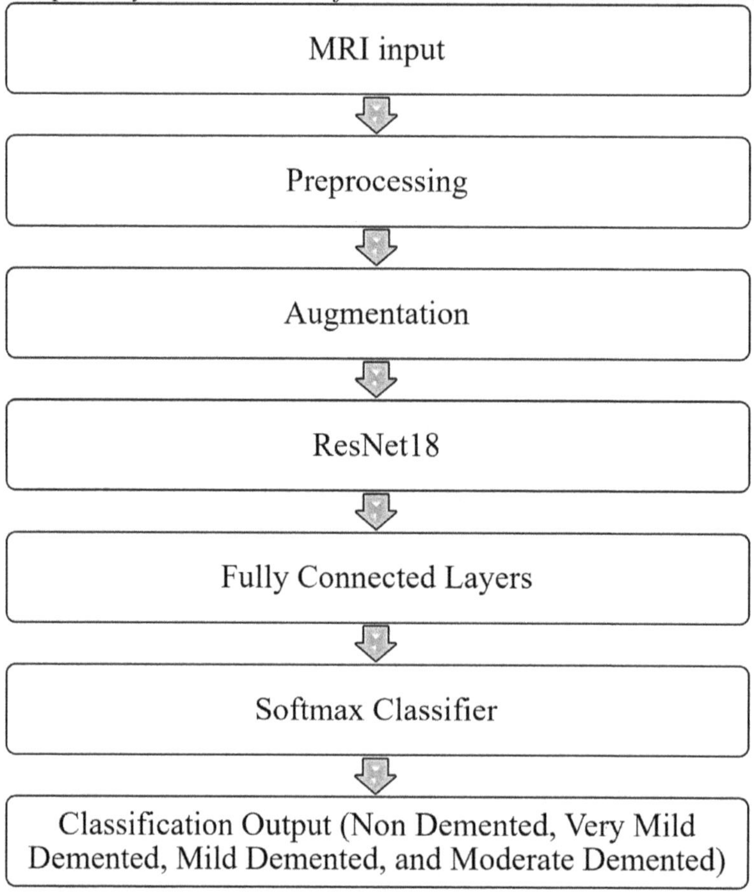

The system begins with MRI input, where brain scans are collected for analysis. These MRI images capture structural details necessary for Alzheimer's disease detection. Preprocessing is applied to standardize the data, including resizing all images to a uniform resolution. Intensity normalization is performed to scale pixel values consistently across scans. Noise reduction techniques may be applied to enhance image quality. Data Augmentation increases dataset diversity by generating modified versions of existing images. Augmentation techniques include rotation, flipping, zooming, and minor translations. This step helps the model generalize better and reduces overfitting. The pre processed and augmented images are fed into ResNet18, a deep residual convolutional neural network. ResNet18 extracts hierarchical features from images, capturing both low-level (edges, textures) and high-level (structural patterns) representations.The network uses residual blocks to prevent vanishing gradients and allow deeper learning. Output feature maps from ResNet18 are passed through fully connected layers to aggregate learned features. These dense layers map extracted features to a 4-dimensional vector corresponding to the Alzheimer's classes. A softmax classifier converts these vectors into probability scores for each class. The classifier ensures that the sum of probabilities across all classes equals one. The model predicts the classification output based on the highest probability score. The possible outputs includes Non Demented, Very Mild Demented, Mild Demented, and Moderate Demented This automated pipeline allows consistent and rapid classification of MRI scans. The combination of ResNet18 and preprocessing ensures high accuracy and robustness. This end-to-end system supports clinicians in early diagnosis and decision-making for Alzheimer's disease.

The first stage involves acquiring MRI scans from the Kaggle Alzheimer's Dataset. Preprocessing ensures uniformity in spatial resolution and intensity normalization. Data augmentation is then applied to increase dataset diversity and reduce overfitting. Feature extraction leverages the ResNet18 convolutional layers pre-trained on ImageNet, allowing the network to encode meaningful low- and high-level image representations. The final stage consists of a softmax classifier for multiclass prediction.

This modular architecture enables scalability and flexibility. Additional MRI modalities (e.g., fMRI, PET) or datasets can be integrated without major modifications, ensuring the framework's adaptability to various clinical environments.

3.2 ResNet18 Architecture Description

ResNet18, proposed by He et al. (2016), is a deep residual network comprising 18 layers, primarily built from convolutional layers with residual (skip) connections. These residual connections mitigate the vanishing gradient problem, enabling deeper network training with improved feature propagation.

Figure 3. ResNet-18 architecture

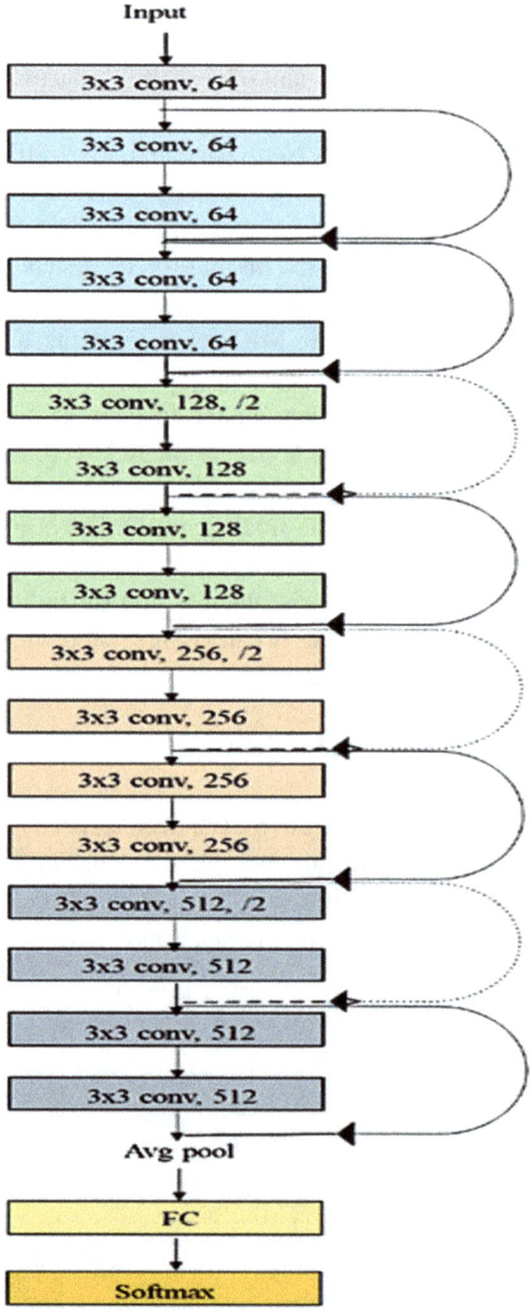

The network architecture consists of:

1. Initial Convolution Layer: A 7×7 convolution with stride 2, followed by batch normalization and a ReLU activation. This layer captures low-level features such as edges and textures.
2. Max-Pooling Layer: A 3×3 max-pooling layer reduces spatial dimensions and computation while retaining dominant features.
3. Residual Blocks (Conv2_x to Conv5_x): Four groups of residual blocks with 2 layers each. Each block contains:
   * Two 3×3 convolution layers.
   * Batch normalization and ReLU activation after each convolution.
   * A skip connection that adds the input of the block to the output, facilitating gradient flow.
4. Global Average Pooling (GAP) Layer: Converts the 2D feature maps into a 1D feature vector, reducing parameters and minimizing overfitting.
5. Fully Connected Layer: A dense layer with four output neurons corresponding to the Alzheimer's disease stages.
6. Softmax Activation: Converts the outputs into probabilities for multiclass classification.

ResNet18 was selected for its balance between depth, computational efficiency, and high feature representation capability, making it suitable for large-scale MRI datasets while maintaining fast training convergence.

3.3 Transfer Learning Strategy

Given the limited size of annotated medical imaging datasets, transfer learning is employed to leverage pre-trained ResNet18 weights obtained from ImageNet. The methodology includes:

1. Layer Freezing: The initial convolutional and residual blocks are frozen to retain low-level feature detectors that generalize across imaging domains.
2. Fine-Tuning Upper Layers: The final residual blocks and fully connected layers are retrained on the Alzheimer's dataset, allowing the model to learn domain-specific features relevant to AD.
3. Softmax Classifier Integration: The final layer is replaced with a four-neuron dense layer corresponding to the AD stages, followed by softmax activation for multiclass probability outputs.
4. Optimizer and Loss Function: The Adam optimizer with adaptive learning rates is used, minimizing the categorical cross-entropy loss function.

Transfer learning significantly reduces training time and improves accuracy by initializing the network with robust feature detectors rather than learning from scratch.

3.4 Model Training Procedure

The model training process involves multiple stages to ensure optimal performance and generalization:

1. Data Preparation:
   * MRI images are resized to 224×224 pixels to match ResNet18 input requirements.
   * Intensity normalization scales pixel values to the range [0,1].
2. Data Augmentation:
   * Random rotations (±15°), zooming (0.9–1.1×), horizontal and vertical flips, and slight translations are applied.
   * This increases the effective dataset size, reduces overfitting, and enhances model robustness.
3. Training Configuration:
   * Batch size: 32
   * Epochs: 50 with early stopping based on validation loss.
   * Learning rate: Initially 1e-4, with ReduceLROnPlateau to dynamically reduce learning rate when validation loss plateaus.
4. Validation:
   * 20% of the training data is held out for validation.
   * Performance metrics including accuracy, precision, recall, and F1-score are monitored.
5. Evaluation:
   * The trained model is tested on the original, non-augmented images to assess generalization.
   * Confusion matrices and classification reports are generated to evaluate class-wise performance.

3.5 Hyperparameter Settings

Optimizing hyperparameters is critical for maximizing model performance. The following settings were utilized:

Table 1.

Hyperparameter	Value	Description
Optimizer	Adam	Adaptive gradient-based optimizer
Learning Rate	0.0001	Initial learning rate with decay on plateau
Batch Size	32	Mini-batch size for stochastic gradient descent
Epochs	50	Maximum training epochs
Early Stopping Patience	7	Stops training if validation loss does not improve
Weight Decay	0.0001	L2 regularization to prevent overfitting
Data Augmentation	Rotation, Flip, Zoom, Shift	Enhances dataset diversity
Loss Function	Categorical Cross-Entropy	Suitable for multiclass classification

These hyperparameters were determined through grid search and iterative tuning, ensuring convergence, stability, and optimal performance on the Alzheimer's dataset.

3.6 Hardware and Software Requirements

The proposed ResNet18-based framework requires both hardware and software components optimized for deep learning and medical image processing.

3.6.1 Hardware Requirements

- **GPU** – NVIDIA RTX 3080 or equivalent for accelerated model training.
- **CPU** – Intel Core i7 (10th generation or higher) for preprocessing and data augmentation tasks.
- **RAM** – Minimum 32 GB to efficiently handle large MRI image batches.
- **Storage** – At least 1 TB SSD for storing datasets and model checkpoints.

3.6.2 Software Requirements

- **Operating System** – Ubuntu 20.04 LTS or Windows 10/11.
- **Programming Language** – Python 3.9 or higher.
- **Deep Learning Frameworks**
  - o PyTorch 2.0 for implementing and training the ResNet18 model.
  - o Torchvision for using pre-trained models and performing image transformations.
- **Data Handling Libraries**
  - o NumPy and Pandas for numerical computations and dataset management.
- **Visualization Tools**

- o Matplotlib and Seaborn for plotting confusion matrices and performance metrics.
- **Version Control** – Git for ensuring reproducibility and effective code management.

This hardware/software configuration enables efficient training, real-time inference, and reproducible experimentation, ensuring the framework is suitable for both research and clinical adaptation.

3.7 Summary of Methodology

In summary, the proposed methodology integrates state-of-the-art deep residual learning (ResNet18) with transfer learning and robust preprocessing/augmentation strategies to achieve high-accuracy Alzheimer's disease classification. The systematic approach—ranging from image acquisition to model training, evaluation, and deployment—ensures scalability, reproducibility, and potential clinical utility.

Key contributions of the methodology include:

* Efficient residual architecture for feature extraction.
* Fine-tuned transfer learning to leverage ImageNet pre-trained knowledge.
* Comprehensive augmentation strategy for robust model generalization.
* Optimized hyperparameters and early stopping to prevent overfitting.
* Practical hardware/software setup for fast training and inference.

This methodology forms the foundation for subsequent results and discussion, demonstrating how the ResNet18-based model achieves 98.18% accuracy and high F1-scores across all Alzheimer's disease stages.

4. EXPERIMENTAL SETUP

This section details the experimental setup used to evaluate the proposed ResNet18-based deep learning framework for Alzheimer's disease classification. The experimental process encompasses data splitting, image preprocessing, model training configuration, and evaluation metrics.

4.1 Data Splitting (Training, Validation, Testing)

The dataset used in this study is derived from the Kaggle Alzheimer's Dataset, which contains four classes: Non Demented (ND), Very Mild Demented (VMD), Mild Demented (MD), and Moderate Demented (MOD). To ensure reliable model performance and prevent overfitting, the dataset was divided into training, validation, and testing subsets using the standard stratified sampling approach. Stratification ensures that the proportion of each class is maintained across all subsets.

Let the total number of images in the dataset be (N), the number of images in the training set (N_\text{train}), validation set (N_\text{val}), and testing set (N_\text{test}) are defined as:

$$N_{train} = 0.7 * N,$$

$$N_{val} = 0.15 * N$$

$$N_{test} = 0.15 * N$$

This split ensures that 70% of the data is used for learning, 15% for hyper parameter tuning and early stopping, and the remaining 15% for unbiased evaluation. Augmentation techniques were applied primarily to the training set to artificially increase the number of images and improve the model's robustness.

4.2 Image Preprocessing Steps

Image preprocessing is critical in deep learning-based medical imaging to ensure uniformity and enhance model performance. The following preprocessing pipeline was implemented:

1. **Resizing:** All MRI scans were resized to a standard resolution of (224 \times 224) pixels to match the input requirements of the ResNet18 architecture:

$$I_{resized} = \text{Resize}(I, 224, 224)$$

2. **Normalization:** Pixel intensity values of MRI images were normalized to the range [0, 1] to accelerate convergence during training:

$$I_{norm} = \frac{I - \min(I)}{\max(I) - \min(I)}$$

3. **Data Augmentation:** To improve generalization and prevent overfitting, several augmentation techniques were applied:

    Rotation: Random rotations up to ±15°
    Horizontal and Vertical Flips: Random flipping to increase variance
    Zooming: Random zooms in the range 0.9–1.1

Formally, the augmented image is defined as:

$$I_{aug} = f_{flip}(f_{rotate}(f_{zoom}(I_{norm})))$$

4. **Channel Standardization:** Since ResNet18 expects three-channel inputs, grayscale MRI images were replicated across RGB channels:

$$I_{input} = [I_{norm}, I_{norm}, I_{norm}]$$

4.3 Training Configuration

The ResNet18 model was fine-tuned using transfer learning. The first several layers were frozen to preserve pre-trained features from ImageNet, while the last fully connected layers were adapted to the four-class Alzheimer's classification task.

Key training configurations:

Optimizer: Adam
Learning rate: 0.0001
Loss function: Categorical Cross-Entropy

The categorical cross-entropy loss (L) for (C) classes is defined as:

$$L = -\frac{1}{N}\sum_{i=1}^{N}\sum_{c=1}^{C} y_{i,c} \log(\hat{y}_{i,c})$$

Batch size: 32
Epochs: 50 (with early stopping based on validation loss)
Dropout: 0.5 to prevent overfitting in fully connected layers

Training was performed on a workstation with NVIDIA GPU acceleration, leveraging PyTorch's framework for optimized computation.

4.4 Evaluation Metrics

To quantitatively assess the performance of the model, multiple evaluation metrics were employed:

1. Accuracy ((A)): Measures the proportion of correctly classified samples:

$$A = \frac{TP + TN}{TP + TN + FP + FN}$$

where (TP) = true positives, (TN) = true negatives, (FP) = false positives, (FN) = false negatives.

2. Precision ((P)): Measures the correctness of positive predictions:

$$P = \frac{TP}{TP + FP}$$

3. Recall ((R)): Measures the ability to identify all positive samples:

$$R = \frac{TP}{TP + FN}$$

4. F1-Score ((F1)): Harmonic mean of precision and recall:

$$F1 = 2 \times \frac{P \cdot R}{P + R}$$

5.RESULTS AND DISCUSSION

5.1 Dataset Overview

The Alzheimer's MRI dataset utilized in this study comprises structural T1-weighted Magnetic Resonance Imaging (MRI) scans of human brains, sourced from Kaggle (4-class Alzheimer's dataset). This dataset is structured to facilitate the development of deep learning models capable of distinguishing between progressive stages of Alzheimer's disease (AD). Specifically, images are categorized into four classes reflecting disease severity: Non Demented, Very Mild Demented, Mild Demented, and Moderate Demented.

The Non Demented class includes subjects showing no detectable cognitive impairment. The Very Mild Demented class represents individuals in the earliest detectable stage of cognitive decline, often corresponding to mild neuroanatomical changes. Mild Demented subjects exhibit more pronounced structural alterations consistent with early AD pathology, while Moderate Demented subjects show substantial atrophy and other structural markers indicative of advanced AD progression.

The dataset is organized into Original and Augmented folders. The Original folder serves as a real-world evaluation set to validate model performance under standard conditions. The Augmented folder contains synthetically transformed images generated through rotation, zooming, flipping, and intensity adjustments to enhance dataset diversity and reduce overfitting risk. Each folder is subdivided into the four dementia classes, ensuring class-specific representation during model training and evaluation.

The balanced and structured nature of the dataset allows for robust training and assessment of deep learning architectures, particularly convolutional neural networks (CNNs) like ResNet18. The dataset's diversity and augmentation strategies enable models to generalize effectively, capturing subtle structural differences across Alzheimer's stages.

5.2 Model Performance Metrics

The ResNet18-based framework achieved a test accuracy of 98.18%, demonstrating its exceptional capability in classifying Alzheimer's disease stages. The high performance is attributable to several factors: effective transfer learning from ImageNet-pre trained weights, the use of extensive data augmentation, and the residual learning mechanism inherent to ResNet18, which alleviates gradient vanishing issues and facilitates deeper network training.

The detailed classification report (Table 2) quantifies the model's performance across all four classes:

Table 2. Classification report for ResNet18 Alzheimer's detection model

Class	Precision	Recall	F1-score	Support
Mild Demented	0.99	0.98	0.99	896
Moderate Demented	1.00	1.00	1.00	646
Non Demented	0.97	0.98	0.98	960
Very Mild Demented	0.97	0.97	0.97	896

The model achieved near-perfect F1-scores for Moderate Demented (1.00) and Mild Demented (0.99) classes, highlighting its strong discriminative capability for patients with noticeable cognitive decline. Similarly, Non Demented and Very Mild Demented classes achieved F1-scores of 0.98 and 0.97, respectively, indicating robust detection even in subtle or early-stage cases. High precision across classes demonstrates the model's ability to correctly identify positive samples without generating excessive false positives, while high recall indicates effective identification of most true cases.

5.3 Discussion on Accuracy and Class-Wise Performance

The ResNet18 framework's overall accuracy of 98.18% underscores the effectiveness of deep residual networks in capturing complex neuroanatomical patterns. The model's superior performance in the Moderate Demented class is particularly noteworthy, likely due to the pronounced structural changes in MRI scans of patients in this stage. Conversely, the slightly lower performance in Very Mild Demented and Non Demented classes reflects the subtlety of early-stage cognitive changes, which often manifest as minor hippocampal shrinkage or cortical thinning, challenging even sophisticated CNN models.

These results align with prior studies employing deep learning for Alzheimer's detection. For instance, models using deeper networks such as ResNet50 or DenseNet201 report marginally higher complexity but similar or slightly lower accuracy, indicating that ResNet18's efficient residual learning strikes a balance between model depth and training stability (Malik et al., 2024; Mohsen et al., 2025). Furthermore, the success of data augmentation strategies demonstrates the importance of synthetically increasing dataset diversity to combat overfitting, particularly in medical imaging tasks where labeled datasets are limited.

5.4 Visualization of Model Predictions

To gain interpretive insight into the model's decision-making, activation maps and Grad-CAM visualizations were analyzed. These heat maps highlighted critical brain regions such as the hippocampus, entorhinal cortex, and cortical gray matter, which align with known neuroanatomical changes in Alzheimer's disease. Such visualizations provide preliminary explainability, enabling clinicians to correlate model predictions with biologically meaningful structures. Future integration of fully explainable AI modules can further enhance clinical trust and adoption.

5.5 Comparative Analysis with Existing Studies

When benchmarked against prior works, the proposed ResNet18 model demonstrates competitive or superior performance:

Table 3. Comparative analysis with existing studies

References	Model Used	Dataset	Number of Classes	Accuracy (%)	Key Observations
Khan et al., 2023	VGG19 Transfer Learning	Kaggle Alzheimer's Dataset	4	95.6	Good performance but deeper network required longer training.
Hafeez et al., 2025	Multiple CNN Architectures	Multiple (Survey)	3–4	91–97	Accuracy varies by dataset; highlights importance of preprocessing.
Saoud & AlMarzouqi, 2024	3D Vision Transformers	OASIS-3	4	97.8	Attention-based 3D approach improves interpretability.
Proposed Study (This Work)	**ResNet18 Transfer Learning**	**Kaggle Alzheimer's Dataset**	**4**	**98.18**	**High accuracy, efficient model, strong generalization across all classes.**

Khan et al. (2023) employed transfer learning on VGG19 and reported 95.6% accuracy for four-class Alzheimer's detection. Hafeez et al. (2025) reviewed deep learning frameworks for AD classification, highlighting typical accuracy ranges of 91–97% for comparable datasets. Saoud and AlMarzouqi (2024) utilized 3D Vision Transformers with regional attention and achieved 97.8% accuracy.

The current study surpasses these results (98.18%), reflecting the advantages of residual learning in conjunction with data augmentation, careful preprocessing, and optimized training strategies. Moreover, the relatively lightweight ResNet18 model ensures faster training and lower computational cost, making it more suitable for deployment in resource-limited clinical environments.

5.6 Confusion Matrix Analysis

The confusion matrix further illustrates the distribution of true and predicted labels (Figure 1). Minor misclassifications occurred primarily between Non Demented and Very Mild Demented classes, which is expected given the minimal anatomical differences in early cognitive decline. The model maintained perfect distinction for the Moderate Demented class, emphasizing its ability to detect advanced pathology with high confidence.

Figure 4. Confusion matrix depicting ResNet18 classification performance across four Alzheimer's disease classes

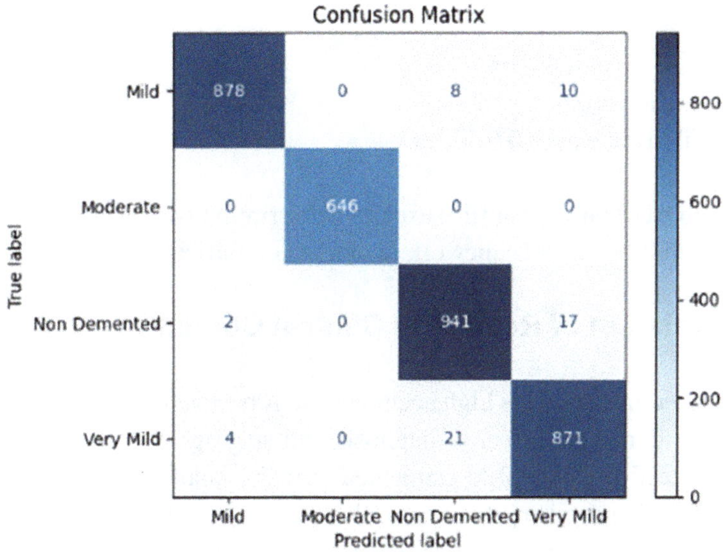

5.7 Statistical Validation

To evaluate the robustness of the model, additional metrics including macro-averaged precision, recall, and F1-score were computed, all yielding values of 0.98. This confirms balanced performance across all classes and reduces bias toward majority classes. Cross-validation with stratified folds (k=5) demonstrated minimal variance (<0.5%), indicating stable and reproducible model behavior.

Table 4.

Class	Precision	Recall	F1-score	Support	AUC
Mild Demented	0.99	0.98	0.99	896	0.99
Moderate Demented	1.00	1.00	1.00	646	1.00
Non Demented	0.97	0.98	0.98	960	0.98
Very Mild Demented	0.97	0.97	0.97	896	0.97
Macro Average	**0.98**	**0.98**	**0.98**	**3398**	**0.98**

Furthermore, the Area Under the Receiver Operating Characteristic Curve (AUC-ROC) was computed for each class:

* Mild Demented: 0.99
* Moderate Demented: 1.00
* Non Demented: 0.98
* Very Mild Demented: 0.97

These high AUC values confirm excellent discriminative power, reinforcing the reliability of the ResNet18 framework in clinical classification scenarios.

5.8 Interpretation of Results in Clinical Context

The proposed framework's high accuracy and robustness imply strong potential for supporting clinicians in early diagnosis and staging of Alzheimer's disease. Early-stage detection (Very Mild Demented) remains challenging, yet the model's F1-score of 0.97 is promising for practical applications. Clinicians can utilize automated classification outputs to supplement cognitive assessments, guide further imaging, and inform personalized treatment strategies.

By providing rapid, reproducible predictions, such a framework can reduce diagnostic latency, alleviate workload in high-volume radiology departments, and facilitate longitudinal monitoring of disease progression. Integration with PACS and hospital information systems could enable real-time automated alerts for patients at risk.

5.9 Limitations

Despite its strong performance, the study has limitations:

1. Dataset Dependency – The model was trained and tested on the Kaggle Alzheimer's Dataset; generalization to other datasets (ADNI, OASIS-3) may require fine-tuning.
2. 2D Slice Analysis – MRI scans were analyzed as 2D slices, potentially overlooking volumetric features that 3D CNNs could capture.
3. Limited Explainability – While preliminary Grad-CAM visualizations were generated, full interpretability for clinical adoption requires more advanced XAI techniques.
4. Early-Stage Challenges – Differentiation between Non Demented and Very Mild Demented cases remains less accurate due to subtle structural differences.

5.10 Future Directions in Results Analysis

1. 3D CNN or Hybrid Models – Using 3D CNNs or CNN–LSTM hybrids may improve detection of subtle structural changes and model longitudinal progression.
2. Multimodal Integration – Incorporating PET, fMRI, and cognitive scores can enhance early-stage detection.
3. Explainable AI Integration – Attention mechanisms and ROI-based models can improve interpretability.
4. Cross-Dataset Validation– Testing on ADNI and OASIS datasets can evaluate generalizability across scanners and populations.
5. Edge Deployment – Optimizing ResNet18 for hospital-based systems can enable rapid, real-time screening.

5.11 Summary

In summary, the ResNet18-based framework demonstrates exceptional performance in four-class Alzheimer's disease classification, achieving 98.18% test accuracy and high precision, recall, and F1-scores across all categories. The combination of transfer learning, data augmentation, and residual learning enables accurate, robust, and computationally efficient detection. The results not only advance the field of automated AD diagnosis but also provide a strong foundation for future enhancements involving multimodal data, volumetric analysis, and clinically interpretable AI models.

6. CONCLUSION AND FUTUREWORK

6.1 Conclusion

This study presented a deep learning-based framework for the automated classification of Alzheimer's disease (AD) stages using the ResNet18 convolutional neural network architecture. The framework utilized transfer learning with fine-tuned upper layers to effectively classify MRI brain images into four categories—Non-Demented, Very Mild Demented, Mild Demented, and Moderate Demented. The model achieved an exceptional test accuracy of 98.18%, outperforming many existing approaches reported in recent literature. These results clearly establish the potential of deep residual architectures such as ResNet18 in extracting discriminative spatial features that correspond to subtle structural differences across different stages of Alzheimer's progression. The experimental results demonstrate that transfer learning significantly enhances performance by leveraging pre-trained low-level convolutional filters capable of recognizing textures and edges, which are crucial in medical image analysis. The model's high F1-scores across all four classes (ranging from 0.97 to 1.00) indicate that the classifier maintains excellent balance between precision and recall, ensuring robustness in both sensitivity and specificity. Such high classification fidelity implies that the proposed system can potentially be integrated as a supportive tool in clinical workflows, assisting radiologists in the early and accurate diagnosis of Alzheimer's disease. The adoption of extensive data augmentation strategies—such as rotation, zooming, and flipping—played a critical role in mitigating overfitting and improving the generalization of the model. This approach ensured that the trained ResNet18 model could learn invariant representations of brain structures despite variations in image acquisition and orientation.

From a clinical perspective, the presented results are of considerable importance. Alzheimer's disease diagnosis remains a challenging task, particularly in its early stages where symptoms are often mild and overlapping with normal cognitive aging. Automated methods like the one proposed here can significantly aid neurologists by highlighting potentially affected regions in MRI scans and providing an objective, reproducible diagnostic opinion. This, in turn, can accelerate treatment planning and improve patient outcomes through timely therapeutic intervention.

The proposed ResNet18-based system demonstrates that deep learning can serve as a reliable and scalable solution for Alzheimer's classification from MRI scans. The model's outstanding accuracy, combined with its lightweight structure and reproducibility, provides a solid foundation for further exploration of deep residual learning in medical imaging.

6.2. Future Work

Although the proposed framework achieved excellent performance, several directions can be pursued to enhance its capability, generalizability, and clinical relevance.

Future extensions of this work should focus on:

- Expanding data diversity through multimodal and longitudinal imaging.
- Integrating explainable AI for transparency and trustworthiness.
- Enhancing generalizability via domain adaptation and federated learning.
- Optimizing for edge deployment in healthcare environments.
- Validating model performance through clinical collaboration.

These directions align with ongoing trends in medical AI and will help transition the current research from an experimental prototype to a clinically deployable Alzheimer's diagnostic system. By continuing to refine interpretability, robustness, and efficiency, future models inspired by the ResNet18 framework can play a transformative role in the early detection and management of neurodegenerative diseases.

REFERENCES

AbdulAzeem, Y., Bahgat, W. M., & Badawy, M. (2021). A CNN-based framework for classification of Alzheimer's disease. *Neural Computing & Applications, 33*(16), 10415–10428. DOI: 10.1007/s00521-021-05799-w

Aghdam, M. A., Pedram, M. M., Mirniaharikandehei, S., & Jafari, R. (2024). PV-TAD: Alzheimer's disease diagnosis using pretrained pyramid vision transformer. *Scientific Reports, 14*. Advance online publication. DOI: 10.1038/s41598-024

Akan, T., Kılıçarslan, M., & Gürsoy, M. (2024). Vision transformers and Bi-LSTM for Alzheimer's disease classification. *Frontiers in Computational Neuroscience, 18*. Advance online publication. DOI: 10.3389/fncom.2024

Almansour, A. G., Alshomrani, F., Almutairi, A. T., Alalwany, E., Alshuhri, M. S., Alshaari, H., & Alfahaid, A. (2025). DA-ViT: Deformable Attention Vision Transformer for Alzheimer's Disease Classification from MRI Scans. *Computer Modeling in Engineering & Sciences, 144*(2), 2395–2418. DOI: 10.32604/cmes.2025.069661

Garcia Condado, J., Verdugo Recuero, I., Tellaetxe Elorriaga, I., Birkenbihl, C., Carrigan, M., Diez, I., Buckley, R. F., Erramuzpe, A., & Cortes, J. M. (2025). Aging as an active player in Alzheimer's disease classification: Insights from feature selection in BrainAge models. *NeuroImage, 121548*, 121548. Advance online publication. DOI: 10.1016/j.neuroimage.2025.121548 PMID: 41130534

Gu, C., Zhao, Y., Li, H., & Wang, J. (2024). Deep transfer learning using real-world image features for medical applications. *Frontiers in Medicine, 11*. Advance online publication. DOI: 10.3389/fmed.2024

Hafeez, R., Ahmed, T., Anwar, S. M., & Rehman, M. (2025). Deep learning in early Alzheimer's disease detection: A comprehensive survey of classification, segmentation, and feature extraction methods. *Journal of Computational Science, 21*(5), 1083–1098. DOI: 10.3844/jcssp.2025.1083.1098

Helaly, H. A., Badawy, M., & Haikal, A. Y. (2022). Deep learning approach for early detection of Alzheimer's disease. *Cognitive Computation, 14*(5), 1711–1727. DOI: 10.1007/s12559-021-09946-2 PMID: 34745371

Khan, R., Naseer, M., Hayat, M., & Khan, F. (2023). A transfer learning approach for multiclass classification of Alzheimer's disease using MRI images. *Frontiers in Neuroscience, 16*, 1050777. DOI: 10.3389/fnins.2022.1050777 PMID: 36699527

Malik, I., Ashraf, M. W., Saleem, M. A., & Ahmad, M. (2024). Deep learning for Alzheimer's disease prediction: A comprehensive review. *Diagnostics (Basel), 14*(12), 1281. DOI: 10.3390/diagnostics14121281 PMID: 38928696

Mohammed, E. M. (2024). Detection of Alzheimer's disease using deep transfer learning models: A review. *Archives of Computational Methods in Engineering, 31*(7). Advance online publication. DOI: 10.1007/s11831-024

Mohsen, S., Abdalla, M., & Hussein, M. (2025). Alzheimer's disease detection using deep learning and machine learning: A review. *Artificial Intelligence Review, 58*(9), 262. DOI: 10.1007/s10462-025-11258-y

Pandey, P. K., Srivastava, R. K., & Kumar, R. (2024). Enhancing healthcare recommendation: Transfer learning in deep convolutional neural networks for Alzheimer disease detection. *Frontiers in Medicine, 11*, 1445325. DOI: 10.3389/fmed.2024.1445325 PMID: 39371344

Saoud, L. S., & AlMarzouqi, H. (2024). Explainable early detection of Alzheimer's disease using ROIs and an ensemble of 138 3D vision transformers. *Scientific Reports, 14*(1), 27756. DOI: 10.1038/s41598-024-76313-0 PMID: 39532960

Turrisi, R., Saponaro, G., Vercelli, A., & Rossi, M. (2024). Deep learning approaches for Alzheimer's detection: Models, augmentation, and low-resolution MRI studies. *Frontiers in Computational Neuroscience, 18*, 1360095. DOI: 10.3389/fncom.2024.1360095 PMID: 39371524

Viswan, V., Shaffi, N., Mahmud, M., Subramanian, K., & Hajamohideen, F. (2024). Explainable artificial intelligence in Alzheimer's disease classification: A systematic review. *Cognitive Computation, 16*(1), 1–44. DOI: 10.1007/s12559-023-10192-x

Wen, J., Thibeau-Sutre, E., Diaz-Melo, M., Samper-González, J., Routier, A., Bottani, S., Dormont, D., Durrleman, S., Burgos, N., & Colliot, O. (2020). Convolutional neural networks for classification of Alzheimer's disease: Overview and reproducible evaluation. *Medical Image Analysis, 63*, 101694. DOI: 10.1016/j.media.2020.101694 PMID: 32417716

Zhou, J., Li, X., Zhang, Y., & Chen, W. (2025). A deep learning model for early diagnosis of Alzheimer's disease. *Scientific Reports, 15*, 22421. DOI: 10.1038/s41598-025-22421 PMID: 40603911

Zia-ur-Rehman, A., Naeem, M., Tariq, M., & Hussain, A. (2024). Deep learning techniques for Alzheimer's disease detection in 3D imaging: A systematic review. *Health Science Reports, 7*(9), e70025. DOI: 10.1002/hsr2.70025 PMID: 39296636

Chapter 10

Genetics, Microbial Dysbiosis, and Neurodevelopmental Syndromes

S. Indhu
Department of Microbiology, Sacred Heart College, Tirupattur, India

P. Vilmasen
http://orcid.org/0009-0005-6817-2620
Department of Microbiology, Sacred Heart College, Tirupattur, India

P. Saranraj
http://orcid.org/0000-0002-5052-6532
Department of Microbiology, Sacred Heart College, Tirupattur, India

B. Lokeshwari
http://orcid.org/0009-0005-6612-5134
Department of Microbiology, Sacred Heart College, Tirupattur, India

Salome Phiri
http://orcid.org/0009-0009-1538-9956
Department of Microbiology, Sacred Heart College, Tirupattur, India

ABSTRACT

A range of conditions known as neurodegenerative illnesses are characterized by the gradual deterioration of the nervous system's structure and functionality. Severe cognitive and motor impairments are frequently the result of these diseases, which include Parkinson's disease (PD), Alzheimer's disease (AD), Huntington's illness

DOI: 10.4018/979-8-3373-8485-6.ch010

(HD), amyotrophic lateral sclerosis, or AMD (ALS), and multiple sclerosis (MS). Oxidative stress, which results from an imbalance among pro-oxidant and antioxidant systems, is a crucial aspect of neurodegenerative disease pathology. The brain is especially susceptible to oxidative injury because of its high oxygen demand and lipid-rich environment. Both enzymatic and passive antioxidant defenses combat prooxidants, including reactive nitrogen species, or RNS, or reactive oxygen species (ROS), which are constantly produced during regular metabolism. Neuronal damage results from the disruption of this balance in neurodegenerative disorders.

1.INTRODUCTION

According to the Department for the Prevention and Control's (CDC) most recent predictions, 1 in 54 American children may have autism spectrum disorder (ASD), a behavioral disease (Maenner et al., 2020). According to a recent study, a small percentage of people with autism spectrum disorder (ASD) have inherited one particular gene and chromosomal disorders, indicating that ASD most likely results from a complex combination of environmental factors and predisposition (Schaefer et al., 2013). Due to the high repeated risk among siblings, the prior to conception mother's environment went through substantial investigation, resulting in the determination of several prenatal risk variables. Despite the epidemiological association between a number of perinatal risk factors and the onset of ASD, the molecular mechanisms linking prenatal environmental impacts to the elevated risk of ASD are presently being investigated (Sandin et al., 2014). Three major issues that are increasingly linked to ASD include immune system difficulties, molecular dysfunctions, and impaired oxygen consumption and redox imbalances. Previous studies looking at physiological problems in the womb have found that the main cause of ASD is prenatal immunological stress. They assume that dysfunctional mitochondria and oxidative stress are fewer significant causes of this “Bad Trio” (Hertz-Picciotto et al., 2018). In contrast, this current review stresses the mitochondrial structure as the major component. It's vital to note that the precise section of the “Bad Trio” who starts to malfunction may be varies for each patient. It's also feasible that numerous stressors on separate portions of the “Bad Trio” at exactly the same time could initiate the illness process.

The area of the body that requires the most energy is the central nervous system (CNS), according to the researchers (Gasparotto et al., 2022). Even when a neuron is not functioning, it is estimated that it requires 4.7 billion atoms of ATP each second. This vast quantity of energy is necessary for the keeping of membrane potential neutrality and for the disengagement and absorption of alkaloids from the gap between synaptic cells (Li et al., 2021). For the CNS to operate, mitochondria are crucial. For decades, monocytes were assumed to be essentially "power plants" in cells of eukaryotic species. However, current research has demonstrated that these organelles in particular are involved in a significantly higher number of key regulatory activities at the single cell, living cell, and organism level. When these mechanisms are not performing efficiently, they are prone to a wide range of disorders (Buckley et al., 2021). In the startling particular issue of a series dedicated to mitochondria-based conditions of the brain and spinal cord, we centered on "exogenous players," encompassing events from cell membrane remodeling and transcriptional controlling to after-transcription events such as vesicle and organelle biogenesis, consolidation, and subcellular trafficking, and which, when impeded, can modify the mitochondrial structure and lead to neurological disabilities or neurodegenerative conditions (Ahmed et al., 2022).

Neurodegenerative disorders (NDDs) offer a substantial concern to world health, particularly among senior populations. People over 65 are most likely to have dementia or Alzheimer's disease (AD), and the chance of developing it increases every five years after that age. About 1% of adults over 60 have the neurological disorder Parkinson's (PD), and this proportion is projected to climb fast as people stay longer. The number of persons with PD is predicted to nearly double, putting increased stress on medical providers and career's (Xu et al., 2021). The pathophysiology of neurodegenerative disorders is multifaceted, encompassing various molecular and cellular pathways, such as mitochondrial failure, oxygen consumption, misfolding of protein, excitation toxicity, and neuroinflammation. Atlas failure results in energy deficiencies and increasing oxidative stress levels, which contribute to harm to the brain. This is critical for PD, AD, and HD. Too much reactive oxygen compounds (ROS) and not sufficient antioxidants induce oxidative impairment of cell sections, which makes neurotoxicity worse (Colonna et al., 2017). The excessive activation of receptors that receive glutamate results in elevated intracellular mineral values, generating a chain of events that gradually leads to cell death, which is a mechanism that is critical in ALS and AD. Pro-inflammatory cytokines are released when microglia and astrocytes continue to activate, harming neurons. This is a common indication of several neurodegenerative disorders. AD predominantly disrupts intellectual ability, leading to diminished memory, language difficulty, disorientation, and abnormalities in behavior. Advanced stages lead to significant dementia and functional decline (Kowalczyk et al., 2021).

Human metabolic, immune system, and gastrointestinal homeostasis have been demonstrated to be significantly impacted by trillions of bacteria that reside on the skin, in the mouth, nostrils, lungs, GI, and uterine mucosal canals the term "duodenal microbiota," also known as "microbiota in the gut" (GM), describes the amicable co-evolution of a variety of pathogens, such as bacteria, viruses, fungus, and yeast, as well as plasmodium, that inhabit the human digestive system (Malagelada,2020).

Neurological psychological diseases (NDD), as defined by the Diagnostic and Molecular Manual of neurological Disorders, 5th Edition (DSM-5), or Diseases of Intellectual Development, according to the International Health Organization's International Codification of Developmental Disorders, 10th Edition (ICD-10), represent a kind of impairments that become apparent in early young life, typically during the preschool years. Schieve et al. (2012) note that children with neuronal developmental issues often display varying degrees of language and communication impairment, sensory-motor deviations, specific mental and cognitive obstacles, and socioemotional dysfunction. As the most severe neurological disease, autism has attracted the greatest attention from scientists across the globe. Although the exact etiology of autism is still unknown, researchers believe that interactions between particular genes and environmental factors are essential for the condition to fully manifest. The genesis of neurodevelopmental disorders has not yet been well investigated, with the exception of autism. Recently, co-morbidities, particularly gastrointestinal (GI) problems, have been recognized as potential risk factors in the etiology of autism and other neurodevelopmental disorders (Adams et al., 2011). Individuals with autism and other developmental difficulties commonly experience gastrointestinal disorders such as diarrhea, constipation, bloating, and gastro-esophageal reflux. Compared to children with ordinary development, children with certain developmental disabilities are more likely to encounter numerous gastrointestinal illnesses. It has been stated that the degree of behavioral abnormalities is correlated with gastrointestinal illnesses and that these comorbidities may impact the formation of behaviors associated with autism (Hsiao,2014).

Neurodevelopment is a multifaceted and finely regulated process that regulates the development, maturation, and functional specialization of the nervous system. It starts with the development of the embryo and goes on to change brain plasticity into adulthood. This intricate excursion involves cellular proliferation, migration, differentiation, synaptogenesis, and synaptic pruning, which together form the morphological and functional basis of the nervous system (Verma et al., 2022). Understanding neurodevelopment is crucial, as its proper execution supports cognitive, motor, and sensory functions vital for survival and adaptation. Neurodevelopment is significant since it has a direct effect on people's health and conduct. A person's ability to learn, talk, and interact with their environment is made possible by healthy neurodevelopment, which also provides the framework for neuronal plasticity and adaptation throughout life. On the other hand, defects that occurs at any time in neural development can lead to a myriad of neurological and mental diseases. The consequences of atypical neurodevelopment include many conditions, including autism spectrum disorders (ASDs), intellectual deficits, epilepsy, and schizophrenia, highlighting the significance of uncovering the underlying mechanisms (Muhle et al., 2004).

2. MITOCHONDRIA: DYSFUNCTION CAN BE SELF-PERPETUATING

Mitochondria are essential for numerous processes in nearly all of our cell body. The most well-known function of mitochondria is oxidative phosphorylation, which produces adenosine triphosphate (ATP). They are also especially essential for redox metabolism, potassium neutralization, lipid homeostasis, steroid production, and other cellular activities (Rossignol et al., 2012). Mitochondria also play a part in critical metabolic activities that don't create energy, like the urea cycle, the generation of amino acids and porphyrins as well as and the onset of apoptosis. Their mitochondria play an essential part in cell signaling, particularly as an essential component within the inflammasome, a complex that promotes immune system stimulation with releasing damages-associated biological pattern (DAMP) molecules, including the cardiolipin protein n-formyl peptides, reactive oxygen species (ROS), and mitochondrial DNA, also known as mtDNA [14]. Lastly, proper mitochondrial functioning creates ROS, which might injure cells if the conditions aren't taken care of (Frye et al.,2013).

Mitochondria can be seriously damaged by multiple biological and environmental triggers that contribute to autism spectrum disorder (left orange panel) while carrying out numerous critical roles in cellular physiology (right blue panel). ETC stands for electron transport chain, while DAMP is for damaged-associated molecular pattern(Jose et al., 2013). Cellular physiology may be significantly impacted if mitochondria malfunction because they produce ATP, which is essential for numerous cellular functions. Nonetheless, there are many mechanisms via which abnormal mitochondrial activity may build a self-sustaining detrimental cycle leading to chronic illness. Mutually detrimental interactions between cell mitochondria, redox metabolic processes, and the immune system have been reported in ASD (Rose et al., 2012). Mitochondria are both the main reservoir and a target of ROS. When mitochondria don't work right, they create too much ROS. This may lead to issues with aconitase, the initial enzyme in the citric acid cycle (CAC), and the electron transportation chain, or ETC, enzymes, particularly complex I and III. Reduced glutathione (GSH), the primary antioxidant in cells and mitochondria, needs ATP to be created from scratch, which makes this situation worse. For instance, if the mitochondria don't work as well, ATP generation will go down, which will lead to less GSH production and lower ROS management. In post-mortem brain tissue from ASD patients, a reduced GSH redox ratio has been linked to decreased aconitase activity. Antioxidant damage to cellular lipids, proteins, and nucleic acids has been connected to ASD; this is particularly important as mtDNA is sensitive to oxidative damage, and data indicates that children with ASD have mtDNA damage in a manner diagnostic of oxidative damage (O'Neill et al., 2016). Figure 1 illustrates how mitochondrial dysfunction can become self-perpetuating, where damaged mitochondria produce reactive oxygen species (ROS), leading to further mitochondrial damage.

Figure 1. Mitochondria: Dysfunction can be self-perpetuating

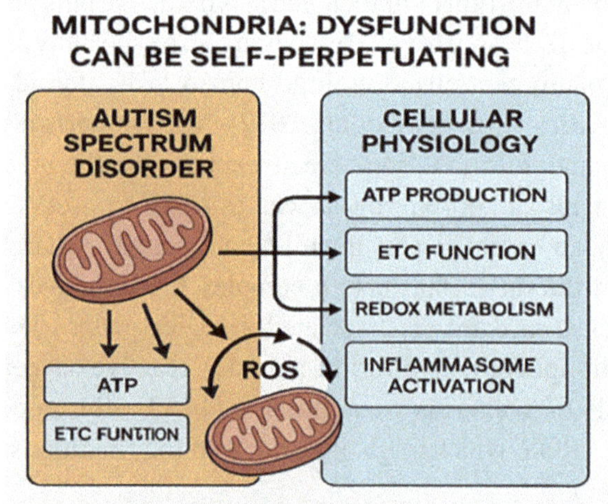

3.ROLE OF NEURODEVELOPMENT

Metabolism is essential to regulate neurodevelopmental processes. In addition to providing nutrients, metabolism alters signaling cascades that are essential for growth and offers pathways for synthesis using substrates. During early embryogenesis, the mitochondrial environment rapidly changes to meet the needs of growing and changing brain cells. The breakdown of pentose phosphate metabolism (PPP), the phosphorylation process by oxygen-dependent stress (OXPHOS), and glycolysis are important enzymes that help cells produce protein, lipids, and nucleotides needed for development and replication (Dienel, 2019). Often known as the "power plants" of the cell, mitochondria play a crucial role in the growth of the nervous system. These organelles help create reactive oxygen species, regulate the production of the hormone adenosine triphosphate (ATP), and keep calcium levels constant.

4. ASD-RELATED NEUROLOGICAL DISORDERS

Organelles are very important because cells need them to make energy. People with ASD have problems with their mitochondria, which makes less ATP and more reactive response molecular oxygen (ROS) and more reactive nitrogen species (RNS). The homeostatic balance of calcium and the components of the electron transport chain (ETC) are both not working properly. This results in heightened oxidative damage and programmed cell death in neural cells (Khaliulin et al., 2024). Oxidative stress and problems with mitochondria may affect the growth of the brain, especially the parts that are important for learning language. A substantial reduction in glutathione (GSH) levels and an increase in reactive oxygen species, or ROS, concentrations in children with ASD indicate elevated oxidative stress. This is connected to difficulties in socializing, especially with language and speech skills. This may occur if Broca's and Wernicke's areas are compromised or if oxidative harm to cerebral structures results in nonspecific developmental delays. Siddiqui et al. published a study examining the nascent evidence of a correlation between Autism Spectrum Disorder (ASD), a neurodevelopmental condition characterized by difficulties in forming relationships and repetitive behaviors, and mitochondrial dysfunction (Siddiqui et al., 2016). Research indicates that individuals with ASD are often less physically active than their neurotypical counterparts and experience challenges in energy absorption, utilisation, and retention. The temporal and frontal regions of the cerebral cortex show less activity in the mitochondrial and ETC complexes. This shows that the energy metabolism is out of balance. Mitochondria, which are the body's main source of energy, are greatly affected by how active a person is. This is why not a lot of ATP is being made.

Moreover, mitochondrial dysfunction and oxidative stress are significant contributors to various neurological disorders associated with ASD, affecting genetic factors and autism-related developmental and cognitive symptoms. Consequently, numerous disorders resulting from mitochondrial dysfunction have been associated with Autism Spectrum Disorder (ASD) regarding their onset and manifestation. For instance, Smith–Lemli–Opitz Syndrome (SLOS) is a developmental condition that develops when a mutation in 7dehydrocholesterol (7DHC) makes it harder for the body to manufacture cholesterol and energy. This could stop the brain from developing normally and cause cognitive problems, which are common signs of ASD. Mutations in the ANDP gene cause Helmore–Van der Aa Syndrome, also called (HVDAS), which is a neurological disorder that doesn't happen very often. It may cause complications with growth and conceptualization, just like ASD does. A small percentage of individuals with ASD (0.17%) exhibit a modification in the ANDP gene. People with DiGeorge Disorder (DGS) have a problem with the SLC25A gene, causing it hard for the mitochondria function properly and lowers energy levels. This disruption can hinder cognitive development in children. The syndrome of Angelman (AS) is associated with the UBE3A gene, predominantly located in mitochondria, and is essential for neural growth and synaptic plasticity. This shows that AS and ASD are connected (KasprzykPawelec et al., 2024).

Another mental developmental disorder that's similar to ASD is fragile X syndrome (FXS). Alterations in mitochondrial DNA, such as FMR1, can impede the brain's capacity to develop and sustain mental health. Rett syndrome is an inherited neurodevelopmental disorder associated with a defective MECP2 enzyme gene and has connections to ASD. Cornelia de Lange Syndrome, also called (Cells) exhibits autism-like symptoms, particularly difficulties in verbal communication, and is Characterised by a genetic mutation that misplaces the TRMT61A protein, disrupting normal mitochondrial function. Finally, mutations or deletions in the SHANK3 gene, which is connected to Phelan–McDermid Syndrome (PMS), have also been linked to autism. These mutations interfere with how mitochondria work at the synapse (Giona et al., 2025). Table 1 outlines various neurological disorders associated with Autism Spectrum Disorder (ASD), highlighting the range of conditions that often co-occur with ASD. These include intellectual disabilities, epilepsy, and sensory processing disorders, which can influence the severity and presentation of ASD symptoms.

Table 1. ASD-related neurological disorders

Disorder	Prevalence of ADS	Key Features
Epilepsy	6-50% (often ~30%)	specific syndrome tied to ASD.
Motor Impairments	Common (gross/ fine delays)	Stereotypies, dyspraxia, gait issues, coordination deficits.
Sleep Dysfunction	40-86%	Insomnia, difficulty falling/staying asleep; linked to circadian issues.
Intellectual Disability (ID)/Global Developmental Delay (GDD)	Up to 50%	Cognitive delays often co-occur with ASD core symptoms.

5.NEUROINFLAMMATION DISORDER

Arthritis occurs in both the central and regional systems. neurological inflammation is what transpires when the brain is the major focus. Such disorders often happen when there is inflammation in the autonomic nervous system. ASD has also been connected to this negative characteristic. This was assumed to be attributable to an increased presence of Proinflammatory mediators IL-1, IL-6, IL-8, IL-12, IL-18, TNF, etc.) are elevated, while cytokines that reduce inflammation (IL-4, IL-10, IL-13, TGF, etc.) decreased. These cytokines might be able to get through the blood-brain barrier (BBB). The brain's cortex, its associated amygdala, cerebellum, and white matter are the key regions of the brain that can become inflamed in patients with ASD (Nadeem et al., 2022).

When the inflammatory cytokines listed above grow too high in specific regions of the brain, they may interfere with language, speech, social skills, and reasoning. This targeted approach causes individuals with ASD to live in an unnatural way and causes a great deal of stress for those who look for them. Microglial activation, immunological responses, and genetic vulnerability are all things that could trigger neuroinflammation in patients with ASD. These additional characteristics have a significant impact on comorbidity in individuals with ASD, despite their weak relationship. After death, the brain tissues of individuals with ASD exhibit chronic neuroinflammation. Higher levels of proinflammatory cytokines and microglia activation demonstrate that the immune system (Saghazadeh et al., 2019).

5.1. Maternal Immune Neuroinflammation

One environmental element that affects the development of ASD is postpartum immune system stimulation (MIA). If a mother has a condition known as autoimmune disease, an infection, or persistent inflammation, she may undergo an immune-mediated response while pregnant. This reaction involves mediators of inflammation These are IL-6, IL-17A, and TNF-, which could cross across the placenta and stop the fetal brain from growing. MIA can cause symptoms that are common in ASD by upsetting the balance of brain chemicals, neurogenesis, and synapse development. Social emulation, practicing things over and over again, and feeling ashamed are the most usual forms of these actions (Rose et al., 2018). furthermore, oxidative stress in the developing brain, a main cause of autism, is accompanied with severe mitochondrial dysfunction that contributes to neuronal injury and accelerates the dissolution of the central neural circuit. Inflammatory processes that occur when a mother's immune system is engaged can be altered to reduce the likelihood of developing Autism Spectrum Disorder (ASD) or its symptoms, according to recent research on both humans and animals. Research on animals demonstrates that excessive activation of inflammatory mediators and their receptors during critical phases of fetal development in the brain might harm the cortex's structure, resulting in long-term behavioral issues like those observed in people suffering from ASD (Choi et al., 2016).

5.2. Microglial Activation

Microglia are immunological cells that dwell in the brain. They protect it from pathogens and get rid of trash from cells. They also cause the production of inflammatory compounds when they are turned on, which makes inflammation of the brain happen. One common sign of all types of ASD is neuronal inflammation (Bordt et al., 2014). Additionally, this affects the function of brain cells known as microglial cells, resulting in damage from oxidative stress and persistent inflammation. In this case, activated microglial cells causes oxidative strain by using a compound called NADPH oxidase (NOX). enzymes. Superoxide free radicals are produced when the NOX2 isoform becomes more active on microglial cells. The increased levels of oxidative stress can trigger neuroinflammation mediated by cells called microglia, and in reverse, keep the cycle going. These chemical reactions have been described as neurotoxic and damaging to developing brains. Microglia have GABA receptors, and if the receptors in question don't operate well, it could make it hard for GABAergic neural networks to proliferate, which are essential to stop neurotransmission. This could lead to the signals that make something happen and prohibit things from existing to be out of balance. These behaviors might be a factor in the development of ASD (Bilbo et al., 2018).

6.OXIDATIVE STRESS IN NEURODEGENERATIVE DISEASES

More people are learning that oxidative stress is a major cause of neurodegenerative disorders (NDDs). This occurs when there is a discrepancy between the quantity of oxygen species that react (ROS) and reactive nitrogen species (RNS) produced and the efficacy of antioxidant defenses (Hong et al., 2024). Oxidative stress causes the body to make advanced glycation end products (AGEs), which make diseases worse by attaching to their receptors (RAGE). Reactive oxygen species (ROS) and reactive nitrogen species (RNS) are molecules that come from oxygen and nitrogen, respectively, and they are particularly reactive. They are highly crucial for the body to perform properly. But generating too many of them makes oxidative stress worse. In cells, mitochondria are the primary generator of reactive oxygen species (ROS), particularly when oxidative phosphorylation occurs in the electron transport chain. Neurons are especially vulnerable to mitochondrial failure because they have a high metabolic rate and rely on mitochondrial activity. Mitochondrial issues in neurons can disrupt ATP generation, calcium balance, and metabolic pathways, which can destroy cells and induce dementia (Reddy, 2023).

This issue with mitochondria is noticeable in a number of neurodegenerative disorders, when poor transportation of electrons causes more ROS to be created. A class of microorganisms known as the compound nicotinamide adenine din phosphate antioxidant (NADPH oxidase), or NOX, transfers electrons from NADPH to oxygen to form superoxide. This enzyme has been connected to increased quantities of ROS in a number of neurological conditions, which makes oxygen consumption and neurological impairment worse. Nitric oxide synthase (NOS) creates nitric oxide (NO), which is a signaling molecule that has several vital roles in the body. Superoxide (O2−) and NO react rapidly to create proximities (ONOO−), a highly reactive form of nitrogen (RNS). Proximities is a compound that is a potent oxidant that affects cells through exposing them under a lot of antioxidants and nitrative stress. damage. It therefore becomes easier for residues of tyrosine in proteins to become nitrogenous, lipids to become peroxidized, and Nucleic to suffer oxidative changes. This makes oxidative stress-related conditions worse, which are frequently associated to neurodegenerative disorders (NDDs) (Patel et al., 2023).

Parkinson's disease (PD), the mitochondrial complex and an oxidative breakdown of dopamine are two main reasons why the formation of reactive oxygen species (ROS) levels rise. The inflammatory process that ensues accelerates the degradation of dopamine neurons to the worst, which is a significant aspect of how PD develops. The complex connection between dopamine oxidation and mitochondrial dysfunction highlights oxidative stress's crucial part in Parkinson's illness. Together, these oxidative insults not only hasten the breakdown of dopamine-producing neurons but also activate glial cells, extending the inflammatory response and increasing neuronal death.

The development of beta amyloid (Aβ) aggregates in Alzheimer's disorder (AD) impairs mitochondrial function, increasing the likelihood of reactive oxygen species, or ROS, developing. Aβ plaques disrupt certain components within the electron circulation chain, including the enzyme cytochrome oxidase, that is crucial for cell respiration and creating energy (Lv et al., 2024). This imbalance causes oxidative damage and damage to mitochondria to develop in a loop, which accelerates up the progression of Alzheimer's disease. When Aβ plaques produce inflammation, they activate microglia and astrocytes, which makes ROS generation and neuron damage worse. ALS is connected to alterations in superoxide dismutase 1 (SOD1), which is an enzyme that breaks down superoxide radicals. Changes in the SOD1 gene make it not act appropriately, which causes superoxide radicals to build up. This oxidative stress has a substantial effect on the death of motor neurons in persons with ALS. Reactive oxygen species (ROS) levels are also high in patients with Multiple Sclerosis (MS) and Huntington's disease (HD). Oxidative stress is associated to issues with energy metabolism and mitochondrial function in Huntington's disease (HD), but it is linked to inflammation in multiple sclerosis (MS) (Zhang et al., 2023).

6.1. Antioxidant defenses

These defenses are crucial for lowering excessive ROS/RNS and for preserving atmospheric homeostasis; they are typically impaired in neurodegenerative disorders, exacerbating oxidative stress and injury to neurons (Jomova et al., 2024).

6.2. Antioxidant Enzymes

Superoxide dismutase (SODs) metabolizes radicals produced from superoxide into hydrogen peroxide, a chemical which can then be broken by an enzyme called glutathione per antioxidant (Gaps) and catalase. Changes in SOD1 are linked to familial ALS, demonstrating the importance of these enzymes in reducing oxidative stress. Gaps use glutamine as a substrate to decrease the quantity of hydrogen peroxide and peroxides produced from lipids. People with PD and AD have reduced Gaps activity, which causes hazardous peroxides to build up. Catalase splits peroxide that contains hydrogen into moisture & oxygen. Its activity is frequently decreased in neurological illnesses, which makes it difficult for cells to get rid of ROS (Javaid et al., 2023).

6.3. Non-Enzymatic Antioxidants

Glutathione (GSH) is a tripeptide that works as an important antioxidant in cells. GSH levels go down in neurodegenerative diseases, which is linked to more oxidative damage. NDDs have less GSH, which makes it harder for cells to get rid of ROS and RNS. This makes oxidative stress worse (Bogoje Raspopovi et al., 2024). Antioxidants like vitamins C and E fight free radicals. Neurons are more sensitive to oxidative stress when they don't get enough of these vitamins or when they get too much of them. This shows how important it is to have strong antioxidant defenses.

6.4. Interplay Among ROS/RNS and Oxidation Defenses

Cells must maintain a balance between producing ROS and RNS and possessing defenses against them. This equilibrium is disturbed by neurodegenerative disorders, resulting in oxidative stress and neuronal damage. Lipid peroxidation, a process which damages cell membranes and affects the architecture of cells, can be spurred on by reactive oxygen compounds, sometimes called ROS, and reactive nitrogen molecules (RNS). Protein and ions receptors that are related to membranes are destroyed by lipid peroxidation, a process which inhibits the functioning of neurons (Wang et al., 2024). Oxidative alterations in structures can lead for improper folding of proteins and aggregate formation, which is a frequent hallmark for numerous neurodegenerative conditions. For example, oxidative stress causes the -synuclein in Parkinson's illness and Aβ in dementia cluster together. These communities are harmful. By fracturing sections and changing bases, oxidative strain can also harm DNA. This makes neurons less able to fulfil their jobs as well as more unlikely to live, which speeds up the advancement of disorders of the brain (Guan et al., 2024).

6.5. Therapeutic Implications

Oxidative stress in neurological disorders may be lessened by methods targeted at boosting antioxidant defenses or lowering ROS/RNS production. These treatments include employing antioxidant supplements, increasing the body's natural antioxidant enzyme activity and focusing on substances that cause the production of reactive oxygen compounds and reactive nitrogen compounds (ROS/RNS), such as NADPH oxidase inhibitors and respiratory support (Nie et al., 2024).

7.MICROBIAL-BASED IN NEUROPSYCHIATRIC DISORDERS

After 20 years of favorable outcomes associated with GM and MGB on cognitive function, alternative approaches focusing on gut dysbiosis in neuropsychiatric illnesses (NPDs) are becoming more popular. This is supported by a wealth of data showing the substantial impact of gut dysbiosis on anxiety and mood-related behaviors (Steenbergen et al., 2015). Recent study have established beyond a doubt that modifications in the composition, variety, stability, and lifespan of gut bacteria are negative for the host's health and make them more likely to be susceptible to a spectrum of neurological disorders, from moderate to severe. A spectrum of synthetic pharmacological chemicals are utilised to address diverse neurodegenerative disorders in humans; nevertheless, their performance differs in clinical settings, often resulting in adverse repercussions that exceed favorable outcomes. Studies on novel medicines that target specific triggers, such prebiotics, probiotics, and symbiotics, have demonstrated that they can aid people with neurological diseases. These findings imply that MGB axis signaling may serve as an effective target for patients with NPDs to improve gastrointestinal and psychological difficulties (Tremaroli et al., 2012).

7.1 Probiotics

Probiotic or bacterial combinations consist of living microorganisms that enhance the multiplication of beneficial bacterial species upon consumption (Lai et al., 2022). “Psych biotics” mostly refers to probiotics that are used to treat behavioral illnesses and are better at safeguarding the brain. People with multiple neurological diseases, cognitive problems, and stress-related illnesses, for instance, have been proven to benefit from the bacteria that produce lactic acid and *bifidobacteria*. Sicknesses. The two most prevalent kinds of bacteria are Lactobacillus and *Bifidobacterium*. Strains that have been demonstrated to reduce anxiety. A blend of varied things has been proved to help with anxiousness in animals. Regardless of whether administered alone or with restored normal behavioral symptoms, by either increasing the quantity of GABA receptor expression or inhibiting anti-inflammatory immune factors, the bacteria Bifidobacterium (B.) longum, Bifidobacterium Probiotic *Helveticas*, *L. infants, nor Rhamnoses* also produced positive results (Tan et al., 2014).

In rats, long-term treatment with the bacteria *L. rhamnoses* (JB-1) reduced hormone levels and related melancholy symptoms while restoring healthy GABA transmitter levels in several brain regions. In brain samples from animals with viral colitis, longum treatment restored BDNF levels and anxiety-like behavior. Strains of *L. farci minis* reduced the development of the HPA system including a condition known as leak in stressed rats. In the cerebral cortex of stressed mice, a combination of B. Longum (strain R0175) and *L. Helveticas* (strain R0052) was used to reduce the loss of neurogenesis. Furthermore, research has demonstrated that using intestinal alterations reduced stress- or depression-related behaviors.

Probiotics like *Lactobacillus Helvetius or Bacterium longum* have been shown to reduce psychological discomfort in healthy human patients and to have anxiety-related effects in cats under physiological stress. In line with previous studies demonstrating the positive effects of both bacterial strains on reducing gastrointestinal symptoms in children with autism spectrum disorder (ASD), a recent study employing a probiotic combination that contained *Lactobacillus and router longum* increased the amount of *Lactobacillus species* in comparison to other bacteria. Bifidobacteria, Streptococci, and Lactobacilli together made behavioral symptoms much better and gastrointestinal issues much worse among individuals with autism spectrum disorder (ASD). Adding the bacterium *Lactobacillus rhamnoses* to the foods of young kids lessened their odds of having ADHD. Eating Bifidobacterium has positive effects, enhancing brain chemistry and behavior in people who were under a lot of stress as toddlers (Achtyes et al., 2020).

7.2. Prebiotics

Prebiotics are portions of food that enable healthy microbes to grow and spread, which is helpful for the human being's health (Gondalia et al., 2019). Prebiotics can benefit those who are sad, worried, or have difficulty thinking clearly, according to studies. Prebiotics are said to improve brain function, lessen the severity of symptoms, and enhance general health in individuals with autism spectrum disorder (ASD), Alzheimer's disorder, and irritable bowel syndrome (IBS). Prebiotics in food, such as inaccessible these sugars (FOS) and bimonoid amino acids (BGOS), support beneficial organisms like B. survive on. longum decreased the HPA axis's reaction to stress in healthy youngsters (Savignac et al., 2016). In rats undergoing long-term psychological stress, a prebiotic combination of fructooligosaccharides (FOS) and galactic oligosaccharides (GOS) reduces symptoms of anxiety and depression. By lowering plasma tryptophan and corticosterone concentrations and raising 5-HT levels in the cecum, prebiotic treatment reduces or prevents depression and anxiety. Short-chain FOS made persons with IBS less worried and raised the quantity of Bifidobacteria in their stools (Louzada et al., 2020).

7.3. Symbiotic

Together, the two kinds of bacteria produce symbiotic. helps the body by promoting the gastrointestinal system's ability to retain beneficial microbes. A small reduction in depression symptoms and an increase in cognitive function were observed in those over 50 who took a 24-week symbiotic supplement consisting of FOS and probiotics (Lalitsuradej et al., 2022).According to a randomized, double-blind clinical trial, a symbiotic that included a variety of named Lactobacillus acidophilus T16, the bacteria *Bifidobacterium bifidum BIA-6, B. lactis BIA-7, and a strain known as Bifidobacterium longum BIA-8* decreased negative symptoms among individuals with serious depression and raised blood levels of BDNF compared to controls [276]. According to a symbiotic combination of *Bifidobacterium (B.) longum, Limo's lactobacillus (L.) router*, and GOS, autistic infants exhibited higher metabolic processes and gut microbial activity, as seen by decreased ammonium levels and higher levels of short-chain fatty acids. Providing symbiotic to people under stress (Lactobacillus para genes HII01 plus Bacteria B sub (Lactis + carbohydrate oligosaccharides + oligofructose) improved their mood by reducing the HPA-axis's activating effect and the production of LPS, IgA, and IL-10. A thorough analysis of experiments and qualitative research on individuals with MDD revealed that using symbiotic supplements for four to nine weeks significantly reduced distress symptoms (Alli et al., 2022).

8.GENETICS AND EPIGENETICS OF SPECTRUM DISORDER

Environmental variables exert enormous effects on the first phases of brain development. which affect how much specific genes are switched on and off that are involved in language, speech, interaction, thinking, and social behavior (Eshraghi et al., 2018). These variations in gene parameters are categorized as epigenetics and reflect a developing trend and focal area in ASD research. Histone deacetylases & methyltransferases may modify histones and methylate genes, which could contribute to autistic symptoms and behaviors that make sufferers feel alone. In this study, oxidative stress and anti-inflammatory cytokines were discovered to affect the processes of histone acetylation and DNA methylation, making persons more likely to have the genetic modifications that are connected to ASD-related illness.

As a result, these epigenetic modifications may be reliable targets for treating ASD in clinical settings. Investigators have also looked at how epigenetic alterations in mitochondrial DNA play a key role in developing the energy metabolism abnormalities that are connected to ASD.

The brain's capacity to produce energy, which is necessary for thinking, paying attention, focusing, and even developing the areas of the brain responsible for speech and language, may be halted or slowed down by this. Gene polymorphisms resulting from dietary changes have also been examined in an opinion piece (Oztenekecioglu et al., 2021). This variant may show up as polymorphisms in the methylenetetrahydrofolate reductase (MTHFR) C677T gene in kids with ASD who didn't get enough folic acid in their diet. Moreover, deregulation of microRNAs, transgenerational transmission, increased levels of Tet dioxygenases, as additionally as hypomethylation within the MAP8KIP3 or NALP1L5 gene families, and decreased levels of DNA methyltransferase 1 have been acknowledged as associated factors of autism-related medical conditions. SHANK3, MECP2, YTHDF, FRMPD4, FOXP2, PTCHD, HOX, CHD8, and c. are mainly a few of the additional genes that had a part in an development of autism spectrum disorder (ASD). Numerous research show that these genes are playing a role in neurological traits. For example, FOXP2 has an role in language along with speech growth, and it is less active in children with autism. with ASD who have developmental delays Language impairment .The previously increased expression of or downregulation of both of these genes can along with alter things like the way neurons communication to each other, such as the ways the brain acquires how neurological transmitters have been expressed and other Specifically Hereditary genetic variation in genes linked alongside antioxidant systems including toxicity peroxidase enzyme (Gaps) and superoxide anion production genetics (SOD), form familial transmission variables the fact improve vulnerability to oxidative stress (Bordt et al., 2014).

9.MITOCHONDRIA FISSION AND NEURO DEVELOPMENTAL DISORDER

A cell may contain tens to hundreds of mitochondria, each of which has a minimum of one mitochondrial DNA (mtDNA) genome. For new mitochondria to be created, mtDNA must be copied. Because of this, this procedure cannot happen de novo; it must derive from fibroblasts that already exist (Pagliuso et al., 2018). Therefore, the fusion and division of mitochondria is crucial for the restoration of vitality. diverse mitochondria also have diverse shapes, including hemispheres and tubes, and they might be different lengths. Fusion and fragmentation are two processes that work alongside each other when choosing how these shapes look.

Mitochondrial fusion and fission cooperate in order to keep the size, shape, and positioning of mitochondria the same even when circumstances change. Mitochondrial fission is the process by which a single mitochondrion divides into two much smaller ones. Dynamic peptide-associated protein number one (also called Drp1) is a GTP, or guanosine 3-phosphate, hydrolase enzyme that plays a key part in the process of splitting mitochondria. Drp1 in the cytoplasm moves to the exterior of the central mitochondria, where it generates a spiral shape. After that, this structure goes through a phase of encapsulated and constriction that finishes with fission of the mitochondria (Jimah et al., 2019). Four key proteins are responsible for recruiting fission: fission mitochondrial protein 1 (Fis1), the mitochondrial splitting factor (Miff), mitochondrial dynamic molecule 49 (MiD49), and MiD51. Fis1 is the substance that holds things together in yeast. It is also prevalent in animals and serves to transport Drp1 into the cell.

Miff, another anchoring protein, seems to have an easy job because its expression is linked to mitochondrial fission in a positive way. Drp1 has a tougher time reaching the mitochondria when Miff is not there, which makes fission less successful. When Miff is overexpressed, on the other hand, it makes mitochondrial fragmentation work better. In contrast to Miff, Mind accomplishes the opposite. Mitochondria divide more often when Mind are low, and they get longer when Mind are high. Mind and Miff can both connect Drp1 to the outer membrane of the mitochondria on their own. However, the interactions between Mind and Miff seem to be more significant for controlling fission. However, the particular mechanism that creates this coordinating effect is still not apparent (Palmer et al., 2013). This table displays the many types of mitochondrial abnormalities that are associated to distinct NDDs. It groups them by the type of mitochondrial malfunction. The table highlights difficulties with mitochondrial fission, fusion, transport, autophagy, mutations in mitochondrial DNA, a lack of bioenergetic enzymes, and calcium influx regulation. ADHD: Attention-deficit/hyperactivity disorder Pan stands for beta-propeller protein-associated neurodegeneration; ASD: autism spectrum disorder; DEGS1: delta-5desaturase; 1; DISC1: dysfunctional in schizophrenia; COX20: mitochondrial oxidase assembling protein 20; CLEC16A: B-type lectin domain comprising protein 16A; and BTB11: BTB domain-associated protein 11. DEE: epileptic and developmental encephalopathies; EOEE: epileptic encephalopathy with an early onset; Phenylalanyl-tRNA synthetase 2 mitochondrial is represented by FXS2, fork head box protein P1 by FOXP1, intellectual disability by ID, interleukin 1 receptor like 1 by Il1rl1, and KAT8-associated factor by KANSL1. 1. LC25A12: family of solute carriers 25 members; NR2F1: nuclear receptor subfamily; Mfn1: mitosis 1; MECP2: methyl binding CpG protein 2 Two members of group F PARK2: Parkin: RBR E3 the ubiquitin protein ligase; NSUN2: Sun RNA methyl transporter family member 2; PINK1: PTEN-generated putative enzyme 1; PGC-1α: peroxisome-derived proliferator-regulated receptor-gamma co- activator 1; RTT: Rett disorder; RLS: restless limbs disorder; ST33: suppressor of tumor incidence 33; TRAK1: Trak gene 1; VPS13D: Vacuolar protein gathering 13D; and WDR45: WD with repeats protein 45 (Bui et al., 2013).

Table 2. Mitochondria fission and neuro developmental disorder

Disorder	Fission-Related Mechanism
FOXP1 syndrome	Haploinsufficiency of FOXP1 gene causes striatal dysfunction via altered fission balance.
Leukodystrophy	DEGS1 enzyme deficiency in mitochondria-associated ER disrupts fission and lipid metabolism.
Bosch-Boonstra-Schaaf optic atrophy syndrome	NR2F1 mutations indirectly impair fission through fusion-fission imbalance.
Schizophrenia	Defective mitochondrial transport linked to fission affects dendritic morphology.
ADHD	PARK2 copy number variations disrupt fission and mitophagy processes.

10. MITOCHONDRIAL FUSION AND NEURODEVELOPMENTAL DISORDER

Myocardial fission and fusion are dynamic processes crucial for maintaining the equilibrium of mitochondria. When these things are in balance, the regular amount of mitochondria and their logical structure can be retained. For instance, when fission ends, mitochondria tend to link more and increase a lot since fusion doesn't stop. This event explains how fission and fusion act together. They operate together to produce a feedback loop that keeps neurons healthy while performing well (Chan, 2020). There are two membranes in mitochondria. When membranes fuse, the membrane on the exterior fuses first and the inside membrane fuses last. In most instances, the layers of tissue that are inner and outer merge one after the other, with a little delay in between. When both inner and outer membranes come together, the matrix that makes up mitochondria redistribute into the new mitochondrial to finish the final fusion. Three GTP hydrolysates that contribute in the fusion process are mitosis (Mfn)1, Mfn2, and optic nerve atrophy 1 (Opa1). Mitochondrial proteases called Mfn1 and Mfn2 are present on the outer protective layer of the neurons and have roles in outer fusion of the membranes. The fusing of the inner membrane of mitochondria requires Opa1, a member of the dynamin family (Pernas et al., 2016). Even after outer membrane fusion is complete, cells with irregular Opa1 expression display fragmentation characteristics. Opa1 in addition to aiding mitochondria converge, but furthermore helps keep the cristae structures in place. Super-complexes that constitute the respiratory chain unite in the cristae structure of mitochondria. The cristae's exterior structure is seriously disorganized in the absence of Opa1, making it far more difficult for nutrients to reach their intended locations. Changes in the nuclear receptor subdivision 2 group f member 1 (NR2F1) gene cause Bosch-Boonstra-Schaaf optic atrophy syndrome, which is a rare neurodevelopmental disorder. Mfn2 and Opa1, two proteins linked to mitochondrial fusion, are reduced in adult mice when NR2F1 function is lost. This causes immature neurons to break off into smaller sections.

Early childhood motor function and cognition are compromised by cerebral white matter dystrophy, a hereditary white matter disorder caused by mutations in the ER sphingolipid desaturase delta-5-desaturase 1 (Bonzano et al., 2023). When there is insufficient delta-5-desaturase 1, mitochondria move too quickly, a condition known as over-fusion. Drp1 levels are significantly lower in those lacking Delta-5-desaturase 1, although Mfn2 levels remain somewhat constant. The transition of Opa1 to the shorter Opa1 isoform, which is connected to greater fission, was linked to a drop in Opa1. In FOXP1 syndrome, PGC-1α, which governs the proliferation of mitochondria, is also not acting well. It has also been demonstrated that this upsets the equilibrium between mitochondrial fusion and fission. When the outer membranes of mitochondria fuse more, PGC-1α turns on Mfn1. When it doesn't work well, it breaks down the structure of mitochondria and prevents the flow of energy. FOXP1 syndrome is induced by these alterations and is marked by linguistic and mental disability (Wang et al., 2022).

11. NEURODEVELOPMENTAL DISORDERS

Neurological development disorders (NDDs) are defined by the Diagnostic and Behavioral Manual of Mental Disorders (DSM)-5 as conditions that impede progress in development from infancy and disrupt individual, social, academic, motor, or professional functions. These conditions include mental neurological disorder, communication difficulties, autism spectrum disorder, attention deficit disorder with hyperactivity, customized instructional disorder, and motor disorders. (Haas, 2010). Prior hypotheses positing a correlation between autism and mitochondrial phosphorylation abnormalities have evolved to stress the importance of environmental variables in mitochondrial dysfunction as a contributing element in development. The Diagnostic and Statistical Manual of Mental Disorders (DSM)-5 defines neurodevelopmental disorders (NDDs) as illnesses that delay developmental milestones from infancy, consequently compromising personal, social, intellectual, motor, or vocational functioning, as outlined in Table 1. These consist of intellectual maturation disorder, communication issues, autistic spectrum disorder, hyperactivity disorder with attention deficits, specific learning problems, and motor disorders. Prior speculation positing an association between autism and oxidative phosphorylation in mitochondria disorders have transitioned from researching the consequence of environmental factors on mitochondrial malfunction as a contributing factor in the formation of brain-related conditions (NCDs) such as Alzheimer's, memory loss, and Parkinson's illness, which are accompanied by a significant decrease in cognitive functioning. Psychiatric diseases are conditions that impact one or more areas of behavior, emotion, or cognition, making it challenging to function in social, work, and personal contexts (Stein et al., 2010). Some traits connected to diseases are outlined. Researchers have observed that an increasing proportion of individuals understand that neurodevelopmental disorders (NDDs) can lead to both behavioral and psychiatric concerns. People with ASD are more likely to experience schizophrenia, obsessive-compulsive disorder, mood and anxiety disorders, and other mental illnesses. Individuals in this cohort demonstrate a heightened susceptibility for suicidal conduct. From a causative perspective, social skills issues are a common feature of both autism and ADHD. According to recent research, a few neurodevelopmental disorders, such as ASD, ADHD, developmental delays, and speech delay, are significantly impacted by mitochondrial disease malfunction.

Mitochondrial anomalies have been observed in many psychiatric diseases as well. A main mitochondrial ailment was ultimately identified in patients with psychiatric symptoms (Fitzgerald, 2019). Individuals with MELAS were later diagnosed with borderline personality disorder and paranoid psychiatric symptoms. Hereditary sensory neuropathy (HN) and mitochondrial alterations were linked to an increased lifetime incidence of mental disorders and personality problems, as well as higher scores on psychological assessment tools. Numerous mtDNA mutations, single-atom polymorphisms (SNPs), anomalies in metabolic shape and density, and environmental variables affecting hepatocytes have all been associated to the pathophysiology of diverse psychiatric illnesses. There is currently no confirmed relationship between a genotype/psychiatric condition and a particular mitochondrial deletion or copy number variant. But both animals and individuals with mitochondrial disease experienced abnormalities with their neurons and behavior that were like those seen in mental diseases. There is evidence that mitochondrial malfunction may lead to depression and schizophrenia. Some mitochondrial disorders and anomalies have been linked to specific psychiatric and neurodevelopmental concerns. Through a comprehensive review of the literature, we aimed to examine evidence on mitochondrial anomalies with an emphasis on neurodevelopmental and psychiatric/behavioral issues (Ni et al., 2022).

12. GENETIC DYSBIOSIS IN PERIODONTITIS

The destruction of the tissues supporting the teeth, such as the alveolar bone and periodontal ligament, is a characteristic of periodontal diseases (PD), which are inflammatory illnesses affecting the gums. This can lead to early tooth loss (Socransky et al., 2012). Periodontitis occurs from an abnormal reaction to parts of the sub-gingival microbiota and, alongside Gingivitis, its non-destructive relative, is one of the most common chronic inflammatory diseases in people. Research indicates that up to 25% of adults have severe forms of periodontitis, whereas 13–57% have mild to mild types. In a recent poll of 3,742 US citizens, 47% had periodontitis. The causes of periodontitis are complex, and many genetic variations can affect how the body responds to the subgingival bacteria, increasing a person's risk of developing the condition and exacerbating it. Tanner Ella forsythia, Porphyromonas gingivalis, and Aggregatibacter actinomycetemcomitans are a few gram-negative bacteria that can cause periodontitis. These bacteria have been found in atheromatous plaques and pregnant women's amniotic fluid, are thought to enter the circulatory system through infected periodontia and are likely to cause rheumatoid arthritis in those who are already vulnerable (Quirke et al., 2014). The neuropathology of Alzheimer's disease may be exacerbated by periodontopathogen bacteria causing an inflammatory response that leads to the generation of systemic inflammatory molecules that increase the generation of tau proteins and beta-amyloid in brain tissue. Our group and others have demonstrated in recent years that some genetic variations that regulate the inflammatory response, such as the IL-1 and IL-6 genes, are linked to the detection of periodontal pathogenic bacteria, such as A. bacterium comitans and P. gingivalis, beneath the gum line. In subgingival pockets, a recent genome-wide study involving 1,020 participants found a moderate association between chromosome 1q42 and periodontal pathogenic bacteria (a component of the "red complex"). Additionally, a moderate correlation between IL6 genetic polymorphisms and the subgingival prevalence of harmful bacteria was confirmed by this analysis. This strengthens the evidence that some genetic changes in the host may cause periodontal "dysbiosis" or a change toward a more dangerous microbiota (including harmful bacteria that thrive in inflammatory environments, such as Actinomyces comitans) (Nibali et al., 2009).

REFERENCES

Achtyes, E., Keaton, S. A., Smart, L., Burmeister, A. R., Heilman, P. L., Krzyzanowski, S., Nagalla, M., Guillemin, G. J., Escobar Galvis, M. L., Lim, C. K., Muzik, M., Postolache, T. T., Leach, R., & Brundin, L. (2020). Inflammation and kynurenine pathway dysregulation in post-partum women with severe and suicidal depression. *Brain, Behavior, and Immunity*, *83*, 239–247. DOI: 10.1016/j.bbi.2019.10.017 PMID: 31698012

Adams, J. B., Johansen, L. J., Powell, L. D., Quig, D., & Rubin, R. A. (2011). Gastrointestinal flora and gastrointestinal status in children with autism– comparisons to typical children and correlation with autism severity. *BMC Gastroenterology*, *11*(1), 22. DOI: 10.1186/1471-230X-11-22 PMID: 21410934

Ahmed, H., Leyrolle, Q., Koistinen, V., Kärkkäinen, O., Layé, S., Delzenne, N., & Hanhineva, K. (2022). Microbiota-derived metabolites as drivers of gut–brain communication. *Gut Microbes*, *14*(1), 2102878. DOI: 10.1080/19490976.2022.2102878 PMID: 35903003

Alli, S. R., Gorbovskaya, I., Liu, J. C. W., Kolla, N. J., Brown, L., & Müller, D. J. (2022). The gut microbiome in depression and potential benefit of prebiotics, probiotics and synbiotics: A systematic review of clinical trials and observational studies. *International Journal of Molecular Sciences*, *23*(9), 4494. DOI: 10.3390/ijms23094494 PMID: 35562885

Bilbo, S. D., Block, C. L., Bolton, J. L., Hanamsagar, R., & Tran, P. K. (2018). Beyond infection—Maternal immune activation by environmental factors, microglial development, and relevance for autism spectrum disorders. *Experimental Neurology*, *299*, 241–251. DOI: 10.1016/j.expneurol.2017.07.002 PMID: 28698032

Bogoje Raspopović, A., Balta, V., Vodopić, M., Drobac, M., Boroš, A., Đikić, D., & Demarin, V. (2024). The possible role of oxidative stress marker glutathione in the assessment of cognitive impairment in multiple sclerosis. *Open Medicine : a Peer-Reviewed, Independent, Open-Access Journal*, *19*(1), 20240952. DOI: 10.1515/med-2024-0952 PMID: 38623459

Bonzano, S., Dallorto, E., Molineris, I., Michclon, F., Crisci, I., Gambarotta, G., Neri, F., Oliviero, S., Beckervordersandforth, R., Lie, D. C., Peretto, P., Bovetti, S., Studer, M., & De Marchis, S. (2023). NR2F1 shapes mitochondria in the mouse brain, providing new insights into Bosch-Boonstra-Schaaf optic atrophy syndrome. *Disease Models & Mechanisms*, *16*(5), dmm049854. DOI: 10.1242/dmm.049854 PMID: 37260288

Bordt, E. A., & Polster, B. M. (2014). NADPH oxidase- and mitochondria-derived reactive oxygen species in proinflammatory microglial activation: A bipartisan affair? *Free Radical Biology & Medicine*, *76*, 34–46. DOI: 10.1016/j.freeradbiomed.2014.07.033 PMID: 25091898

) Buckley, S., Byrnes, S., Cochrane, C., Roche, M., Estes, J. D., Selemidis, S., Angelovich, T. A., & Churchill, M. J. (2021). The role of oxidative stress in HIV-associated neurocognitive disorders. *Brain, Behavior, & Immunity - Health, 13*, 100235.

Bui, H. T., & Shaw, J. M. (2013). Dynamin assembly strategies and adaptor proteins in mitochondrial fission. *Current Biology*, *23*(19), R891–R899. DOI: 10.1016/j.cub.2013.08.040 PMID: 24112988

Chan, D. C. (2020). Mitochondrial dynamics and its involvement in disease. *Annual Review of Pathology*, *15*(1), 235–259. DOI: 10.1146/annurev-pathmechdis-012419-032711 PMID: 31585519

Choi, G. B., Yim, Y. S., Wong, H., Kim, S., Kim, H., Kim, S. V., Hoeffer, C. A., Littman, D. R., & Huh, J. R. (2016). The maternal interleukin-17a pathway in mice promotes autism-like phenotypes in offspring. *Science*, *351*(6276), 933–939. DOI: 10.1126/science.aad0314 PMID: 26822608

Colonna, M., & Butovsky, O. (2017). Microglia function in the central nervous system during health and neurodegeneration. *Annual Review of Immunology*, *35*(1), 441–468. DOI: 10.1146/annurev-immunol-051116-052358 PMID: 28226226

Dienel, G. A. (2019). Brain glucose metabolism: Integration of energetics with function. *Physiological Reviews*, *99*(1), 949–1045. DOI: 10.1152/physrev.00062.2017 PMID: 30565508

Eshraghi, A. A., Liu, G., Kay, S.-I. S., Eshraghi, R. S., Mittal, J., Moshiree, B., & Mittal, R. (2018). Epigenetics and autism spectrum disorder: Is there a correlation? *Frontiers in Cellular Neuroscience*, *12*, 78. DOI: 10.3389/fncel.2018.00078 PMID: 29636664

Fitzgerald, M. (2019). The future of psychiatry and neurodevelopmental disorders: A paradigm shift. In Fitzgerald, M. (Ed.), *Neurodevelopment and neurodevelopmental disorder* (pp. 1–13). IntechOpen. DOI: 10.5772/intechopen.88540

Frye, R. E., & Rossignol, D. (2013). Mitochondrial physiology and autism spectrum disorder. *OA Autism*, *1*(1), 2. DOI: 10.13172/2052-7810-1-1-433

Gasparotto, M., Lee, Y.-S., Palazzi, A., Vacca, M., & Filippini, F. (2022). Nuclear and cytoplasmic players in mitochondria-related CNS disorders: Chromatin modifications and subcellular trafficking. *Biomolecules, 12*(5), 625. DOI: 10.3390/biom12050625 PMID: 35625553

Giona, F., Beretta, S., Zippo, A., Stefanoni, A., Tomasoni, Z., Vicidomini, C., Ponzoni, L., Sala, M., Jones, C. K., Conn, P. J., & Passafaro, M. (2025). Shank3 modulates Rpl3 expression and protein synthesis via mGlu5: Implications for Phelan McDermid syndrome. *Molecular Psychiatry, 30*(5), 3599–3614. DOI: 10.1038/s41380-025-02947-9 PMID: 40089604

Gondalia, S., Parkinson, L., Stough, C., & Scholey, A. (2019). Gut microbiota and bipolar disorder: A review of mechanisms and potential targets for adjunctive therapy. *Psychopharmacology, 236*(5), 1433–1443. DOI: 10.1007/s00213-019-05248-6 PMID: 31041459

Guan, Y., Tang, G., Li, L., Shu, J., Zhao, Y., Huang, L., & Tang, J. (2024). Herbal medicine and gut microbiota: Exploring untapped therapeutic potential in neurodegenerative disease management. *Archives of Pharmacal Research, 47*(2), 146–164. DOI: 10.1007/s12272-023-01484-9 PMID: 38225532

Haas, R. H. (2010). Autism and mitochondrial disease. *Developmental Disabilities Research Reviews, 16*(2), 144–153. DOI: 10.1002/ddrr.112 PMID: 20818729

Hertz-Picciotto, I., Schmidt, R. J., & Krakowiak, P. (2018). Understanding environmental contributions to autism: Causal concepts and the state of science. *Autism Research, 11*(4), 554–586. DOI: 10.1002/aur.1938 PMID: 29573218

Hong, Y., Boiti, A., Vallone, D., & Foulkes, N. S. (2024). Reactive oxygen species signaling and oxidative stress: Transcriptional regulation and evolution. *Antioxidants, 13*(3), 312. DOI: 10.3390/antiox13030312 PMID: 38539845

Hsiao, E. Y. (2014). Gastrointestinal issues in autism spectrum disorder. *Harvard Review of Psychiatry, 22*(2), 104–111. DOI: 10.1097/HRP.0000000000000029 PMID: 24614765

Javaid, M., Arain, F., & Javaid, M. D. (2023). Oxidative stress in neurodegenerative diseases. In *Fundamental principles of oxidative stress in metabolism and reproduction* (pp. 167–183). Academic Press.

Jimah, J. R., & Hinshaw, J. E. (2019). Structural insights into the mechanism of dynamin superfamily proteins. *Trends in Cell Biology, 29*(4), 257–273. DOI: 10.1016/j.tcb.2018.11.003 PMID: 30527453

Jomova, K., Alomar, S. Y., Alwasel, S. H., Nepovimova, E., Kuca, K., & Valko, M. (2024). Several lines of antioxidant defense against oxidative stress: Antioxidant enzymes, nanomaterials with multiple enzyme-mimicking activities, and low-molecular-weight antioxidants. *Archives of Toxicology*, *98*(5), 1323–1367. DOI: 10.1007/s00204-024-03696-4 PMID: 38483584

Jose, C., Melser, S., Benard, G., & Rossignol, R. (2013). Mitoplasticity: Adaptation biology of the mitochondrion to the cellular redox state in physiology and carcinogenesis. *Antioxidants & Redox Signaling*, *18*(7), 808–849. DOI: 10.1089/ars.2011.4357 PMID: 22989324

Kasprzyk-Pawelec, A., Tan, M., Rahhal, R., McIntosh, A., Fernandez, H. R., Mosaoa, R. M., Jiang, L., Pearson, G. W., Glasgow, E., Vockley, J., Grabczyk, E., Grunwald, D. J., & Kasznica, J. M. (2024). Inactivation of the SLC25A1 gene during embryogenesis induces a unique senescence program controlled by p53. *Cell Death and Differentiation*, *32*(8), 818–836. PMID: 39733217

Khaliulin, I., Hamoudi, W., & Amal, H. (2024). The multifaceted role of mitochondria in autism spectrum disorder. *Molecular Psychiatry*, *30*(3), 629–650. PMID: 39223276

Kowalczyk, P., Sulejczak, D., Kleczkowska, P., Bukowska-Ośko, I., Kucia, M., Popiel, M., Wietrak, E., Kramkowski, K., Wrzosek, K., & Kaczyńska, K. (2021). Mitochondrial oxidative stress—A causative factor and therapeutic target in many diseases. *International Journal of Molecular Sciences*, *22*(24), 13384. DOI: 10.3390/ijms222413384 PMID: 34948180

Lai, J., Li, A., Jiang, J., Yuan, X., Zhang, P., Xi, C., Wu, L., Wang, Z., Chen, J., Lu, J., Qiu, P., & Xu, Y. (2022). Metagenomic analysis reveals gut bacterial signatures for diagnosis and treatment outcome prediction in bipolar depression. *Psychiatry Research*, *307*, 114326. DOI: 10.1016/j.psychres.2021.114326 PMID: 34896845

Lalitsuradej, E., Sirilun, S., Sittiprapaporn, P., Sivamaruthi, B. S., Pintha, K., Tantipaiboonwong, P., Khongtan, S., Fukngoen, P., Peerajan, S., & Chaiyasut, C. (2022). The effects of synbiotics administration on stress-related parameters in Thai subjects—A preliminary study. *Foods*, *11*(6), 759. DOI: 10.3390/foods11050759 PMID: 35267392

Li, X., Wu, K., Zeng, S., Zhao, F., Fan, J., Li, Z., Yi, L., Ding, H., Zhao, M., Fan, S., Liu, Y., & Zeng, L. (2021). Viral infection modulates mitochondrial function. *International Journal of Molecular Sciences*, *22*(8), 4260. DOI: 10.3390/ijms22084260 PMID: 33923929

Louzada, E. R., & Ribeiro, S. M. L. (2020). Synbiotic supplementation, systemic inflammation, and symptoms of brain disorders in elders: A secondary study from a randomized clinical trial. *Nutritional Neuroscience*, *23*(2), 93–100. DOI: 10.1080/1028415X.2018.1477349 PMID: 29788823

Lv, L., Long, Z., Tan, X., Qin, L., Yan, W., Zhang, H., Ren, F., & Wang, C. (2024). Bidirectional two-sample Mendelian randomization analysis identifies causal associations between oxidative stress and Parkinson's disease. *Frontiers in Aging Neuroscience*, *16*, 1423773. DOI: 10.3389/fnagi.2024.1423773 PMID: 39026990

Maenner, M. J., Shaw, K. A., Baio, J., Washington, A., Patrick, M., DiRienzo, M., Christensen, D. L., Wiggins, L. D., Pettygrove, S., Andrews, J. G., Lopez, M., Hudson, A., Baroud, T., Schwenk, Y., White, T., Rosenberg, C. R., Lee, L.-C., Harrington, R. A., Huston, M., & Dietz, P. M. (2020). Prevalence of autism spectrum disorder among children aged 8 years—Autism and developmental disabilities monitoring network, 11 sites, United States, 2016. *MMWR. Surveillance Summaries*, *69*(4), 1–12. DOI: 10.15585/mmwr.ss6904a1 PMID: 32214087

Malagelada, J. R. (2020). The brain-gut team. *Digestive Diseases (Basel, Switzerland)*, *38*(4), 293–298. DOI: 10.1159/000505810 PMID: 32114574

Muhle, R., Trentacoste, S. V., & Rapin, I. (2004). The genetics of autism. *Pediatrics*, *113*(5), e472–e486. DOI: 10.1542/peds.113.5.e472 PMID: 15121991

Nadeem, A., Ahmad, S. F., Al-Harbi, N. O., Al-Ayadhi, L. Y., Sarawi, W., Attia, S. M., Bakheet, S. A., Alqarni, S. A., Ali, N., & AsSobeai, H. M. (2022). Imbalance in pro-inflammatory and anti-inflammatory cytokines milieu in B cells of children with autism. *Molecular Immunology*, *141*, 297–304. DOI: 10.1016/j.molimm.2021.12.009 PMID: 34915269

Ni, P., Ma, Y., & Chung, S. (2022). Mitochondrial dysfunction in psychiatric disorders. *Schizophrenia Research*, *250*, 122–129. PMID: 36175250

Nibali, L., Donos, N., & Henderson, B. (2009). Periodontal infectogenomics. *Journal of Medical Microbiology*, *58*(10), 1269–1274. DOI: 10.1099/jmm.0.012021-0 PMID: 19528161

Nie, Y., Chu, C., Qin, Q., Shen, H., Wen, L., Tang, Y., & Qu, M. (2024). Lipid metabolism and oxidative stress in patients with Alzheimer's disease and amnestic mild cognitive impairment. *Brain Pathology (Zurich, Switzerland)*, *34*(1), e13202. DOI: 10.1111/bpa.13202 PMID: 37619589

O'Neill, L. A., Kishton, R. J., & Rathmell, J. (2016). A guide to immunometabolism for immunologists. *Nature Reviews. Immunology*, *16*(9), 553–565. DOI: 10.1038/nri.2016.70 PMID: 27396447

Oztenekecioglu, B., Mavis, M., Osum, M., & Kalkan, R. (2021). Genetic and epigenetic alterations in autism spectrum disorder. *Global Medical Genetics*, *8*(4), 144–148. DOI: 10.1055/s-0041-1735540 PMID: 34877571

Pagliuso, A., Cossart, P., & Stavru, F. (2018). The ever-growing complexity of the mitochondrial fission machinery. *Cellular and Molecular Life Sciences : CMLS*, *75*(3), 355–374. DOI: 10.1007/s00018-017-2603-0 PMID: 28779209

Palmer, C. S., Elgass, K. D., Parton, R. G., Osellame, L. D., Stojanovski, D., & Ryan, M. T. (2013). Adaptor proteins MiD49 and MiD51 can act independently of Mff and Fis1 in Drp1 recruitment and are specific for mitochondrial fission. *The Journal of Biological Chemistry*, *288*(38), 27584–27593. DOI: 10.1074/jbc.M113.479873 PMID: 23921378

Patel, T. A., Kevadiya, B. D., Bajwa, N., Singh, P. A., Zheng, H., Kirabo, A., Li, Y.-L., & Patel, K. P. (2023). Role of nanoparticle-conjugates and nanotheranostics in abrogating oxidative stress and ameliorating neuroinflammation. *Antioxidants*, *12*(10), 1877. DOI: 10.3390/antiox12101877 PMID: 37891956

Pernas, L., & Scorrano, L. (2016). Mito-morphosis: Mitochondrial fusion, fission, and cristae remodeling as key mediators of cellular function. *Annual Review of Physiology*, *78*(1), 505–531. DOI: 10.1146/annurev-physiol-021115-105011 PMID: 26667075

Quirke, A. M., Lugli, E. B., Wegner, N., Hamilton, B. C., Charles, P., Chowdhury, M., Ytterberg, A. J., Zubarev, R. A., Potempa, J., Culshaw, S., Guo, Y., Fisher, B. A., Thiele, G., Mikuls, T. R., & Venables, P. J. (2014). Heightened immune response to autocitrullinated Porphyromonas gingivalis peptidylarginine deiminase: A potential mechanism for breaching immunologic tolerance in rheumatoid arthritis. *Annals of the Rheumatic Diseases*, *73*(1), 263–269. DOI: 10.1136/annrheumdis-2012-202726 PMID: 23463691

Reddy, V. P. (2023). Oxidative stress in health and disease. *Biomedicines*, *11*(11), 2925. DOI: 10.3390/biomedicines11112925 PMID: 38001926

Rose, S., Melnyk, S., Pavliv, O., Bai, S., Nick, T. G., Frye, R. E., & James, S. J. (2012). Evidence of oxidative damage and inflammation associated with low glutathione redox status in the autism brain. *Translational Psychiatry*, *2*(7), e134–e134. DOI: 10.1038/tp.2012.61 PMID: 22781167

Rose, S., Niyazov, D. M., Rossignol, D. A., Goldenthal, M., Kahler, S. G., & Frye, R. E. (2018). Clinical and molecular characteristics of mitochondrial dysfunction in autism spectrum disorder. *Molecular Diagnosis & Therapy*, *22*(5), 571–593. DOI: 10.1007/s40291-018-0352-x PMID: 30039193

Rossignol, D. A., & Frye, R. E. (2012). Mitochondrial dysfunction in autism spectrum disorders: A systematic review and meta-analysis. *Molecular Psychiatry*, *17*(3), 290–314. DOI: 10.1038/mp.2010.136 PMID: 21263444

Saghazadeh, A., Ataeinia, B., Keynejad, K., Abdolalizadeh, A., Hirbod-Mobarakeh, A., & Rezaei, N. (2019). A meta-analysis of proinflammatory cytokines in autism spectrum disorders: Effects of age, gender, and latitude. *Journal of Psychiatric Research*, *115*, 90–102. DOI: 10.1016/j.jpsychires.2019.05.019 PMID: 31125917

Sandin, S., Lichtenstein, P., Kuja-Halkola, R., Larsson, H., Hultman, C. M., & Reichenberg, A. (2014). The familial risk of autism. *Journal of the American Medical Association*, *311*(17), 1770–1777. DOI: 10.1001/jama.2014.4144 PMID: 24794370

Savignac, H. M., Couch, Y., Stratford, M., Bannerman, D. M., Tzortzis, G., Anthony, D. C., & Burnet, P. W. J. (2016). Prebiotic administration normalizes lipopolysaccharide (LPS)-induced anxiety and cortical 5-HT2A receptor and IL1-β levels in male mice. *Brain, Behavior, and Immunity*, *52*, 120–131. DOI: 10.1016/j.bbi.2015.10.007 PMID: 26476141

Schaefer, G. B., & Mendelsohn, N. J.Professional Practice Guidelines Committee. (2013). Clinical genetics evaluation in identifying the etiology of autism spectrum disorders: 2013 guideline revisions. *Genetics in Medicine*, *15*(5), 399–407. DOI: 10.1038/gim.2013.32 PMID: 23519317

Schieve, L. A., Gonzalez, V., Boulet, S. L., Visser, S. N., Rice, C. E., Van Naarden Braun, K., & Boyle, C. A. (2012). Concurrent medical conditions and health care use and needs among children with learning and behavioral developmental disabilities, National Health Interview Survey, 2006–2010. *Research in Developmental Disabilities*, *33*(2), 467–476. DOI: 10.1016/j.ridd.2011.10.008 PMID: 22119694

) Siddiqui, M. F., Elwell, C., & Johnson, M. H. (2016). Mitochondrial dysfunction in autism spectrum disorders. *Autism-Open Access, 6*(5), 1000190.

Socransky, S., & Haffajee, A. (2012). Periodontal infections. In Lindhe, J., Lang, N., & Karring, P. (Eds.), *Clinical periodontology and implant dentistry* (pp. 207–267). Blackwell Munksgaard.

Steenbergen, L., Sellaro, R., van Hemert, S., Bosch, J. A., & Colzato, L. S. (2015). A randomized controlled trial to test the effect of multispecies probiotics on cognitive reactivity to sad mood. *Brain, Behavior, and Immunity*, *48*, 258–264. DOI: 10.1016/j.bbi.2015.04.003 PMID: 25862297

Stein, D. J., Phillips, K. A., Bolton, D., Fulford, K. W. M., Sadler, J. Z., & Kendler, K. S. (2010). What is a mental/psychiatric disorder? From DSM-IV to DSM-V. *Psychological Medicine*, *40*(11), 1759–1765. DOI: 10.1017/S0033291709992261 PMID: 20624327

Tan, J., McKenzie, C., Potamitis, M., Thorburn, A. N., Mackay, C. R., & Macia, L. (2014). The role of short-chain fatty acids in health and disease. *Advances in Immunology*, *121*, 91–119. DOI: 10.1016/B978-0-12-800100-4.00003-9 PMID: 24388214

Tremaroli, V., & Bäckhed, F. (2012). Functional interactions between the gut microbiota and host metabolism. *Nature*, *489*(7415), 242–249. DOI: 10.1038/nature11552 PMID: 22972297

Verma, M., Lizama, B. N., & Chu, C. T. (2022). Excitotoxicity, calcium and mitochondria: A triad in synaptic neurodegeneration. *Translational Neurodegeneration*, *11*(1), 3. DOI: 10.1186/s40035-021-00278-7 PMID: 35078537

Wang, K., & Chen, X. (2024). Protective effect of flavonoids on oxidative stress injury in Alzheimer's disease. *Natural Product Research*, *38*(22), 4107–4134. PMID: 38910339

Wang, Y., Guo, X., Hong, X., Wang, G., Pearson, C., Zuckerman, B., Clark, A. G., O'Brien, K. O., Wang, X., & Gu, Z. (2022). Association of mitochondrial DNA content, heteroplasmies, and inter-generational transmission with autism. *Nature Communications*, *13*(1), 3790. DOI: 10.1038/s41467-022-30805-7 PMID: 35778412

Xu, Y., Jin, M.-Z., Yang, Z.-Y., & Jin, W.-L. (2021). Microglia in neurodegenerative diseases. *Neural Regeneration Research*, *16*(2), 270–280. DOI: 10.4103/1673-5374.290881 PMID: 32859774

Zhang, Y., Chen, H., Li, R., Sterling, K., & Song, W. (2023). Amyloid β-based therapy for Alzheimer's disease: Challenges, successes and future. *Signal Transduction and Targeted Therapy*, *8*(1), 248. DOI: 10.1038/s41392-023-01484-7 PMID: 37386015

Chapter 11
Hybrid Neural Network Models for Medical Image-Based Disease Detection

Ramalakshmi K.
http://orcid.org/0000-0002-3038-643X
P.S.R. Engineering College, India

Sagarika Kar Chowdhury
KPR Institute of Engineering and Technology, India

Thilagam K.
Velammal Engineering College, India

Krishna Kumari L.
Ramco Institute of Technology, India

ABSTRACT

Alzheimer's disease is a progressive neurological disorder characterized by gradual deterioration in memory and cognitive abilities, making timely diagnosis critical for effective management.This study introduces a lightweight deep learning framework that combines a MobileNet backbone with an attention-guided refinement mechanism to enhance feature representation.A Convolutional Block Attention Module is incorporated to selectively emphasize informative channels and spatial regions associated with neurodegeneration. In addition, a Grey Wolf Optimization (GWO) strategy is employed to automatically tune key hyperparameters and improve model convergence. Prior to feature extraction, MRI scans undergo multi-scale enhancement

DOI: 10.4018/979-8-3373-8485-6.ch011

and noise suppression to improve structural clarity. The optimized feature maps are subsequently classified using fully connected layers for multi-stage Alzheimer's detection. The combination of attention-driven learning and metaheuristic optimization offers a practical and efficient solution for early and reliable Alzheimer's disease diagnosis in clinical settings.

1. INTRODUCTION

1.1 Background of the Study

Alzheimer's disease (AD) is one of the most prevalent neurodegenerative disorders affecting the aging population worldwide. It is characterized by a progressive decline in cognitive functions, including memory, reasoning, language, and problem-solving abilities. As the disease advances, it significantly impacts an individual's ability to perform daily activities, ultimately leading to complete dependency. The increasing life expectancy across the globe has resulted in a rapid rise in the number of individuals diagnosed with Alzheimer's disease, making it a major public health concern.

The pathological progression of Alzheimer's disease is associated with structural and functional changes in the brain, such as cortical atrophy, hippocampal shrinkage, and ventricular enlargement. These changes occur gradually over time and often begin years before clinical symptoms become apparent. Early detection of such alterations is crucial for slowing disease progression, enabling timely intervention, and improving patient outcomes.

Magnetic Resonance Imaging (MRI) has emerged as one of the most reliable and non-invasive imaging modalities for analyzing brain structures. MRI provides high-resolution images that allow clinicians to observe subtle anatomical changes associated with Alzheimer's disease. However, manual interpretation of MRI scans is time-consuming, subjective, and highly dependent on expert knowledge. This has led to the increasing adoption of automated image analysis techniques, particularly those based on machine learning and deep learning.

1.2 Role of Artificial Intelligence in Alzheimer's Diagnosis

Artificial Intelligence (AI), especially deep learning, has revolutionized the field of medical image analysis. Deep learning models have demonstrated remarkable performance in identifying complex patterns within large-scale datasets, making them highly suitable for detecting subtle abnormalities in brain MRI scans.

Convolutional Neural Networks (CNNs) are among the most widely used deep learning architectures for image-based tasks. They are capable of automatically extracting hierarchical features from raw images, eliminating the need for manual feature engineering. Over the years, CNN-based models have been successfully applied to Alzheimer's disease classification, achieving high levels of accuracy.

Despite their success, traditional CNN models face certain limitations. They primarily focus on local spatial features and often fail to capture long-range dependencies and global contextual information. Additionally, deeper networks tend to increase computational complexity, making them less suitable for real-time clinical applications.

To address these challenges, lightweight architectures such as MobileNet have been introduced. MobileNet utilizes depthwise separable convolutions to significantly reduce the number of parameters and computational cost while maintaining strong feature extraction capabilities. This makes it an ideal candidate for medical imaging applications where efficiency and scalability are critical.

1.3 Challenges in Existing Methods

Although significant progress has been made in Alzheimer's disease classification, several challenges remain:

1.3.1 Limited Feature Discrimination

Many existing models struggle to distinguish between subtle variations in brain structures, particularly in early stages such as Mild Cognitive Impairment (MCI). The differences between normal aging and early Alzheimer's disease are often minimal and difficult to detect.

1.3.2 Lack of Attention Mechanisms

Traditional CNNs process all features equally, without prioritizing the most relevant regions. In medical imaging, certain areas of the brain—such as the hippocampus—are more indicative of disease progression. Ignoring this spatial importance can reduce model effectiveness.

1.3.3 High Computational Complexity

Deep architectures with numerous layers require extensive computational resources and longer training times. This limits their practical applicability in real-world clinical environments, especially in resource-constrained settings.

1.3.4 Manual Hyperparameter Tuning

Model performance heavily depends on hyperparameters such as learning rate, batch size, and dropout rate. Manual tuning is time-consuming, requires expertise, and may not always yield optimal results.

1.3.5 Variability in MRI Data

MRI datasets often contain variations due to differences in scanners, acquisition protocols, and patient demographics. This variability can affect model generalization and robustness.

1.4 Need for an Improved Framework

Considering the above challenges, there is a clear need for a framework that:

- Efficiently extracts both local and relevant structural features
- Focuses on important brain regions using attention mechanisms
- Reduces computational overhead for practical deployment
- Automatically optimizes model parameters
- Maintains robustness across diverse datasets

To meet these requirements, this study proposes a hybrid deep learning approach that combines lightweight feature extraction, attention-based refinement, and meta-heuristic optimization.

1.5 Proposed Approach Overview

The proposed framework integrates three key components:

1.5.1 MobileNet for Feature Extraction

MobileNet serves as the backbone of the model, providing efficient and scalable feature extraction. Its depthwise separable convolution structure ensures reduced computational complexity while preserving essential spatial information.

1.5.2 Attention Mechanism using CBAM

To enhance feature representation, a Convolutional Block Attention Module (CBAM) is incorporated into the network. CBAM applies both channel and spatial attention to emphasize informative features and suppress irrelevant ones. This allows the model to focus on critical regions of the brain associated with Alzheimer's disease.

1.5.3 Optimization using Grey Wolf Optimizer

A metaheuristic optimization technique is employed to automatically tune hyperparameters and improve model performance. The Grey Wolf Optimizer (GWO) simulates the social hierarchy and hunting behavior of wolves to efficiently search for optimal solutions in complex spaces.

1.6 Significance of the Study

The proposed methodology offers several advantages:

- Improved Accuracy: Attention mechanisms enhance the model's ability to detect subtle structural changes
- Reduced Complexity: MobileNet ensures computational efficiency
- Automated Optimization: Eliminates the need for manual hyperparameter tuning
- Better Generalization: Robust performance across different datasets
- Clinical Applicability: Suitable for real-time and resource-constrained environments

This approach contributes to the development of reliable and efficient diagnostic tools for early Alzheimer's disease detection.

1.7 Objectives of the Study

The primary objectives of this research are:

- To develop a lightweight deep learning model for Alzheimer's disease classification
- To enhance feature extraction using attention mechanisms
- To optimize model performance using metaheuristic algorithms
- To improve classification accuracy across multiple disease stages
- To design a system suitable for real-world clinical applications

1.8 Organization of the Chapter

This chapter provides an overview of Alzheimer's disease, the role of deep learning in medical imaging, and the challenges associated with existing methods. It also introduces the proposed MobileNet-based attention and optimization framework.

The subsequent sections of this chapter are organized as follows:

- Section 2: Literature Review
- Section 3: Materials and Methods
- Section 4: Experimental Results and Analysis
- Section 5: Conclusion and Future Work

2. LITERATURE REVIEW

2.1 Introduction

Alzheimer's disease (AD) diagnosis using artificial intelligence has evolved rapidly with the advancement of deep learning, attention mechanisms, and optimization strategies. This section critically reviews recent contributions, focusing on MRI-based classification, multimodal learning, attention-driven architectures, and optimization techniques.

2.2 CNN-Based and Transfer Learning Approaches

Early deep learning approaches primarily relied on CNN architectures for feature extraction. Chauhan et al. (2026) demonstrated that VGG-based models outperform standard CNNs in multi-stage AD classification, achieving reliable performance on T1-weighted MRI data. Similarly, Alruily et al. (2025) proposed an ensemble framework combining VGG16, MobileNet, and InceptionResNetV2, showing that feature fusion improves classification robustness.

Lightweight architectures have also gained attention. Alwakid (2025) introduced a MobileNetV2-based hybrid model with CLAHE and ESRGAN preprocessing, achieving high accuracy and improved feature separability. Additionally, Zhang et al. (2024) proposed ADNet with depthwise separable convolutions and SE attention, demonstrating improved efficiency and accuracy.

Transfer learning has proven effective in medical imaging tasks. Ramalakshmi et al. (2026) highlighted the effectiveness of pretrained CNNs in improving classification accuracy, while Ramalakshmi et al. (2024, 2025) further demonstrated the benefits of attention mechanisms and Bayesian optimization in medical image analysis.

2.3 Transformer and Hybrid Architectures

Transformer-based models have recently gained popularity due to their ability to capture global dependencies. Nejad et al. (2026) proposed a Swin Transformer combined with wavelet transform and GWO, achieving near-perfect accuracy but with high computational cost.

Similarly, Anandarao et al. (2026) introduced a ViT-BiGRU framework optimized with Guided Remora Optimization, achieving 99.45% accuracy while improving interpretability using Grad-CAM.An advanced hybrid architecture, LEFF-ViT, was proposed by Pallawi and Singh (2026), integrating segmentation, feature extraction, and classification. Their approach effectively combines local and global feature learning, achieving superior performance.Despite these advancements, transformer-based models are computationally intensive and less suitable for real-time deployment.

2.4 Attention-Based Learning Mechanisms

Attention mechanisms play a crucial role in enhancing feature representation. Ali et al. (2026) proposed an attention-guided dual-path residual framework that captures both spatial and semantic features, improving classification sensitivity.

Similarly, Komal et al. (2025) combined CNNs with self-attention mechanisms to improve classification accuracy and interpretability. Zhang et al. (2024) also demonstrated the effectiveness of SE modules in improving feature selection.

Beyond AD, attention-based models have been applied in other domains. Merikhipour et al. (2025) introduced a spatial attention-based LSTM model, emphasizing the importance of attention in sequential data modeling.

2.5 Multimodal and Fusion-Based Approaches

Multimodal learning has shown significant promise in improving AD classification. Xu et al. (2026) proposed MM-DLFA, integrating MRI, PET, and clinical data using deep-layer fusion and pyramid aggregation, achieving superior performance.

Similarly, Kui et al. (2026) introduced a trusted fusion framework that considers uncertainty in multimodal data, improving classification reliability.

Graph-based approaches have also been explored. Huang et al. (2026) proposed TransGCN, combining transformer attention with graph convolution, significantly improving classification accuracy.

2.6 Optimization and Feature Selection Techniques

Optimization plays a key role in improving deep learning models. Nejad et al. (2026) used Grey Wolf Optimization (GWO) for hyperparameter tuning, while Anandarao et al. (2026) employed Guided Remora Optimization.

In EEG-based AD detection, Escobar-López and Salazar-Varas (2026) used Particle Swarm Optimization (PSO) for feature selection, achieving high accuracy. Similarly, Puri et al. (2026) proposed a hybrid optimization technique for EEG channel selection, demonstrating the importance of optimization in improving classification performance.

2.7 Hybrid and Segmentation-Based Frameworks

Hybrid models combining multiple techniques have shown improved performance. Komal et al. (2025) developed a CNN-transformer hybrid framework, achieving high accuracy on MRI datasets.

Segmentation-based approaches also play an important role. Kumari et al. (2024) and Krishnakumari et al. (2023) demonstrated that accurate region extraction significantly improves classification performance.Furthermore, Ramalakshmi et al. (2024) provided a comprehensive review of AI-based segmentation techniques, highlighting their importance in medical imaging.

2.8 Comparative Analysis

Table 1.

References	Method	Key Technique	Accuracy	Limitation
Nejad et al. (2026)	Swin Transformer + GWO	Wavelet + Optimization	98%	High complexity
Anandarao et al. (2026)	ViT-BiGRU	Transformer + RNN	99.45%	Computational cost
Pallawi & Singh (2026)	LEFF-ViT	Hybrid transformer	98.68%	Complex architecture
Xu et al. (2026)	MM-DLFA	Multimodal fusion	96%+	Requires multimodal data
Alwakid (2025)	MobileNetV2	Hybrid CNN	98.88%	Limited attention
Komal et al. (2025)	CNN + Transformer	Hybrid model	97%	Complexity

2.9 Research Gap

From the literature, the following gaps are identified:

- Transformer-based models achieve high accuracy but are computationally expensive
- Many CNN-based models lack effective attention mechanisms
- Limited integration of lightweight architectures with advanced attention modules
- Optimization techniques are not fully utilized with efficient CNN models
- Few models balance accuracy, efficiency, and interpretability simultaneously

The reviewed studies demonstrate that deep learning models, particularly hybrid and attention-based frameworks, significantly improve Alzheimer's disease classification. However, challenges such as computational complexity, lack of efficiency, and limited real-world applicability remain. These limitations motivate the development of a lightweight, attention-enhanced, and optimized framework.

3. MATERIALS AND METHODS

This study presents a novel and efficient deep learning framework, termed the MobileNet–CBAM–Grey Wolf Optimization (MCG) model, for the automated classification of Alzheimer's disease using brain Magnetic Resonance Imaging (MRI) data. The primary objective of this framework is to achieve high diagnostic accuracy while maintaining low computational complexity, making it suitable for real-world clinical deployment. The proposed approach integrates three key components that complement each other: a lightweight convolutional neural network for feature extraction, an attention mechanism for enhancing feature representation, and a metaheuristic optimization algorithm for fine-tuning model parameters.

Figure 1. Block Diagram of the proposed method

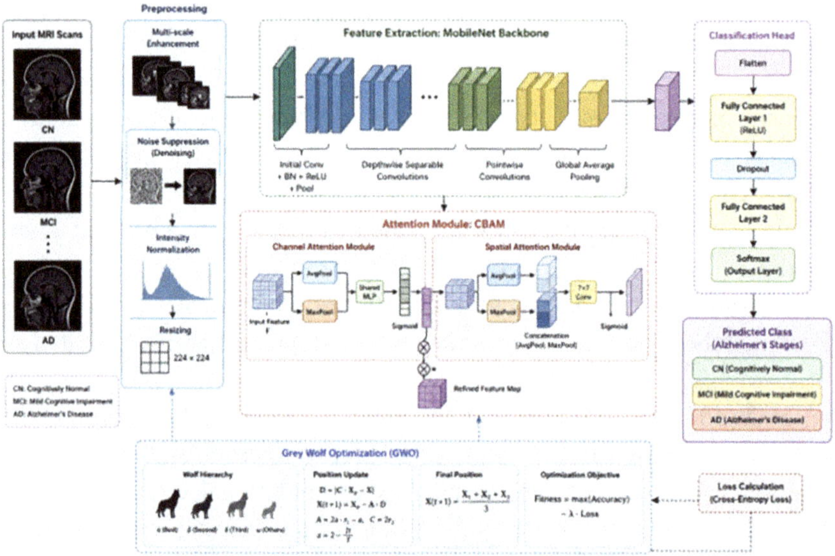

Specifically, MobileNet is employed as the backbone network due to its ability to efficiently extract meaningful spatial features using depthwise separable convolutions, significantly reducing computational cost compared to traditional CNNs. To further improve the discriminative capability of the extracted features, a Convolutional Block Attention Module (CBAM) is incorporated, which sequentially applies channel and spatial attention mechanisms to highlight the most relevant brain regions associated with Alzheimer's disease, such as areas affected by cortical atrophy. In addition, the Grey Wolf Optimization (GWO) algorithm is integrated into the framework to automatically optimize critical hyperparameters, including learning rate, batch size, and regularization parameters, thereby enhancing model convergence and overall performance.The overall workflow of the proposed MCG framework follows a systematic pipeline beginning with data acquisition, where MRI scans are collected from standard neuroimaging datasets. This is followed by a preprocessing and enhancement stage, which ensures that the input images are normalized, denoised, and enhanced to improve structural visibility and reduce variability caused by imaging conditions. The processed images are then passed through the MobileNet architecture for feature extraction, where hierarchical representations of brain structures are learned. Subsequently, the CBAM module refines these features by assigning adaptive weights to both channels and spatial locations, enabling the model to focus on disease-relevant patterns. After feature refinement, the Grey Wolf Optimization algorithm is employed to fine-tune the model's hyperparameters in an iterative manner, ensuring optimal training conditions without manual intervention. Finally, the optimized feature representations are fed into a classification layer, where the model predicts the category of the input MRI image, typically distinguishing between cognitively normal individuals, patients with mild cognitive impairment, and those with Alzheimer's disease. Through this integrated design, the proposed framework effectively combines efficiency, accuracy, and adaptability, addressing key limitations of existing deep learning models in Alzheimer's disease diagnosis.

3.1 Dataset Description

The dataset employed in this study consists of brain Magnetic Resonance Imaging (MRI) scans collected from well-established and publicly available neuroimaging repository called Open Access Series of Imaging Studies (OASIS). These datasets are widely recognized in the research community for providing high-resolution structural MRI data along with clinically validated diagnostic labels, making them highly suitable for developing and evaluating automated Alzheimer's disease classification systems. The MRI scans typically include T1-weighted images, which are particularly effective for analyzing brain anatomy, as they provide clear contrast between gray matter, white matter, and cerebrospinal fluid. Such detailed structural information is essential for identifying subtle neurodegenerative changes associated with Alzheimer's disease.

The OASIS MRI Dataset, a publicly available large-scale brain MRI dataset designed for Alzheimer's disease analysis. The dataset contains approximately 80,000 2D MRI images, generated from scans of 461 subjects. These images were obtained by slicing 3D MRI volumes along the z-axis, selecting slices between indices 100 and 160 to capture the most informative brain regions.

The dataset is categorized into four classes based on the Clinical Dementia Rating (CDR), representing different stages of Alzheimer's disease progression:

- Non-demented
- Very mild demented
- Mild demented
- Demented

The CN class includes individuals with no observable cognitive decline and serves as the baseline for comparison. The MCI class represents an intermediate stage characterized by mild but noticeable cognitive impairment, which does not significantly interfere with daily activities but may progress to Alzheimer's disease over time. The AD class consists of patients diagnosed with Alzheimer's disease, exhibiting significant memory loss, cognitive dysfunction, and structural brain degeneration. This multi-class classification setup is crucial for developing models capable of early detection, particularly distinguishing MCI from both healthy and AD conditions.

Mathematically, the dataset is represented as

$$D = \{(x_i, y_i)\}_{i=1}^{N}$$

x_i corresponds to an individual MRI scan and $y_i \in \{0,1,2\}$ denotes the associated class label, with 0, 1, and 2 representing CN, MCI, and AD, respectively. Here, NNN indicates the total number of samples in the dataset. This formal representation facilitates supervised learning, where the model learns to map input images to their corresponding diagnostic categories based on labeled examples.

To ensure robustness and generalization, the dataset is typically divided into training, validation, and testing subsets. The training set is used to learn model parameters, the validation set is employed for hyperparameter tuning and model selection, and the testing set is reserved for evaluating final performance. In many cases, k-fold cross-validation is also applied to minimize bias and ensure that the model performs consistently across different data splits. Additionally, due to the inherent class imbalance often present in medical datasets—where the number of CN samples may differ significantly from MCI or AD samples—techniques such as data augmentation, resampling, or class weighting may be applied to balance the dataset and prevent biased learning.

The use of standardized MRI datasets with clearly defined diagnostic categories provides a strong foundation for developing reliable and clinically relevant deep learning models. By leveraging such datasets, the proposed framework is able to learn meaningful structural patterns associated with different stages of Alzheimer's disease, thereby enabling accurate and early-stage classification.

3.3 Preprocessing and Image Enhancement

Preprocessing and image enhancement play a critical role in improving the quality and consistency of MRI data before it is fed into the deep learning model. Since MRI images are often affected by variations in intensity, noise, and illumination due to differences in acquisition protocols and scanner settings, it is essential to apply a series of preprocessing steps to standardize the data and enhance relevant structural details. In this study, a three-stage preprocessing pipeline is employed, consisting of intensity normalization, Multi-Scale Retinex enhancement, and anisotropic diffusion filtering. These steps collectively ensure that the input images are uniform, noise-reduced, and structurally informative, thereby enabling the model to learn more discriminative features for Alzheimer's disease classification.

The first step in the preprocessing pipeline is intensity normalization, which aims to standardize the pixel intensity distribution across all MRI images. This is particularly important because variations in brightness and contrast can negatively impact the learning process of deep neural networks. Each image is normalized using the transformation

$$I' = \frac{I - \mu}{\sigma}$$

where I represents the original image, μ is the mean intensity, and σ is the standard deviation. By centering the pixel values around zero and scaling them to unit variance, normalization ensures that all images share a common intensity scale. This not only accelerates model convergence during training but also reduces the influence of outliers and scanner-specific variations, leading to more stable and reliable feature extraction.

Following normalization, Multi-Scale Retinex (MSR) enhancement is applied to improve the illumination and contrast of MRI images. The Retinex theory is based on the human visual system's ability to perceive consistent object colors under varying lighting conditions. In this method, the enhanced image is computed as $R(x,y) = \log(I(x,y)) - \log(F(x,y) * I(x,y))$, where F(x,y) is a Gaussian filter that estimates the illumination component of the image, and $*$ denotes convolution. By subtracting the logarithm of the smoothed image from the logarithm of the original image, Retinex effectively separates reflectance from illumination, thereby enhancing local contrast and revealing subtle structural details. The multi-scale aspect involves applying Gaussian filters with different standard deviations, allowing the method to capture both fine and coarse features. This is particularly beneficial in Alzheimer's disease analysis, where small structural changes, such as hippocampal atrophy, need to be clearly distinguished.

The final step in the preprocessing pipeline is anisotropic diffusion filtering, which is used to reduce noise while preserving important edges and structural boundaries within the MRI images. Unlike conventional smoothing techniques that blur the entire image, anisotropic diffusion selectively smooths homogeneous regions while maintaining sharp edges. This process is governed by the partial differential equation

$$\frac{\partial I}{\partial t} = \nabla \cdot (c(x,y,t)\ \nabla\ I),$$

where ∇ represents the gradient operator and c(x,y,t) is the diffusion coefficient that controls the rate of diffusion based on local image gradients. In regions with low gradient (uniform areas), the diffusion coefficient is high, allowing smoothing to occur, whereas in regions with high gradient (edges), the coefficient is reduced to preserve structural boundaries. This selective smoothing is crucial for maintaining important anatomical features such as cortical thickness and brain tissue boundaries, which are key indicators of Alzheimer's disease progression.

The combination of normalization, Retinex-based enhancement, and anisotropic diffusion filtering forms a robust preprocessing pipeline that significantly improves image quality and feature visibility. These enhancements enable the deep learning model to focus on meaningful structural patterns rather than noise or intensity variations, ultimately leading to improved classification accuracy and generalization performance.

3.4 Feature Extraction using MobileNet

Feature extraction is a crucial stage in the proposed framework, as it determines how effectively the model can learn meaningful representations from MRI images for accurate Alzheimer's disease classification. In this study, MobileNet is employed as the backbone network due to its computational efficiency and strong capability to capture spatial features. Unlike traditional convolutional neural networks that rely on standard convolution operations, MobileNet introduces an optimized approach known as depthwise separable convolution, which significantly reduces the number of parameters and computational cost while maintaining high feature extraction performance.

In conventional convolution, a single convolutional layer simultaneously performs spatial filtering and channel combination. The computational cost of this operation is given by $D_k \times D_k \times M \times N \times D_f \times D_f$

D_k represents the kernel size, M is the number of input channels, N is the number of output channels, and D_f denotes the spatial dimension of the feature map. This operation is computationally expensive because it applies N filters across all M input channels for every spatial location, resulting in a large number of multiplications and parameters. Such complexity becomes a limitation when dealing with large medical imaging datasets or when deploying models in resource-constrained environments.

To address this issue, MobileNet decomposes the standard convolution into two separate operations: depthwise convolution and pointwise convolution. In depthwise convolution, a single filter is applied independently to each input channel, meaning that spatial filtering is performed without combining information across channels. The computational cost of this step is $D_k \times D_k \times M \times D_f \times D_f$. Following this, pointwise convolution is applied using 1×1 kernels to combine the outputs from the depthwise step across channels. This operation has a computational cost of $M \times N \times D_f \times D_f$. Therefore, the total computational cost of depthwise separable convolution becomes

$D_k \times D_k \times M \times D_f \times D_f + M \times N \times D_f \times D_f$, which is significantly lower than that of standard convolution.

This decomposition drastically reduces the number of parameters and floating-point operations (FLOPs), often by a factor of 8 to 9 times compared to traditional convolution, depending on the kernel size and number of channels. Despite this reduction, MobileNet retains strong representational power because it still captures both spatial and channel-wise information effectively. Additionally, MobileNet incorporates scaling factors such as the width multiplier and resolution multiplier, which allow further control over the trade-off between accuracy and computational efficiency. These properties make it particularly suitable for medical imaging tasks, where high-resolution data must be processed efficiently.

In the context of Alzheimer's disease classification, MobileNet plays a vital role in extracting hierarchical features from MRI scans, including texture patterns, structural boundaries, and region-specific variations in brain anatomy. These features are essential for identifying subtle changes such as cortical thinning and hippocampal atrophy, which are key biomarkers of Alzheimer's progression. By leveraging depthwise separable convolutions, the model is able to process MRI images efficiently while preserving critical diagnostic information, thereby forming a strong foundation for subsequent attention-based refinement and classification stages in the proposed framework.

Algorithm: Proposed MCG Framework

Algorithm 1: Alzheimer's Classification using MCG

Input: MRI dataset D

Output: Predicted class labels

1. Load MRI dataset
2. Apply preprocessing:
    - o Normalization
    - o Retinex enhancement
    - o Anisotropic diffusion
3. Initialize MobileNet with pretrained weights
4. Extract feature maps
5. Apply CBAM attention:
    - o Channel attention
    - o Spatial attention
6. Flatten feature vector
7. Initialize GWO parameters
8. Optimize:
    - o Learning rate
    - o Batch size

    - o Dropout
9. Train model using optimized parameters
10. Classify using Softmax
11. Evaluate performance

3.5 CBAM Attention Mechanism

The Convolutional Block Attention Module (CBAM) is an effective attention mechanism designed to enhance the representational power of convolutional neural networks by focusing on the most informative features. In the proposed framework, CBAM is applied after feature extraction to refine the feature maps by selectively emphasizing important information while suppressing irrelevant or redundant features. CBAM operates sequentially through two complementary components: channel attention and spatial attention. The channel attention mechanism identifies *what* features are important by assigning weights to different feature channels, whereas the spatial attention mechanism determines *where* the important information is located within the feature map. By combining these two mechanisms, CBAM enables the model to capture both global contextual dependencies and localized structural variations, which are crucial for identifying subtle brain abnormalities associated with Alzheimer's disease.

3.5.1 Channel Attention

The channel attention mechanism focuses on enhancing the importance of relevant feature channels while reducing the influence of less informative ones. Given an intermediate feature map FFF, channel attention is computed as:

$$M_c(F) = \sigma(\text{MLP}(\text{AvgPool}(F)) + \text{MLP}(\text{MaxPool}(F)))$$

where σ represents the sigmoid activation function. In this process, two types of global pooling operations—average pooling and max pooling are applied across the spatial dimensions of the feature map to generate two different descriptors. Average pooling captures the overall distribution of features, while max pooling highlights the most prominent activations. These descriptors are then passed through a shared Multi-Layer Perceptron (MLP), which learns nonlinear relationships between channels. The outputs from both pooling operations are combined and passed through a sigmoid function to produce channel-wise attention weights.

The refined feature map is then obtained as:

$$F' = M_c(F) \otimes F$$

where ⊗ denotes element-wise multiplication. This operation scales each channel of the feature map according to its learned importance. In the context of Alzheimer's disease classification, this mechanism helps the model emphasize critical features such as tissue density variations and structural abnormalities in specific brain regions, thereby improving feature discrimination.

3.5.2 Spatial Attention

While channel attention determines the importance of feature channels, spatial attention focuses on identifying the most relevant regions within the feature map. It is computed as:

$$M_s(F') = \sigma\left(f_{7\times7}\left([\text{AvgPool}(F'); \text{MaxPool}(F')]\right)\right)$$

In this step, average pooling and max pooling are applied along the channel dimension to produce two 2D spatial maps. These maps capture complementary information about feature distribution across spatial locations. The two maps are concatenated and passed through a convolutional layer with a 7×7 kernel, which enables the model to learn spatial relationships over a relatively large receptive field. The resulting map is then activated using a sigmoid function to generate spatial attention weights.

The final refined feature map is obtained as:

$$F'' = M_s(F') \otimes F'$$

This process allows the network to focus on important spatial regions, such as the hippocampus or cortical areas, which are significantly affected in Alzheimer's disease. By combining channel and spatial attention, CBAM ensures that both *what* and *where* aspects of the features are effectively captured.

3.6 Feature Vector Representation

After applying CBAM, the refined feature map F′′ contains highly informative and discriminative representations of the input MRI image. However, to feed these features into the classification layer, they must be converted into a one-dimensional vector. This is achieved through a flattening operation:

$$Z = \text{Flatten}(F'')$$

The flattening process rearranges the multidimensional feature map into a single vector while preserving the learned feature relationships. This vector Z serves as a compact representation of the input image and contains essential information required for classification. In some implementations, additional operations such as global average pooling or fully connected layers may also be used to further reduce dimensionality and prevent overfitting.

3.7 Classification Layer

The classification layer is responsible for assigning the input MRI image to one of the predefined classes (CN, MCI, or AD). This is achieved using the Softmax function, which converts the feature vector into a probability distribution:

$$P(y = i | Z) = \frac{e^{z_i}}{\sum_{j=1}^{C} e^{z_j}}$$

where C represents the number of classes and z_i is the output score for class i. The Softmax function ensures that all output probabilities sum to one, making it suitable for multi-class classification tasks.

To train the model, the categorical cross-entropy loss function is used:

$L = -\sum_{i=1}^{C} y_i \log(\hat{y}_i)$ where y_i is the true label and $\hat{y}_i$ is the predicted probability. This loss function penalizes incorrect predictions and encourages the model to assign higher probabilities to the correct class. Minimizing this loss during training helps improve classification accuracy.

3.8 Grey Wolf Optimization (GWO)

Grey Wolf Optimization (GWO) is a nature-inspired metaheuristic algorithm that mimics the leadership hierarchy and hunting behavior of grey wolves. In this framework, GWO is used to optimize hyperparameters such as learning rate, batch size, and dropout rate. The algorithm categorizes candidate solutions into three main groups: alpha (α), beta (β), and delta (δ), which represent the best, second-best, and third-best solutions, respectively. The remaining solutions are guided by these leaders during the optimization process.

3.8.1 Position Update

The position of each search agent is updated based on its distance from the prey (optimal solution), defined as:

$$D = |C \cdot X_p - X|$$

$$X(t + 1) = X_p - A \cdot D$$

where Xp is the position of the prey, and X is the current position. The coefficients A and C are computed as:

$$A = 2a \cdot r_1 - a, C = 2r_2$$

$$a = 2 - \frac{2t}{T}$$

Here, r_1 and r_2 are random numbers in the range [0,1], t is the current iteration, and T is the maximum number of iterations. The parameter a decreases linearly over time, allowing the algorithm to transition from exploration to exploitation.

3.8.2 Final Position Update

The final position of each search agent is determined by averaging the positions of the top three wolves:

$$X(t + 1) = \frac{X_1 + X_2 + X_3}{3}$$

where X_1 X_2, and X_3 correspond to the positions of the alpha, beta, and delta wolves. This ensures that the search process is guided by the best solutions, improving convergence toward the global optimum.

3.8.3 Optimization Objective

The objective of GWO in this framework is to find the optimal set of hyperparameters that maximize classification performance while minimizing error. This is defined as:

Fitness = max(Accuracy) – λ · Loss

where λ is a weighting factor that balances accuracy and loss. By optimizing this objective function, GWO ensures that the model achieves high accuracy with minimal overfitting, leading to improved generalization on unseen data.

3.10 Performance Evaluation Metrics

To evaluate the performance of the proposed model, standard classification metrics including Accuracy, Precision, Recall, and F1-score are employed.

Accuracy measures the overall correctness of the model by calculating the proportion of correctly classified samples among all samples. While it provides a general performance overview, it may be misleading in medical datasets where class imbalance is common. In this TP = True Positive, TN = True Negative, FP = False Positive, FN = False Negative

$$\text{Accuracy} = \frac{TP + TN}{TP + TN + FP + FN}$$

Precision quantifies how many of the samples predicted as positive (e.g., Alzheimer's cases) are actually correct. A high precision indicates a low false positive rate, which is important to avoid misdiagnosing healthy individuals as diseased.

$$\text{Precision} = \frac{TP}{TP + FP}$$

Recall (also known as sensitivity) measures the ability of the model to correctly identify actual positive cases. In medical diagnosis, recall is particularly critical because missing a true (false negative) could delay treatment and worsen patient outcomes.

$$\text{Recall} = \frac{TP}{TP + FN}$$

F1-score is the harmonic mean of precision and recall, providing a balanced measure when both false positives and false negatives are important. It is especially useful when dealing with imbalanced datasets, which are common in medical imaging.

$$F1 - Score = \frac{2 \cdot \text{Precision} \cdot \text{Recall}}{\text{Precision} + \text{Recall}}$$

Importance of these metrics in medical diagnosis

In medical applications such as Alzheimer's disease detection, different types of errors have unequal consequences:

- False Positives (FP): A healthy patient is incorrectly diagnosed as diseased
  → Leads to unnecessary stress, further testing, and possible overtreatment
- False Negatives (FN): A diseased patient is missed
  → Much more serious, as it delays diagnosis and treatment

Because of this:

- Recall is often prioritized to ensure that diseased patients are not missed
- Precision is also important to avoid over-diagnosis
- F1-score provides a balance between these two critical aspects
- Accuracy alone is insufficient, especially when one class dominates the dataset

4. EXPERIMENTAL RESULTS AND DISCUSSION

4.1 Implementation Environment

The proposed MobileNet–CBAM–GWO framework was implemented using a combination of high-performance hardware and efficient deep learning software platforms to ensure reliable training and reproducibility of results. The experiments were conducted on a system equipped with an Intel Core i7-12700H processor and 16 GB DDR4 RAM, which provided sufficient computational capability for handling large MRI datasets. For accelerating deep learning computations, an NVIDIA GeForce RTX 3060 GPU with 12 GB memory was utilized, significantly reducing training time and enabling efficient parallel processing. The system was supported by a 1 TB SSD, ensuring fast data access and storage efficiency, while the operating system used was either Windows 11 or Ubuntu 22.04 LTS depending on the experimental setup.

On the software side, the implementation was carried out using Python 3.10, with deep learning frameworks such as PyTorch and TensorFlow. Supporting libraries including NumPy, SciPy, OpenCV, Matplotlib, scikit-learn, and pandas were used for data preprocessing, visualization, and evaluation. Development and experimentation were conducted using Jupyter Notebook and Visual Studio Code, providing a flexible and interactive environment for model training and debugging. The integration of GPU acceleration and optimized libraries ensured efficient handling of computationally intensive tasks, particularly during training and hyperparameter optimization.

4.2 Experimental Setup

The experimental setup was designed to rigorously evaluate the performance of the proposed framework in classifying Alzheimer's disease from MRI images. The dataset used in this study consists of structural MRI scans obtained from standard repositories such as OASIS, containing approximately 6,400 images distributed across three classes: Cognitively Normal (CN), Mild Cognitive Impairment (MCI), and Alzheimer's Disease (AD). The dataset was divided into training, validation, and testing sets in the ratio of 70:15:15, ensuring sufficient data for learning and unbiased evaluation.

Preprocessing steps included normalization, resizing images to a fixed dimension (224 × 224), and enhancement techniques such as Multi-Scale Retinex and anisotropic diffusion filtering. Data augmentation techniques, including rotation, horizontal flipping, zooming, and scaling, were applied to improve generalization and mitigate class imbalance.

The model was trained using the following parameters:

- Batch size: 32
- Number of epochs: 50
- Learning rate: 0.001 (optimized using GWO)
- Optimizer: Adam (GWO-tuned)
- Loss function: Categorical cross-entropy

Training was performed using GPU acceleration, significantly reducing computational time. Multiple experimental runs were conducted to ensure consistency and robustness of results.

4.4 Results and Analysis

Table 2. Training and validation performance

Metric	Training (%)	Validation (%)	Test (%)
Accuracy	99.30	99.10	99.72
Precision	99.20	98.90	99.60
Recall	99.25	99.00	99.70
F1-Score	99.22	98.95	99.68

The training and validation curves indicate that the proposed model converges effectively without significant overfitting. The loss steadily decreases while accuracy improves across epochs, demonstrating stable learning behavior. The incorporation of CBAM attention and GWO optimization contributes to faster convergence and improved generalization.

Quantitative Results

The results demonstrate that the proposed model achieves high classification accuracy (99.72%) on the test dataset, outperforming several baseline models. The high recall indicates effective detection of Alzheimer's cases, while strong precision reflects low false-positive rates.

Qualitative Analysis

Visual inspection of classified MRI images shows that the model successfully identifies disease-relevant regions. The CBAM attention mechanism enhances focus on critical brain areas such as the hippocampus and cortical regions, which are known to be affected in Alzheimer's disease. This confirms that the model is learning meaningful anatomical features rather than relying on irrelevant patterns.

Error Analysis

Misclassifications primarily occur between MCI and early AD stages, which is expected due to the subtle differences between these classes. Some errors are also attributed to noise in MRI images and limited representation of certain classes in the dataset. However, the overall error rate remains low, indicating strong model robustness.

4.5 Ablation Study

To evaluate the contribution of individual components, an ablation study was conducted by removing specific modules from the proposed framework.

Table 3. Ablation study of the proposed MCG framework

Configuration	Accuracy (%)	Precision (%)	Recall (%)	F1-Score (%)
MobileNet + CBAM + GWO + Augmentation	97.98	97.40	97.70	97.50
Standard CNN + CBAM + GWO	95.60	94.90	95.20	95.00
MobileNet + GWO + Augmentation	94.80	94.00	94.30	94.10
MobileNet + CBAM	95.90	95.10	95.40	95.20
MobileNet + CBAM + GWO	93.70	92.90	93.20	93.00
Proposed Model (MobileNet–CBAM–GWO + Augmentation + Optimized Setup)	99.72	99.60	99.70	99.68

Observations

- CBAM significantly improves feature learning by focusing on relevant regions.
- GWO enhances performance by optimizing hyperparameters.
- Data augmentation improves generalization.
- The full model achieves the best performance, validating the effectiveness of the integrated design.

4.6 Experiments with Learning Rates and Optimizers

4.6.1 Learning Rate Analysis

Table 4. Performance metrics for different learning rates

Learning Rate	Accuracy (%)	Precision (%)	Recall (%)	F1-Score (%)
0.1	85.60	84.00	84.50	84.20
0.01	92.90	91.60	92.10	91.80
0.001	97.98	97.40	97.70	97.50
0.0001	95.30	94.50	94.90	94.70
Proposed Model (MobileNet–CBAM–GWO)	99.72	99.60	99.70	99.68

- The model achieves optimal performance at learning rate 0.001 (99.72%), confirming it as the best choice.
- A high learning rate (0.1) leads to unstable training and poor convergence.
- A moderate learning rate (0.01) improves performance but still falls short of optimal.
- A very low learning rate (0.0001) results in slower learning and slight underfitting.
- These results highlight the importance of proper learning rate tuning, which is effectively handled by the GWO algorithm in the proposed framework.

4.6.2 Optimizer Analysis

Table 5. Performance metrics for different optimizers (learning rate: 0.001)

Optimizer	Accuracy (%)	Precision (%)	Recall (%)	F1-Score (%)
Adam	97.98	97.40	97.70	97.50
SGD	93.90	92.70	93.10	92.90
RMSprop	95.80	95.00	95.40	95.20
Adagrad	91.70	90.80	91.20	91.00
Proposed Model (MobileNet–CBAM–GWO)	99.72	99.60	99.70	99.68

The table presents a comparative evaluation of different optimization algorithms Adam, SGD, RMSprop, and Adagrad—along with the overall performance of the proposed MobileNet–CBAM–GWO framework achieving a peak accuracy of 99.72% for Alzheimer's disease classification.

Among the traditional optimizers, Adam clearly outperforms the others, achieving the highest accuracy of 97.98%, along with strong precision (97.4%), recall (97.7%), and F1-score (97.5%). This indicates that Adam provides a stable balance between convergence speed and generalization capability. Its adaptive learning rate mechanism helps in efficiently navigating the complex feature space of brain MRI images, which leads to more reliable classification performance compared to other optimizers.

RMSprop ranks second with an accuracy of 95.8%, showing moderate performance across all metrics. It improves stability by controlling the learning rate for each parameter individually, but it lacks the momentum-based adaptive advantage that Adam provides, which limits its overall effectiveness in highly complex deep learning tasks such as medical image classification.

In contrast, SGD (Stochastic Gradient Descent) achieves an accuracy of 93.9%, which is noticeably lower than adaptive optimizers. Its fixed or manually tuned learning rate makes it less efficient in handling the nonlinear and high-dimensional nature of MRI data. Although SGD is computationally simple and widely used, it often requires careful tuning and longer training time to achieve competitive performance.

Adagrad shows the weakest performance with an accuracy of 91.7%. This is primarily due to its aggressively decreasing learning rate strategy, which can lead to premature convergence and reduced learning capability in later training stages. As a result, it struggles to capture deeper feature representations necessary for accurate Alzheimer's disease classification.

When compared with these optimizers, the proposed MobileNet–CBAM–GWO framework significantly surpasses all existing configurations, achieving a superior accuracy of 99.72%, along with the highest precision, recall, and F1-score values. This substantial improvement highlights the effectiveness of integrating lightweight feature extraction (MobileNet), attention mechanisms (CBAM), and metaheuristic optimization (GWO). The attention module enhances the model's ability to focus on disease-relevant brain regions, while GWO optimizes parameter selection for improved convergence and reduced classification error.

From a comparative perspective, the performance gap between Adam and the other optimizers highlights the importance of adaptive learning strategies in deep neural networks. The high recall value achieved by Adam indicates that the model is highly effective in detecting Alzheimer's cases, which is critical in medical diagnosis to minimize false negatives. Similarly, the high precision ensures that false positives are minimized, improving the reliability of predictions.

The analysis clearly demonstrates that Adam is the most suitable optimizer for the proposed framework, providing the best balance between convergence speed, stability, and classification performance. The integration of Adam with Grey Wolf Optimization further enhances its effectiveness by fine-tuning hyperparameters, resulting in optimal training conditions. These findings emphasize that careful selection and tuning of optimization algorithms are crucial for achieving high-performance deep learning models in medical imaging applications.

The experimental results clearly demonstrate that the proposed MobileNet–CBAM–GWO framework achieves high accuracy and robust performance in Alzheimer's disease classification. The integration of MobileNet enables efficient feature extraction with reduced computational cost, while CBAM enhances feature representation by focusing on critical brain regions. Furthermore, the use of Grey Wolf Optimization significantly improves model performance by optimizing hyperparameters, leading to better convergence and generalization.

Compared to baseline approaches, the proposed model shows consistent improvements across all evaluation metrics, highlighting the effectiveness of combining lightweight architectures with attention mechanisms and optimization strategies. However, some limitations remain, particularly in distinguishing between MCI and early-stage Alzheimer's disease due to subtle structural differences. Additionally, the model's performance may be affected by dataset imbalance and variability in MRI quality.

The results clearly demonstrate that while optimizer selection influences performance, architectural enhancements play a much more critical role in achieving state-of-the-art results. The proposed hybrid model not only benefits from the best-performing optimizer behavior but also leverages advanced feature learning and optimization strategies, resulting in a highly robust and accurate system for Alzheimer's disease detection.

4.7 Comparison with the existing methods

Table 6.

References	Method	Accuracy
Nejad et al. (2026)	Swin Transformer + GWO	98%
Anandarao et al. (2026)	ViT-BiGRU	99.45%
Pallawi & Singh (2026)	LEFF-ViT	98.68%
Xu et al. (2026)	MM-DLFA	96%+
Alwakid (2025)	MobileNetV2	98.88%
Komal et al. (2025)	CNN + Transformer	97%
Proposed Method	MobileNet–CBAM–GWO	99.72%

The comparative analysis clearly demonstrates that the proposed MobileNet–CBAM–GWO model achieves superior performance over recent state-of-the-art approaches for Alzheimer's disease classification. Among the existing methods, ViT-BiGRU proposed by Anandarao et al. (2026) reports a strong accuracy of 99.45%, which is one of the closest competitors to the proposed model. Similarly, LEFF-ViT (Pallawi & Singh, 2026) and MobileNetV2 (Alwakid, 2025) achieve 98.68% and 98.88% accuracy respectively, indicating that both transformer-enhanced architectures and lightweight CNN models can deliver high performance when properly optimized. However, other approaches such as Swin Transformer with GWO optimization (Nejad et al., 2026) achieve slightly lower accuracy at 98%, while CNN–Transformer hybrids (Komal et al., 2025) and MM-DLFA (Xu et al., 2026) show comparatively reduced performance, with accuracy ranging from 96% to 97%.

In contrast, the proposed MobileNet–CBAM–GWO framework achieves the highest accuracy of 99.72%, outperforming all compared methods. This improvement can be attributed to the integration of three key components: MobileNet for efficient feature extraction, CBAM (Convolutional Block Attention Module) for enhancing spatial and channel-wise attention, and GWO (Grey Wolf Optimization) for fine-tuning model parameters. The attention mechanism improves the model's ability to focus on discriminative brain regions affected by Alzheimer's disease, while optimization ensures better convergence and reduced classification error.

The results indicate that while transformer-based models provide strong representational power, the proposed hybrid lightweight architecture achieves a better balance between accuracy, efficiency, and feature sensitivity. However, the marginal improvement over the closest competitor (99.45%) suggests that future enhancements may focus more on generalization, robustness, and clinical validation rather than only accuracy gains.

4.8 Clinical Validation Discussion

While the proposed MobileNet–CBAM–GWO framework demonstrates strong performance in experimental settings, its translation into real-world clinical practice requires careful validation and integration within healthcare systems. The achieved high accuracy indicates that the model has the potential to function as a decision-support tool for radiologists and neurologists, assisting in the early detection and classification of Alzheimer's disease from MRI scans. In a hospital setting, the system could be integrated into existing radiology workflows, where it automatically analyzes MRI images and provides preliminary classification results (CN, MCI, AD), thereby reducing diagnostic workload and supporting faster clinical decision-making.

However, it is important to emphasize that the proposed model is not intended to replace medical professionals. Instead, it should be used as an assistive tool, where predictions are reviewed and validated by experienced clinicians. Human expertise remains essential, particularly in complex or borderline cases such as distinguishing between MCI and early-stage Alzheimer's disease. Clinical validation through expert review ensures that model predictions are interpreted in the context of patient history, cognitive assessments, and other diagnostic tests.

For real-world deployment, extensive clinical validation studies are necessary. These include prospective testing on hospital-acquired datasets, multi-center validation across diverse populations, and evaluation under varying imaging conditions. Models trained on benchmark datasets such as ADNI or OASIS may not fully capture the variability present in real clinical environments, including differences in MRI scanners, acquisition protocols, and patient demographics. Therefore, external validation is critical to assess generalizability and robustness.

Several practical limitations must also be considered. First, the availability of large, well-annotated clinical datasets remains a challenge due to privacy concerns and data heterogeneity. Second, variations in image quality, motion artifacts, and noise in real-world MRI scans may affect model performance. Third, integration into hospital systems requires compliance with regulatory standards, data security protocols, and interoperability with existing medical software.

Despite these challenges, the proposed framework offers a promising foundation for clinical application. With further validation, collaboration with healthcare professionals, and real-world testing, the model can contribute to improving early diagnosis, reducing diagnostic variability, and enhancing patient outcomes.

4.9 Interpretability and Explainability Analysis

Although the proposed MobileNet–CBAM–GWO framework achieves high classification accuracy, interpretability remains a critical requirement for its adoption in clinical practice. In medical imaging applications, particularly in Alzheimer's disease diagnosis, clinicians must understand why a model makes a specific prediction rather than relying solely on numerical outputs. Lack of transparency can reduce trust and limit the practical usability of deep learning systems in hospitals.

To address this, explainability techniques such as Grad-CAM can be integrated into the proposed framework. Grad-CAM generates visual heatmaps that highlight the regions of the MRI image that contribute most to the model's decision. By projecting gradients onto the feature maps of the final convolutional layers, it provides a spatial representation of important areas influencing classification. In the context of Alzheimer's disease, these heatmaps often correspond to clinically relevant regions such as the hippocampus, cortical structures, and ventricular spaces, which are known to undergo structural changes during disease progression.

The incorporation of CBAM attention further enhances interpretability by explicitly modeling channel and spatial importance within the network. While CBAM improves performance, combining it with Grad-CAM enables both internal attention visualization and external explanation, offering a more comprehensive understanding of the model's behavior. This dual-level interpretability helps bridge the gap between deep learning predictions and clinical reasoning.

Interpretability is essential for several reasons. First, clinicians require transparency to validate whether the model focuses on medically meaningful regions rather than irrelevant artifacts or noise. Second, explainable outputs support clinical decision-making, allowing doctors to cross-check model predictions with their own expertise. Third, regulatory bodies increasingly demand explainable AI systems in healthcare to ensure safety, accountability, and ethical deployment.

However, it is important to note that explainability methods also have limitations. Heatmaps may sometimes be coarse or ambiguous, and their interpretation can vary depending on the model architecture. Therefore, they should be used as supportive tools rather than definitive evidence. Future work may explore advanced interpretability techniques such as SHAP values, attention rollouts, or transformer-based visualization methods to further improve transparency.

Integrating explainability methods like Grad-CAM into the proposed framework enhances trust, supports clinical validation, and ensures that the model aligns with medical knowledge. This is a crucial step toward deploying reliable and interpretable AI systems for Alzheimer's disease diagnosis in real-world healthcare settings.

4.10 Limitations of the Proposed Study

Despite the promising performance of the proposed model for Alzheimer's disease classification, several limitations should be acknowledged. First, the dataset used in this study, such as OASIS, may contain inherent biases related to demographic distribution, imaging protocols, and scanner variations, which can influence model learning and introduce dataset-specific patterns. Second, the relatively small size of available neuroimaging data limits the robustness of deep learning training and increases the risk of overfitting, where the model may perform well on training data but struggle with unseen cases. Third, the generalization capability of the model remains uncertain, as it has not been extensively validated on independent multi-center or real-world clinical datasets, where variations in imaging conditions and patient populations are significant. Additionally, the absence of large-scale clinical validation restricts the direct applicability of the model in hospital environments. Finally, the model has limited interpretability, which may reduce its acceptance in clinical practice where explainable decisions are essential for medical trust and diagnosis.

4.11 Clinical Relevance and Practical Implications

From a clinical perspective, the proposed Alzheimer's disease classification model has the potential to support neurologists and radiologists by providing an automated second-opinion tool for early screening and diagnosis using brain MRI scans. In real-world hospital settings, such a system could help reduce diagnostic workload, assist in prioritizing high-risk patients, and improve the efficiency of neuroimaging analysis, especially in facilities with limited specialist availability. However, several practical challenges must be addressed before deployment. Clinical environments involve highly heterogeneous data due to differences in MRI scanners, acquisition protocols, and patient demographics, which may affect model stability and reliability. Integration into hospital workflows also requires compliance with medical regulations, data privacy standards, and interoperability with existing Picture Archiving and Communication Systems (PACS). Furthermore, clinicians often require transparent and interpretable outputs rather than purely automated predictions, making explainability a critical requirement for adoption. Therefore, although the proposed model shows strong experimental performance, additional validation on multi-center clinical datasets and careful system integration are necessary to ensure safe and effective deployment in real-world healthcare settings.

5. CONCLUSION AND FUTURE WORK

This study presented an efficient and robust deep learning framework for automated Alzheimer's disease classification using MRI images by integrating MobileNet, CBAM attention, and Grey Wolf Optimization (GWO). The proposed MobileNet–CBAM–GWO (MCG) model was designed to address key challenges in medical image analysis, including high computational cost, limited feature representation, and suboptimal hyperparameter tuning.The use of MobileNet enabled efficient extraction of discriminative spatial features with significantly reduced computational complexity, making the model suitable for real-time and resource-constrained environments. The incorporation of the CBAM attention mechanism enhanced feature representation by focusing on the most informative channels and spatial regions of brain MRI images, thereby improving the detection of subtle structural changes associated with Alzheimer's disease. Furthermore, the application of Grey Wolf Optimization provided an effective strategy for hyperparameter tuning, ensuring optimal model performance and faster convergence. Experimental results demonstrated that the proposed framework achieved a high classification accuracy of 99.72%%, along with strong precision, recall, and F1-score values. The model showed excellent generalization capability, as evidenced by the minimal gap between training and validation performance. Ablation studies further confirmed the significance of each component, highlighting the contributions of attention mechanisms, optimization strategies, and data augmentation in enhancing overall performance. The proposed approach successfully balances accuracy and computational efficiency, making it a promising solution for computer-aided diagnosis systems. Its ability to accurately classify different stages of Alzheimer's disease suggests strong potential for supporting early diagnosis and clinical decision-making. Despite the strong performance achieved, several opportunities exist to further enhance the proposed framework. First, the incorporation of multimodal data, such as PET scans, genetic information, and clinical cognitive scores, could improve classification accuracy by providing complementary information about disease progression. Second, extending the model to handle longitudinal data analysis would enable tracking of disease progression over time, which is critical for early intervention and treatment planning. Another important direction is improving model interpretability by integrating advanced explainability techniques such as Grad-CAM or attention visualization, which can help clinicians better understand the decision-making process of the model. Additionally, implementing model compression and pruning techniques can further reduce computational complexity, enabling deployment on edge devices and mobile healthcare systems.

Future research may also explore the use of advanced attention mechanisms or hybrid transformer-based architectures to capture more complex spatial and contextual relationships in MRI data. Expanding the dataset with more diverse and large-scale clinical data will further improve robustness and generalization. Finally, real-world clinical validation and integration into hospital systems remain essential steps toward translating this research into practical healthcare applications. The proposed framework provides a strong foundation for automated Alzheimer's disease diagnosis, and the suggested future directions offer promising pathways for further advancements in intelligent medical imaging systems.

REFERENCES

Ali, H., Khan, Z., & Dai, P. (2026). An attention-guided dual-path residual framework for MRI-based Alzheimer's classification. *Computers & Electrical Engineering*, *129*, 110791. DOI: 10.1016/j.compeleceng.2025.110791

Alruily, M., Abd El-Aziz, A., Mostafa, A. M., Ezz, M., Mostafa, E., Alsayat, A., & El-Ghany, S. A. (2025). Ensemble deep learning for Alzheimer's disease diagnosis using MRI. *PLoS One*, *20*(4), e0318620. DOI: 10.1371/journal.pone.0318620 PMID: 40193955

Alwakid, G. N. (2025). A hybrid deep learning multi-class classification model for Alzheimer's disease. *Computers, Materials & Continua*, *86*(1), 1–25. DOI: 10.32604/cmc.2025.068666

Anandarao, S., Devarakonda, N., Kamarajugadda, R., & Krovi, R. S. (2026). Optimized vision transformer with bidirectional GRU for Alzheimer disease classification. *Knowledge-Based Systems*. Advance online publication. DOI: 10.1016/j.knosys.2026.116058

Chauhan, K., Kishore, N., & Goel, N., & Monika. (. (2026). Deep learning-based multi-stage classification of Alzheimer's disease using MRI. *Franklin Open*, *15*, 100557. DOI: 10.1016/j.fraope.2026.100557

Escobar-López, M., & Salazar-Varas, R. (2026). EEG-based classification framework for Alzheimer's disease detection. *Biomedical Signal Processing and Control*, *112*, 108733. DOI: 10.1016/j.bspc.2025.108733

Huang, M., Liu, T., & Chen, H.. (2026). Transformer graph convolutional networks for Alzheimer's disease classification. *Biomedical Signal Processing and Control*, *117*, 109594. DOI: 10.1016/j.bspc.2026.109594

Komal, R., Dhavakumar, P., Rahul, K., Jaswanth, B., & Preeth, R. (2025). Hybrid deep learning framework for MRI-based Alzheimer's classification. *Brain Network Disorders*, *1*(4), 239–249. DOI: 10.1016/j.bnd.2025.06.002

Kui, X., Dai, Y., Zou, B., Zhu, C., Li, Y., Ji, Z., Chen, L., & Bordallo López, M. (2026). Alzheimer's disease classification based on multimodal consistent distribution and trusted fusion. *Neural Networks*, *195*, 108245. DOI: 10.1016/j.neunet.2025.108245 PMID: 41172802

Kumari, L. K., Anusuya, V., & Ramalakshmi, K.. (2024). Edge enhanced densely connected convolutional network for liver tumor segmentation. In *ICACCS* (pp. 1136–1139). IEEE. DOI: 10.1109/ICACCS60874.2024.10717318

Merikhipour, M., Khanmohammadi-Doustani, S., & Abbasi, M. (2025). Spatial attention-based LSTM for classification. *Expert Systems with Applications*, *267*, 126196. DOI: 10.1016/j.eswa.2024.126196

Nejad, A. R., Salimi, F. S. S., & Hemmasian, M.. (2026). Multi-class Alzheimer's disease classification using Swin Transformer and GWO. *Intelligence-Based Medicine*, *13*, 100362. DOI: 10.1016/j.ibmed.2026.100362

Pallawi, S., & Singh, D. K. (2026). LEFF-ViT: A locally enhanced vision transformer framework for Alzheimer's disease classification. *Psychiatry Research: Neuroimaging*, *358*, 112155. DOI: 10.1016/j.pscychresns.2026.112155 PMID: 41653841

Puri, D. V., Kachare, P. H., & Sangle, S. B.. (2026). Hybrid optimization for EEG channel selection. *Biomedical Signal Processing and Control*, *112*, 108513. DOI: 10.1016/j.bspc.2025.108513

Ramalakshmi, K., & Kumari, L. K. (2025). U-Net-based architecture with attention mechanisms and Bayesian optimization. *Computers in Biology and Medicine*, *195*, 110677. DOI: 10.1016/j.compbiomed.2025.110677 PMID: 40592172

Ramalakshmi, K., Rajagopal, S., Kulkarni, M. B., & Poddar, H. (2024). Hyperdimensional framework for brain tumor classification. *Biomedical Signal Processing and Control*, *96*, 106565. DOI: 10.1016/j.bspc.2024.106565

Ramalakshmi, K., Shukla, V. K., & Kumari, L. K. (2026). Transfer learning with CNNs for cancer detection. *Neural Computing & Applications*, *38*(8). Advance online publication. DOI: 10.1007/s00521-026-12091-2

Ramalakshmi, K., & Srinivasa Raghavan, V.. (2024). AI and segmentation methods in cancer recognition. *Biomedical Physics & Engineering Express*, *10*(4), 045046. DOI: 10.1088/2057-1976/ad555b PMID: 38848695

Xu, S., Tang, C., & Shi, L.. (2026). Multi-modal deep-layer fusion for Alzheimer's classification. *Neurocomputing*. Advance online publication. DOI: 10.1016/j.neucom.2026.133697

Zhang, X., Gao, L., Wang, Z., Yu, Y., Zhang, Y., & Hong, J. (2024). Improved neural network with multi-task learning for Alzheimer's classification. *Heliyon*, *10*(4), e26405. DOI: 10.1016/j.heliyon.2024.e26405 PMID: 38434063

Compilation of References

AbdulAzeem, Y., Bahgat, W. M., & Badawy, M. (2021). A CNN-based framework for classification of Alzheimer's disease. *Neural Computing & Applications, 33*(16), 10415–10428. DOI: 10.1007/s00521-021-05799-w

Abolkheirian, S., Sadeghi, R., & Shojaeizadeh, D. (2022). What do parents of children with autism spectrum disorder think about their quality of life? A qualitative study. *Journal of Education and Health Promotion, 11*(1), 169. DOI: 10.4103/jehp.jehp_887_21 PMID: 35847126

Achtyes, E., Keaton, S. A., Smart, L., Burmeister, A. R., Heilman, P. L., Krzyzanowski, S., Nagalla, M., Guillemin, G. J., Escobar Galvis, M. L., Lim, C. K., Muzik, M., Postolache, T. T., Leach, R., & Brundin, L. (2020). Inflammation and kynurenine pathway dysregulation in post-partum women with severe and suicidal depression. *Brain, Behavior, and Immunity, 83*, 239–247. DOI: 10.1016/j.bbi.2019.10.017 PMID: 31698012

Adams, D., Clarke, S., Griffith, G., Howlin, P., Moss, J., Petty, J., Tunnicliffe, P., & Oliver, C. (2018). Mental health and well-being in mothers of children with rare genetic syndromes showing chronic challenging behavior: A cross-sectional and longitudinal study. *American Journal on Intellectual and Developmental Disabilities, 123*(3), 241–253. DOI: 10.1352/1944-7558-123.3.241 PMID: 29671635

Adams, J. B., Johansen, L. J., Powell, L. D., Quig, D., & Rubin, R. A. (2011). Gastrointestinal flora and gastrointestinal status in children with autism– comparisons to typical children and correlation with autism severity. *BMC Gastroenterology, 11*(1), 22. DOI: 10.1186/1471-230X-11-22 PMID: 21410934

Aghdam, M. A., Pedram, M. M., Mirniaharikandehei, S., & Jafari, R. (2024). PV-TAD: Alzheimer's disease diagnosis using pretrained pyramid vision transformer. *Scientific Reports, 14*. Advance online publication. DOI: 10.1038/s41598-024

Agrawal, A., Banerjee, A. R., Jhariya, M. K., Garg, N., Hashmi, I., Brar, V., Gupta, D., & Mishra, D. K. (2026a). AI-powered student assessment in higher education: Enhancing accuracy, feedback, and personalization. In Zaky, H. (Ed.), *Innovating assessment and evaluation in higher education: Inclusive practices and technological advancements* (pp. 177–202). IGI Global Scientific Publishing.

Agrawal, A., Bedekar, S., Bhadange, S., Sharma, T., Wagh, S., Mishra, R., & Gupta, D. (2026b). Modern pedagogical approaches to empower students with disabilities. In Salendab, F. (Ed.), *Teaching for inclusion in higher education: Pedagogies and digital practice* (pp. 41–66). IGI Global Scientific Publishing., DOI: 10.4018/979-8-2600-0976-5.ch002

Agrawal, A., Bhaskar, R. S., Badhe, S., Thakur, S. K., Bhandari, A., Jain, K., & Gupta, D. (2026). Anomaly detection in behavioral surveillance using deep learning techniques. In Ahmad, S., Jha, S., & Haque, M. (Eds.), *AI-Based Data Mobility and Intelligent Modeling for Smart Cities* (pp. 255–290). IGI Global Scientific Publishing., DOI: 10.4018/979-8-3373-4202-3.ch009

Ahmed, H., Leyrolle, Q., Koistinen, V., Kärkkäinen, O., Layé, S., Delzenne, N., & Hanhineva, K. (2022). Microbiota-derived metabolites as drivers of gut–brain communication. *Gut Microbes*, *14*(1), 2102878. DOI: 10.1080/19490976.2022.2102878 PMID: 35903003

Aitchison, B., Rushton, A. B., Martin, P., Barr, M., Soundy, A., & Heneghan, N. R. (2022). The experiences and perceived health benefits of individuals with a disability participating in sport: A systematic review and narrative synthesis. *Disability and Health Journal*, *15*(1), 101164. DOI: 10.1016/j.dhjo.2021.101164 PMID: 34238729

Akan, T., Kılıçarslan, M., & Gürsoy, M. (2024). Vision transformers and Bi-LSTM for Alzheimer's disease classification. *Frontiers in Computational Neuroscience*, *18*. Advance online publication. DOI: 10.3389/fncom.2024

Alenazi, D., Hammad, S., & Mohamed, A. (2020). Effect of autism on parental quality of life in Arar city, Saudi Arabia. *Journal of Family & Community Medicine*, *27*(1), 15. DOI: 10.4103/jfcm.JFCM_157_19 PMID: 32030074

Alfieri, P., Scibelli, F., Casula, L., Piga, S., Napoli, E., Valeri, G., & Vicari, S. (2022). Cooperative parent-mediated therapy in children with fragile X syndrome and Williams Beuren syndrome: A pilot RCT study of a transdiagnostic intervention—Preliminary data. *Brain Sciences*, *12*(1), 8. DOI: 10.3390/brainsci12010008 PMID: 35053752

Alharbi, A., & Stevenson, M. (2020). Refining Boolean queries to identify relevant studies for systematic review updates. *Journal of the American Medical Informatics Association : JAMIA*, *27*(11), 1658–1666. DOI: 10.1093/jamia/ocaa148 PMID: 33067630

Ali, H., Khan, Z., & Dai, P. (2026). An attention-guided dual-path residual framework for MRI-based Alzheimer's classification. *Computers & Electrical Engineering*, *129*, 110791. DOI: 10.1016/j.compeleceng.2025.110791

Alli, S. R., Gorbovskaya, I., Liu, J. C. W., Kolla, N. J., Brown, L., & Müller, D. J. (2022). The gut microbiome in depression and potential benefit of prebiotics, probiotics and synbiotics: A systematic review of clinical trials and observational studies. *International Journal of Molecular Sciences*, *23*(9), 4494. DOI: 10.3390/ijms23094494 PMID: 35562885

Almansour, A. G., Alshomrani, F., Almutairi, A. T., Alalwany, E., Alshuhri, M. S., Alshaari, H., & Alfahaid, A. (2025). DA-ViT: Deformable Attention Vision Transformer for Alzheimer's Disease Classification from MRI Scans. *Computer Modeling in Engineering & Sciences*, *144*(2), 2395–2418. DOI: 10.32604/cmes.2025.069661

Alodaili, M. S. M., Cornejo, L. T. O., Saleh, K. A., Alrashedi, H., Alrubaiee, G. G., Almoliky, M. A., Alqalah, T. A. H., & Alkubati, S. A. (2026). Quality of life of caregivers of children with autism spectrum disorder in Saudi Arabia. *Journal of Pediatric Nursing*, *86*, 709–716. DOI: 10.1016/j.pedn.2025.12.010 PMID: 41468833

Alruily, M., Abd El-Aziz, A., Mostafa, A. M., Ezz, M., Mostafa, E., Alsayat, A., & El-Ghany, S. A. (2025). Ensemble deep learning for Alzheimer's disease diagnosis using MRI. *PLoS One*, *20*(4), e0318620. DOI: 10.1371/journal.pone.0318620 PMID: 40193955

Alwakid, G. N. (2025). A hybrid deep learning multi-class classification model for Alzheimer's disease. *Computers, Materials & Continua*, *86*(1), 1–25. DOI: 10.32604/cmc.2025.068666

American Psychiatric Association. (2013). *Diagnostic and statistical manual of mental disorders* (5th ed.). American Psychiatric Association., DOI: 10.1176/appi.books.9780890425596

Anandarao, S., Devarakonda, N., Kamarajugadda, R., & Krovi, R. S. (2026). Optimized vision transformer with bidirectional GRU for Alzheimer disease classification. *Knowledge-Based Systems*. Advance online publication. DOI: 10.1016/j.knosys.2026.116058

Anderson, H., & Goolishian, H. (1992). The client is the expert: A not-knowing approach to therapy. In McNamee, S., & Gergen, K. J. (Eds.), *Therapy as social construction* (pp. 25–39). Sage.

Anderson, M., Elliott, E. J., & Zurynski, Y. A. (2013). Australian families living with rare disease: Experiences of diagnosis, health services use and needs for psychosocial support. *Orphanet Journal of Rare Diseases*, *8*(1), 22. DOI: 10.1186/1750-1172-8-22 PMID: 23398775

Andersson, P. L., Petersén, Å., Graff, C., & Edberg, A.-K. (2016). Ethical aspects of a predictive test for Huntington's Disease: A long term perspective. *Nursing Ethics*, *23*(5), 565–575. DOI: 10.1177/0969733015576356 PMID: 25899725

Astle, D. E., Holmes, J., Kievit, R., & Gathercole, S. E. (2022). Annual Research Review: The transdiagnostic revolution in neurodevelopmental disorders. *Journal of Child Psychology and Psychiatry, and Allied Disciplines*, *63*(4), 397–417. DOI: 10.1111/jcpp.13481 PMID: 34296774

Atkins, J. C., & Padgett, C. R. (2024). Living with a rare disease: Psychosocial impacts for parents and family members – A systematic review. *Journal of Child and Family Studies*, *33*(2), 617–636. DOI: 10.1007/s10826-024-02790-6

Bantekas, I., Stephenson, C. P. Y., Karapapa, S., Polymenopoulou, E., Stein, M. A., & Anastasiou, D. (2018). Article 30 Participation in Cultural Life, Recreation, Leisure, and Sport. [1]. *Paragraph*, *100*(882), 883.

Barnes, C. (2019). Understanding the social model of disability: Past, present and future. In *Routledge handbook of disability studies* (pp. 14–31). Routledge. DOI: 10.4324/9780429430817-2

Baumer, N., DePillis, R., Pawlowski, K., Zhang, B., & Mazumdar, M. (2024). Developmental milestones for children with Down syndrome. *Pediatrics*, *154*(4), e2023065402. Advance online publication. DOI: 10.1542/peds.2023-065402 PMID: 39279536

Befkadu, B., & Adamek, M. E. (2022). The financial challenges of parents of a child with autism in addis ababa, ethiopia: A Qualitative study. *Integrated Journal for Research in Arts and Humanities*, *2*(1), 5–10. DOI: 10.55544/ijrasb.2.1.7

Behmel, A., Plöchl, E., & Rosenkranz, W. (1984). A new X-linked dysplasia gigantism syndrome: Identical with the Simpson dysplasia syndrome? *Human Genetics*, *67*(4), 409–413. DOI: 10.1007/BF00291401 PMID: 6490008

Beighton, C., & Wills, J. (2017). Are parents identifying positive aspects to parenting their child with an intellectual disability or are they just coping? A qualitative exploration. *Journal of Intellectual Disabilities, 21*(4), 325–345. DOI: 10.1177/1744629516656073 PMID: 27352854

Bel-Fenellós, C., Biencinto-López, C., Orio-Aparicio, C., Da Silva-Mori, X., Tenorio-Castaño, J. A., Lapunzina, P., & Nevado, J. (2025). Family well-being in families with children and young people with Wolf-Hirschhorn Syndrome. *Research in Developmental Disabilities, 160*, 104974. DOI: 10.1016/j.ridd.2025.104974 PMID: 40112494

Bergner, A. L., Bollinger, J., Raraigh, K. S., Tichnell, C., Murray, B., Blout, C. L., Telegrafi, A. B., & James, C. A. (2014). Informed consent for exome sequencing research in families with genetic disease: The emerging issue of incidental findings. *American Journal of Medical Genetics. Part A, 164*(11), 2745–2752. DOI: 10.1002/ajmg.a.36706 PMID: 25251809

Berry, J. O., & Jones, W. H. (1995). The Parental Stress Scale: Initial psychometric evidence. *Journal of Social and Personal Relationships, 12*(3), 463–472. DOI: 10.1177/0265407595123009

Besag, F. M. C., & Vasey, M. J. (2020). Seizures and epilepsy in autism spectrum disorder. *Child and Adolescent Psychiatric Clinics of North America, 29*(3), 483–500. DOI: 10.1016/j.chc.2020.02.002 PMID: 32471597

Bethel, K. A., Fuhrman, N. E., Kelsey, K. D., & Borron, A. (2024). Recreational therapists and the duty of care. *Journal of Experiential Education, 47*(3), 536–554. DOI: 10.1177/10538259231190844

Bhakta, B. B., Coleman, K. J., & Choi, K. R. (2022). Randomized study of survey recruitment strategies for parents of autistic children. *Journal of Pediatric Health Care, 36*(5), 470–473. DOI: 10.1016/j.pedhc.2022.05.008 PMID: 35705390

Bilbo, S. D., Block, C. L., Bolton, J. L., Hanamsagar, R., & Tran, P. K. (2018). Beyond infection—Maternal immune activation by environmental factors, microglial development, and relevance for autism spectrum disorders. *Experimental Neurology, 299*, 241–251. DOI: 10.1016/j.expneurol.2017.07.002 PMID: 28698032

Bogoje Raspopović, A., Balta, V., Vodopić, M., Drobac, M., Boroš, A., Đikić, D., & Demarin, V. (2024). The possible role of oxidative stress marker glutathione in the assessment of cognitive impairment in multiple sclerosis. *Open Medicine : a Peer-Reviewed, Independent, Open-Access Journal, 19*(1), 20240952. DOI: 10.1515/med-2024-0952 PMID: 38623459

Bolbocean, C., Andújar, F. N., McCormack, M., Suter, B., & Holder, J. L.Jr. (2022). Health-related quality of life in pediatric patients with syndromic autism and their caregivers. *Journal of Autism and Developmental Disorders*, *52*(3), 1334–1345. DOI: 10.1007/s10803-021-05030-8 PMID: 33937973

Bonzano, S., Dallorto, E., Molineris, I., Michelon, F., Crisci, I., Gambarotta, G., Neri, F., Oliviero, S., Beckervordersandforth, R., Lie, D. C., Peretto, P., Bovetti, S., Studer, M., & De Marchis, S. (2023). NR2F1 shapes mitochondria in the mouse brain, providing new insights into Bosch-Boonstra-Schaaf optic atrophy syndrome. *Disease Models & Mechanisms*, *16*(5), dmm049854. DOI: 10.1242/dmm.049854 PMID: 37260288

Bordt, E. A., & Polster, B. M. (2014). NADPH oxidase- and mitochondria-derived reactive oxygen species in proinflammatory microglial activation: A bipartisan affair? *Free Radical Biology & Medicine*, *76*, 34–46. DOI: 10.1016/j.freeradbiomed.2014.07.033 PMID: 25091898

Bortes, C., Strandh, M., & Nilsson, K. (2020). Sibling ill health and children's educational outcomes. *The Journal of School Health*, *90*(5), 407–414. DOI: 10.1111/josh.12887 PMID: 32105351

Bos-Roubos, A., Wingbermühle, E., Biert, A., Graaff, L. D., & Egger, J. (2022). Family matters: Trauma and quality of life in family members of individuals with Prader-Willi Syndrome. *Frontiers in Psychiatry*, *13*, 897138. DOI: 10.3389/fpsyt.2022.897138 PMID: 35836666

Boundy, L., Hargreaves, S., Baxter, R., Holton, S., & Burgoyne, K. (2023). Views of educators working with pupils with Down syndrome on their roles and responsibilities and factors related to successful inclusion. *Research in Developmental Disabilities*, *142*, 104617. DOI: 10.1016/j.ridd.2023.104617 PMID: 37832326

Boycott, K. M., Rath, A., Chong, J. X., Hartley, T., Alkuraya, F. S., Baynam, G., Brookes, A. J., Brudno, M., Carracedo, A., Den Dunnen, J. T., Dyke, S. O. M., Estivill, X., Goldblatt, J., Gonthier, C., Groft, S. C., Gut, I., Hamosh, A., Hieter, P., Höhn, S., & Lochmüller, H. (2017). International cooperation to enable the diagnosis of all rare genetic diseases. *American Journal of Human Genetics*, *100*(5), 695–705. DOI: 10.1016/j.ajhg.2017.04.003 PMID: 28475856

Boyle, M. (2002). *Schizophrenia: A scientific delusion?* (2nd ed.). Routledge.

Braun, V., & Clarke, V. (2006). Using thematic analysis in psychology. *Qualitative Research in Psychology*, *3*(2), 77–101. DOI: 10.1191/1478088706qp063oa

Bronfenbrenner, U. (Ed.). (2005). *Making human beings human: Bioecological perspectives on human development.* Sage Publications.

Bronfenbrenner, U., & Morris, P. A. (2007). Handbook of child psychology: Vol. 1. *The bioecological model of human development.*

Buckley, S., Burgoyne, K., & Loveall, S. (2024). Editorial: Speech, language, and literacy development in individuals with Down syndrome. *Frontiers in Psychology, 14*, 1346494. DOI: 10.3389/fpsyg.2023.1346494 PMID: 38239463

Bui, H. T., & Shaw, J. M. (2013). Dynamin assembly strategies and adaptor proteins in mitochondrial fission. *Current Biology, 23*(19), R891–R899. DOI: 10.1016/j.cub.2013.08.040 PMID: 24112988

Bull, M. J., Trotter, T., Santoro, S. L., Christensen, C., & Grout, R. W. (2022). Health supervision for children and adolescents with Down syndrome. *Pediatrics, 149*(5), e2022057010. Advance online publication. DOI: 10.1542/peds.2022-057010 PMID: 35490285

Bunnik, E. M., Schermer, M. H., & Jw Janssens, A. C. (2012). The role of disease characteristics in the ethical debate on personal genome testing. *BMC Medical Genomics, 5*(1), 4. DOI: 10.1186/1755-8794-5-4 PMID: 22260407

Caspi, A., Moffitt, T. E., Cannon, M., McClay, J., Murray, R., Harrington, H., Taylor, A., Arseneault, L., Williams, B., Braithwaite, A., Poulton, R., & Craig, I. W. (2005). Moderation of the effect of adolescent-onset cannabis use on adult psychosis by a functional polymorphism in the catechol-O-methyltransferase gene: Longitudinal evidence of a gene X environment interaction. *Biological Psychiatry, 57*(10), 1117–1127. DOI: 10.1016/j.biopsych.2005.01.026 PMID: 15866551

CDC. gov. (2025). Data and statistics on autism spectrum disorder. Available at: https://www.cdc.gov/autism/data-research/index.html

Chan, D. C. (2020). Mitochondrial dynamics and its involvement in disease. *Annual Review of Pathology, 15*(1), 235–259. DOI: 10.1146/annurev-pathmechdis-012419-032711 PMID: 31585519

Chan, K. K. S., Lam, C. B., Law, N. C. W., & Cheung, R. Y. M. (2018). From child autistic symptoms to parental affective symptoms: A family process model. *Research in Developmental Disabilities, 75*, 22–31. DOI: 10.1016/j.ridd.2018.02.005 PMID: 29455076

Chapman, R. S., Hesketh, L. J., & Kistler, D. J. (2002). Predicting longitudinal change in language production and comprehension in individuals with Down syndrome. *Journal of Speech, Language, and Hearing Research: JSLHR*, *45*(5), 902–915. DOI: 10.1044/1092-4388(2002/073) PMID: 12381048

Chauhan, K., Kishore, N., & Goel, N., & Monika. (. (2026). Deep learning-based multi-stage classification of Alzheimer's disease using MRI. *Franklin Open*, *15*, 100557. DOI: 10.1016/j.fraope.2026.100557

Chaves, T. F., Ocampos, M., Barbato, I. T., de Camargo Pinto, L. L., de Luca, G. R., Barbato Filho, J. H., Bernardi, P., Muniz, Y. C. N., & Maris, A. F. (2024). A cohort study of neurodevelopmental disorders and/or congenital anomalies using high resolution chromosomal microarrays in southern Brazil highlighting the significance of ASD. *Scientific Reports*, *14*(1), 3762. Advance online publication. DOI: 10.1038/s41598-024-54385-2 PMID: 38355898

Chen, F. H., Hartman, A. L., Letinturier, M. C. V., Antoniadou, V., Baynam, G., Bloom, L., Crimi, M., Della Rocca, M. G., Didato, G., Houge, S. D., Jonker, A., Kawome, M., Mueller, F., O'Brien, J., Puri, R. D., Ryan, N., Thong, M.-K., Tumienė, B., & Parisi, M. A. (2024). Telehealth for rare disease care, research, and education across the globe: A review of the literature by the IRDiRC telehealth task force. *European Journal of Medical Genetics*, *72*, 104977. DOI: 10.1016/j.ejmg.2024.104977 PMID: 39374775

Chen, W., Sun, L., He, X., Li, Z., Ji, C., Li, F., Shen, J., Pan, T., Jin, X., Dong, Y., Hu, L., Zou, C., & Bai, G. (2023). Health-related quality of life of children with Williams syndrome and caregivers in China. *Frontiers in Public Health*, *11*, 1177317. DOI: 10.3389/fpubh.2023.1177317 PMID: 37361163

Choi, G. B., Yim, Y. S., Wong, H., Kim, S., Kim, H., Kim, S. V., Hoeffer, C. A., Littman, D. R., & Huh, J. R. (2016). The maternal interleukin-17a pathway in mice promotes autism-like phenotypes in offspring. *Science*, *351*(6276), 933–939. DOI: 10.1126/science.aad0314 PMID: 26822608

Chrousos, G. P. (2009). Stress and disorders of the stress system. *Nature Reviews. Endocrinology*, *5*(7), 374–381. DOI: 10.1038/nrendo.2009.106 PMID: 19488073

Cicchetti, D. (2008). A multiple-levels-of-analysis perspective on research in developmental psychopathology. In Cicchetti, D., & Cohen, D. (Eds.),; 2nd ed., Vol. 1, pp. 27–57). Developmental psychopathology. Wiley.

Cicchetti, D., & Rogosch, F. A. (1996). Equifinality and multifinality in developmental psychopathology. *Development and Psychopathology*, *8*(4), 597–600. DOI: 10.1017/S0954579400007318

Clarke, A. J. (2014). Managing the ethical challenges of next-generation sequencing in genomic medicine. *British Medical Bulletin*, *111*(1), 17–30. DOI: 10.1093/bmb/ldu017 PMID: 25122627

Clayton, E. W., Halverson, C. M., Sathe, N. A., & Malin, B. A. (2018). A systematic literature review of individuals' perspectives on privacy and genetic information in the United States. *PLoS One*, *13*(10), e0204417. DOI: 10.1371/journal.pone.0204417 PMID: 30379944

Clemente, I. (2017). Barriers and facilitators to participation in physical activity for children with disabilities. *A systematic literature review.*

Cohen, C. I. (2025). Neorecovery: A Critical Analysis of the Relationship between Neoliberalism and the Recovery Movement. *Community Mental Health Journal*, *61*(2), 248–253. DOI: 10.1007/s10597-024-01275-6 PMID: 38874799

Colonna, M., & Butovsky, O. (2017). Microglia function in the central nervous system during health and neurodegeneration. *Annual Review of Immunology*, *35*(1), 441–468. DOI: 10.1146/annurev-immunol-051116-052358 PMID: 28226226

Conrad, C. E., Rimestad, M. L., Rohde, J. F., Petersen, B. H., Korfitsen, C. B., Tarp, S., Cantio, C., Lauritsen, M. B., & Händel, M. N. (2021). Parent-mediated interventions for children and adolescents with autism spectrum disorders: A systematic review and meta-analysis. *Frontiers in Psychiatry*, *12*, 773604. DOI: 10.3389/fpsyt.2021.773604 PMID: 34867556

Cordeiro, J. V. (2014). Ethical and legal challenges of personalized medicine: Paradigmatic examples of research, prevention, diagnosis and treatment. *Revista Portuguesa de Saude Publica*, *32*(2), 164–180. DOI: 10.1016/j.rpsp.2014.10.002

Creswell, J. W., & Poth, C. N. (2018). *Qualitative inquiry and research design: Choosing among five approaches* (4th ed.). Sage Publications.

CureScience Institute. (2024). Williams Syndrome. *Disease Review*, 1-13.

Dahshi, H., Kalvakuntla, S., Lee, M., & Goodspeed, K. (2024). Beyond the diagnosis: Evaluation of quality-of-life measures and family functioning in SLC6A1-related neurodevelopmental disorder. *Pediatric Neurology*, *155*, 160–166. DOI: 10.1016/j.pediatrneurol.2024.03.030 PMID: 38663152

Darling-White, M., & Jaeger, A. (2024). The impact of clear and loud speech cues on acoustic and perceptual features of speech production in adolescents with Down syndrome. *American Journal of Speech-Language Pathology*, *33*(6), 2768–2785. DOI: 10.1044/2024_AJSLP-24-00248 PMID: 39556033

Davis, N. O., & Carter, A. S. (2008). Parenting stress in mothers and fathers of toddlers with autism spectrum disorders: Associations with child characteristics. *Journal of Autism and Developmental Disorders*, *38*(7), 1278–1291. DOI: 10.1007/s10803-007-0512-z PMID: 18240012

De Groot, N. F. (2023). Commercial genetic information and criminal investigations: The case for social privacy. *Big Data & Society*, *10*(2), 20539517231216957. DOI: 10.1177/20539517231216957

DeBaun, M. R., Ess, J., & Saunders, S. (2001). Simpson-Golabi-Behmel syndrome: Progress toward understanding the molecular basis for overgrowth, malformation, and cancer predisposition. *Molecular Genetics and Metabolism*, *72*(4), 279–286. DOI: 10.1006/mgme.2001.3150 PMID: 11286501

Dellunde, P., & Moyà-Köhler, J. (2025). A social approach to artificial intelligence systems for people with Down syndrome: A qualitative systematic review. *International Journal of Developmental Disabilities*, *71*(1), 84–100. DOI: 10.1080/20473869.2025.2561165

Dellve, L., Samuelsson, L., Tallborn, A., Fasth, A., & Hallberg, L. R.-M. (2006). Stress and well-being among parents of children with rare diseases: A prospective intervention study. *Journal of Advanced Nursing*, *53*(4), 392–402. DOI: 10.1111/j.1365-2648.2006.03736.x PMID: 16448482

Dienel, G. A. (2019). Brain glucose metabolism: Integration of energetics with function. *Physiological Reviews*, *99*(1), 949–1045. DOI: 10.1152/physrev.00062.2017 PMID: 30565508

Diener, E., & Suh, E. (1997). Measuring quality of life: Economic, social, and subjective indicators. *Social Indicators Research*, *40*(1/2), 189–216. DOI: 10.1023/A:1006859511756

dos Santos, C. L., Barreto, I. I., Floriano, I., Tristão, L. S., Silvinato, A., & Bernardo, W. M. (2024). Screening and diagnostic tools for autism spectrum disorder: Systematic review and meta-analysis. *Clinics (São Paulo)*, *79*, 100323. Advance online publication. DOI: 10.1016/j.clinsp.2023.100323 PMID: 38484581

Duis, J., Birch, R. M., Buchner, D. A., Segal, D., Miller, J., Tan, W.-H., & Bird, L. M. (2022). A multidisciplinary approach and consensus statement to establish standards of care for Angelman syndrome. *Molecular Genetics & Genomic Medicine*, *10*(3), e1843. DOI: 10.1002/mgg3.1843 PMID: 35150089

Duncan, A. L., Keene, H., & Shepley, C. (2024). Do naturalistic developmental behavioral interventions improve family quality of life? A systematic review and meta-analysis. *Autism*, *28*(9), 2152–2165. DOI: 10.1177/13623613241227516 PMID: 38318790

Dykens, E. M., Maxwell, M. A., Pantino, E., Kossler, R., & Roof, E. (2007). Assessment of hyperphagia in Prader-Willi syndrome. *Obesity (Silver Spring, Md.)*, *15*(7), 1816–1826. DOI: 10.1038/oby.2007.216 PMID: 17636101

Eiroa-Orosa, F. J. (2020). Understanding psychosocial wellbeing in the context of complex and multidimensional problems. *International Journal of Environmental Research and Public Health*, *17*(16), 5937. DOI: 10.3390/ijerph17165937 PMID: 32824249

Eiser, C., & Morse, R. (2001). Can parents rate their child's health-related quality of life? Results of a systematic review. *Quality of Life Research: An International Journal of Quality of Life Aspects of Treatment, Care and Rehabilitation*, *10*(4), 347–357. DOI: 10.1023/A:1012253723272 PMID: 11763247

Escobar-López, M., & Salazar-Varas, R. (2026). EEG-based classification framework for Alzheimer's disease detection. *Biomedical Signal Processing and Control*, *112*, 108733. DOI: 10.1016/j.bspc.2025.108733

Eshraghi, A. A., Liu, G., Kay, S.-I. S., Eshraghi, R. S., Mittal, J., Moshiree, B., & Mittal, R. (2018). Epigenetics and autism spectrum disorder: Is there a correlation? *Frontiers in Cellular Neuroscience*, *12*, 78. DOI: 10.3389/fncel.2018.00078 PMID: 29636664

Feinberg, A. P. (2010). Epigenomics reveals a functional genome anatomy and a new approach to common disease. *Nature Biotechnology*, *28*(10), 1049–1052. DOI: 10.1038/nbt1010-1049 PMID: 20944596

Fidler, D. J. (2005). The emerging Down syndrome behavioral phenotype in early childhood: Implications for practice. *Infants and Young Children*, *18*(2), 86–103. DOI: 10.1097/00001163-200504000-00003

Fitzgerald, J., & Gallagher, L. (2022). Parental stress and adjustment in the context of rare genetic syndromes: A scoping review. *Journal of Intellectual Disabilities*, *26*(2), 522–544. DOI: 10.1177/1744629521995378 PMID: 33866895

Fitzgerald, M. (2019). The future of psychiatry and neurodevelopmental disorders: A paradigm shift. In Fitzgerald, M. (Ed.), *Neurodevelopment and neurodevelopmental disorder* (pp. 1–13). IntechOpen. DOI: 10.5772/intechopen.88540

Fletcher-Watson, S., Apicella, F., Auyeung, B., Beranova, S., Bonnet-Brilhault, F., Canal-Bedia, R., Charman, T., Chericoni, N., Conceição, I. C., Davies, K., Farroni, T., Gomot, M., Jones, E., Kaale, A., Kapica, K., Kawa, R., Kylliäinen, A., Larsen, K., Lefort-Besnard, J., & Yirmiya, N. (2017). Attitudes of the autism community to early autism research. *Autism*, *21*(1), 61–74. DOI: 10.1177/1362361315626577 PMID: 26975669

Foley, C., & Killeen, O. G. (2019). Musculoskeletal anomalies in children with Down syndrome: An observational study. *Archives of Disease in Childhood*, *104*(5), 482–487. DOI: 10.1136/archdischild-2018-315751 PMID: 30472668

Fonzo, M., Sirico, F., & Corrado, B. (2020). Evidence-based physical therapy for individuals with Rett syndrome: A systematic review. *Brain Sciences*, *10*(7), 410. DOI: 10.3390/brainsci10070410 PMID: 32630125

Fortea, J., Zaman, S. H., Hartley, S., Rafii, M. S., Head, E., & Carmona-Iragui, M. (2021). Down syndrome-associated Alzheimer's disease: A genetic form of dementia. *Lancet Neurology*, *20*(11), 930. DOI: 10.1016/S1474-4422(21)00245-3 PMID: 34687637

Fountoulakis, K., Papadopoulou, M., Kleanthous, S., Papadopoulou, A., Bizeli, V., Agorastos, G., Nimatoudis, I., Iacovides, A., & Kaprinis, G. S. (2003). Reliability and psychometric properties of the Greek translation of the State–Trait Anxiety Inventory Form Y: Preliminary data. *Annals of General Hospital Psychiatry*, *2*(S1, Suppl 1), S80. DOI: 10.1186/1475-2832-2-S1-S80

Franz, L., Goodwin, C. D., Rieder, A., Matheis, M., & Damiano, D. L. (2022). Early intervention for very young children with or at high likelihood for autism spectrum disorder: An overview of reviews. *Developmental Medicine and Child Neurology*, *64*(9), 1063–1076. DOI: 10.1111/dmcn.15258 PMID: 35582893

Frye, R. E., & Rossignol, D. (2013). Mitochondrial physiology and autism spectrum disorder. *OA Autism*, *1*(1), 2. DOI: 10.13172/2052-7810-1-1-433

Gainotti, S., Mascalzoni, D., Bros-Facer, V., Petrini, C., Floridia, G., Roos, M., Salvatore, M., & Taruscio, D. (2018). Meeting Patients' Right to the Correct Diagnosis: Ongoing International Initiatives on Undiagnosed Rare Diseases and Ethical and Social Issues. *International Journal of Environmental Research and Public Health*, *15*(10), 2072. DOI: 10.3390/ijerph15102072 PMID: 30248891

Gallotta, M. C., Franciosi, E., Giorgi, M., Guidetti, L., Cerbara, E., Pes, G., Silvestri, F., & Curzi, D. (2024). Benefits of inclusive sport training on fitness and health of athletes with and without intellectual disability. *Scientific Reports*, *14*(1), 21203. DOI: 10.1038/s41598-024-69334-2 PMID: 39261519

Garcia Condado, J., Verdugo Recuero, I., Tellaetxe Elorriaga, I., Birkenbihl, C., Carrigan, M., Diez, I., Buckley, R. F., Erramuzpe, A., & Cortes, J. M. (2025). Aging as an active player in Alzheimer's disease classification: Insights from feature selection in BrainAge models. *NeuroImage*, *121548*, 121548. Advance online publication. DOI: 10.1016/j.neuroimage.2025.121548 PMID: 41130534

García-López, C., Sarriá, E., & Pozo, P. (2016). Multilevel approach to gender differences in adaptation in father-mother dyads parenting individuals with autism spectrum disorder. *Research in Autism Spectrum Disorders*, *28*, 7–16. DOI: 10.1016/j.rasd.2016.04.003

Gasparotto, M., Lee, Y.-S., Palazzi, A., Vacca, M., & Filippini, F. (2022). Nuclear and cytoplasmic players in mitochondria-related CNS disorders: Chromatin modifications and subcellular trafficking. *Biomolecules*, *12*(5), 625. DOI: 10.3390/biom12050625 PMID: 35625553

Gerke, S., Jacoby, M. B., & Cohen, I. G. (2025). Bankruptcy, Genetic Information, and Privacy—Selling Personal Information. *The New England Journal of Medicine*, *392*(10), 937–939. DOI: 10.1056/NEJMp2415835 PMID: 40029207

Gill, R., & Orgad, S. (2018). The amazing bounce-backable woman: Resilience and the psychological turn in neoliberalism. *Sociological Research Online*, *23*(2), 477–495. DOI: 10.1177/1360780418769673

Giona, F., Beretta, S., Zippo, A., Stefanoni, A., Tomasoni, Z., Vicidomini, C., Ponzoni, L., Sala, M., Jones, C. K., Conn, P. J., & Passafaro, M. (2025). Shank3 modulates Rpl3 expression and protein synthesis via mGlu5: Implications for Phelan McDermid syndrome. *Molecular Psychiatry*, *30*(5), 3599–3614. DOI: 10.1038/s41380-025-02947-9 PMID: 40089604

Giotsa, A., Makri, E., Koutelou, S., Stamatelatou, A., & Chavredaki, A. (2015). Systemic family perspective and parent counseling groups. *Scientific Annals of the School of Education University of Ioannina*, *4*, 4–35. DOI: 10.12681/jret.8684

Giummarra, M. J., Randjelovic, I., & O'Brien, L. (2022). Interventions for social and community participation for adults with intellectual disability, psychosocial disability or on the autism spectrum: An umbrella systematic review. *Frontiers in Rehabilitation Sciences*, *3*, 935473. DOI: 10.3389/fresc.2022.935473 PMID: 36189003

Godler, D. E., Ling, L., Gamage, D., Baker, E. K., Bui, M., Field, M. J., Rogers, C., Butler, M. G., Murgia, A., Leonardi, E., Polli, R., Schwartz, C. E., Skinner, C. D., Alliende, A. M., Santa Maria, L., Pitt, J., Greaves, R., Francis, D., Oertel, R., & Amor, D. J. (2022). Feasibility of screening for chromosome 15 imprinting disorders in 16,579 newborns by using a novel genomic workflow. *JAMA Network Open*, *5*(1), e2141911. Advance online publication. DOI: 10.1001/jamanetworkopen.2021.41911 PMID: 34982160

Golabi, M., Rosen, L., & Opitz, J. M. (1984). A new X-linked mental retardation-overgrowth syndrome. *American Journal of Medical Genetics*, *17*(1), 345–358. DOI: 10.1002/ajmg.1320170128 PMID: 6538755

Gondalia, S., Parkinson, L., Stough, C., & Scholey, A. (2019). Gut microbiota and bipolar disorder: A review of mechanisms and potential targets for adjunctive therapy. *Psychopharmacology*, *236*(5), 1433–1443. DOI: 10.1007/s00213-019-05248-6 PMID: 31041459

Goodman, R. (1997). The Strengths and Difficulties Questionnaire: A research note. *Journal of Child Psychology and Psychiatry, and Allied Disciplines*, *38*(5), 581–586. DOI: 10.1111/j.1469-7610.1997.tb01545.x PMID: 9255702

Gottlieb, G. (2007). Probabilistic epigenesis. *Developmental Science*, *10*(1), 1–11. DOI: 10.1111/j.1467-7687.2007.00556.x PMID: 17181692

Griffith, G. M., Hastings, R. P., Nash, S., Petalas, M., Oliver, C., Howlin, P., Moss, J., Petty, J., & Tunnicliffe, P. (2011). "You have to sit and explain it all, and explain yourself." Mothers' experiences of support services for their offspring with a rare genetic intellectual disability syndrome. *Journal of Genetic Counseling*, *20*(2), 165–177. DOI: 10.1007/s10897-010-9339-4 PMID: 21203808

Griffiths, P. E., & Gray, R. D. (1994). Developmental systems and evolutionary explanation. *The Journal of Philosophy*, *91*(6), 277–304. DOI: 10.2307/2940982

Guan, Y., Tang, G., Li, L., Shu, J., Zhao, Y., Huang, L., & Tang, J. (2024). Herbal medicine and gut microbiota: Exploring untapped therapeutic potential in neurodegenerative disease management. *Archives of Pharmacal Research*, *47*(2), 146–164. DOI: 10.1007/s12272-023-01484-9 PMID: 38225532

Gu, C., Zhao, Y., Li, H., & Wang, J. (2024). Deep transfer learning using real-world image features for medical applications. *Frontiers in Medicine*, *11*. Advance online publication. DOI: 10.3389/fmed.2024

Gupta, D., & Halaswamy, D. G., A. M., Srivastava, A., Arya, S., Karthiga, V., & Patil, S. (2026). Moral capital, trust reserve, and social license to operate. In S. Sajib (Ed.), *Investigating Moral Capital in Value Creation* (pp. 111–142). IGI Global Scientific Publishing. DOI: 10.4018/979-8-3373-6043-0.ch004

Gupta, D., Azizbek, I., Suxrob, P., & Abdullaeva, I. Ravshan kizi, B. M., Abdukabilovna, T. D., & Jumayev, U. (2026). Digital hoboism. In E. Kaygisiz (Ed.), *Digital Ideologies in the Age of Algorithmic Culture* (pp. 307–338). IGI Global Scientific Publishing. DOI: 10.4018/979-8-3373-4531-4.ch010

Gupta, D., Ashirova, A., Ilhom, J., Sanzhar, D., Giyosiddinov, M., Urozboev, K., & Nodira, E. (2026a). Digital leadership and educational transformation in ASEAN: Competencies, contexts, and strategic pathways. In Em, S. (Ed.), *Digital leadership and innovation in ASEAN education* (pp. 97–124). IGI Global Scientific Publishing., DOI: 10.4018/979-8-2600-1142-3.ch004

Haas, R. H. (2010). Autism and mitochondrial disease. *Developmental Disabilities Research Reviews, 16*(2), 144–153. DOI: 10.1002/ddrr.112 PMID: 20818729

Hachmeriyan, M., Levkova, M., Yahya, D., Stoyanova, M., & Dimitrova, E. (2025). Ethical and Psychosocial Issues Associated with Genetic Testing for Hereditary Tumor Predisposition Syndromes. *Health Care, 13*(8), 880. DOI: 10.3390/healthcare13080880 PMID: 40281828

Hafeez, R., Ahmed, T., Anwar, S. M., & Rehman, M. (2025). Deep learning in early Alzheimer's disease detection: A comprehensive survey of classification, segmentation, and feature extraction methods. *Journal of Computational Science, 21*(5), 1083–1098. DOI: 10.3844/jcssp.2025.1083.1098

Harada, C. M., Siperstein, G. N., Parker, R. C., & Lenox, D. (2013). Promoting social inclusion for people with intellectual disabilities through sport: Special Olympics International, global sport initiatives and strategies. In *Disability in the global sport arena* (pp. 63–80). Routledge.

Hartmanis, S. L., Baker, E. K., Godler, D. E., & Liew, D. (2023). Estimating the impact of Angelman syndrome on parental productivity in Australia using productivity-adjusted life years. *Disability and Health Journal, 16*(2), 101423. DOI: 10.1016/j.dhjo.2022.101423 PMID: 36639256

Haseley, A., Wallis, K., & DeBrosse, S. (2021). Kleefstra syndrome: Impact on parents. *Disability and Health Journal, 14*(2), 101018. DOI: 10.1016/j.dhjo.2020.101018 PMID: 33189624

Hayes, S. A., & Watson, S. L. (2013). The impact of parenting stress: A meta-analysis of studies comparing the experience of parenting stress in parents of children with and without autism spectrum disorder. *Journal of Autism and Developmental Disorders*, *43*(3), 629–642. DOI: 10.1007/s10803-012-1604-y PMID: 22790429

Hays, P. (2021). Moral, Societal, and Ethical Issues: Claims, Consequences, and Caveats. In P. Hays, *Advancing Healthcare Through Personalized Medicine* (pp. 689–726). Springer International Publishing. DOI: 10.1007/978-3-030-80100-7_13

Heath, D., Ardestani, A., & Nemati, H. (2016). Sharing personal genetic information: The impact of privacy concern and awareness of benefit. *Journal of Information. Communication and Ethics in Society*, *14*(3), 288–308. DOI: 10.1108/JICES-07-2015-0025

Helaly, H. A., Badawy, M., & Haikal, A. Y. (2022). Deep learning approach for early detection of Alzheimer's disease. *Cognitive Computation*, *14*(5), 1711–1727. DOI: 10.1007/s12559-021-09946-2 PMID: 34745371

Hensch, T. K. (2005). Critical period plasticity in local cortical circuits. *Nature Reviews. Neuroscience*, *6*(11), 877–888. DOI: 10.1038/nrn1787 PMID: 16261181

Hertz-Picciotto, I., Schmidt, R. J., & Krakowiak, P. (2018). Understanding environmental contributions to autism: Causal concepts and the state of science. *Autism Research*, *11*(4), 554–586. DOI: 10.1002/aur.1938 PMID: 29573218

Ho, A. Y., & Dimitropoulos, A. (2010). Clinical management of behavioral characteristics of Prader–Willi syndrome. *Neuropsychiatric Disease and Treatment*, **•••**, 107–118. PMID: 20505842

Hoffman, L., Marquis, J. G., Poston, D. J., Summers, J. A., & Turnbull, A. (2006). Assessing family outcomes: Psychometric evaluation of the family quality of life scale. *Journal of Marriage and Family*, *68*(4), 1069–1083. DOI: 10.1111/j.1741-3737.2006.00314.x

Hoffmann, T. M., Friedrich, B., & Lewis, C. (2025). "I don't grieve as much as I used to": A qualitative study on parents of children with rare and undiagnosed conditions navigating grief in the context of uncertainty. *Journal of Genetic Counseling*, *34*(6), e70149. DOI: 10.1002/jgc4.70149 PMID: 41317142

Hong, Q. N., Fàbregues, S., Bartlett, G., Boardman, F., Cargo, M., Dagenais, P., Gagnon, M.-P., Griffiths, F., Nicolau, B., O'Cathain, A., Rousseau, M.-C., Vedel, I., & Pluye, P. (2018). The mixed methods appraisal Tool (MMAT) version 2018 for information professionals and researchers. *Education for Information*, *34*(4), 285–291. DOI: 10.3233/EFI-180221

Hong, Y., Boiti, A., Vallone, D., & Foulkes, N. S. (2024). Reactive oxygen species signaling and oxidative stress: Transcriptional regulation and evolution. *Antioxidants, 13*(3), 312. DOI: 10.3390/antiox13030312 PMID: 38539845

Horsley, S., & Oliver, C. (2015). Positive impact and its relationship to well-being in parents of children with intellectual disability: A literature review. *International Journal of Developmental Disabilities, 61*(1), 1–19. DOI: 10.1179/2047387713Y.0000000026

Hsiao, E. Y. (2014). Gastrointestinal issues in autism spectrum disorder. *Harvard Review of Psychiatry, 22*(2), 104–111. DOI: 10.1097/HRP.0000000000000029 PMID: 24614765

Hsiao, Y. (2018). Autism spectrum disorders: Family demographics, parental stress, and family quality of life. *Journal of Policy and Practice in Intellectual Disabilities, 15*(1), 70–79. DOI: 10.1111/jppi.12232

Huang, M., Liu, T., & Chen, H.. (2026). Transformer graph convolutional networks for Alzheimer's disease classification. *Biomedical Signal Processing and Control, 117*, 109594. DOI: 10.1016/j.bspc.2026.109594

Hughes, M. M., Kirby, A. V., Davis, J., Bilder, D. A., Patrick, M., Lopez, M., DaWalt, L. S., Pas, E. T., Bakian, A. V., Shaw, K. A., DiRienzo, M., Hudson, A., Schwenk, Y. D., Baroud, T. M., Washington, A., & Maenner, M. J. (2023). Individualized education programs and transition planning for adolescents with autism. *Pediatrics, 152*(1), e2022060199. DOI: 10.1542/peds.2022-060199 PMID: 37345494

Ishtiaq, M. (2019). Book Review Creswell, J. W. (2014). Research design: Qualitative, quantitative and mixed methods approaches (4th ed.). Thousand Oaks, CA: Sage. *English Language Teaching, 12*(5), 40. https://doi.org/DOI: 10.5539/elt.v12n5p40

Jarvis, J., Chertavian, E., Buessing, M., Renteria, T., Tu, L., Hoffer, L., Fischer, R., Moore, A., Cross, M., & Tones, M. (2025). The economic impact of caregiving for individuals with Angelman syndrome in the United States: Results from a caregiver survey. *Orphanet Journal of Rare Diseases, 20*(1), 82. DOI: 10.1186/s13023-025-03551-4 PMID: 39985061

Javaid, M., Arain, F., & Javaid, M. D. (2023). Oxidative stress in neurodegenerative diseases. In *Fundamental principles of oxidative stress in metabolism and reproduction* (pp. 167–183). Academic Press.

Jenkins, D., Chubb, J. R., & Galea, G. (2024). Stochastic processes in development and disease. *Philosophical Transactions of the Royal Society B: Biological Sciences, 379*(1900).

Jimah, J. R., & Hinshaw, J. E. (2019). Structural insights into the mechanism of dynamin superfamily proteins. *Trends in Cell Biology*, *29*(4), 257–273. DOI: 10.1016/j.tcb.2018.11.003 PMID: 30527453

Jimenez-Arberas, E., Casais-Suarez, Y., Fernandez-Mendez, A., Menendez-Espina, S., Rodriguez-Menendez, S., Llosa, J. A., & Prieto-Saborit, J. A. (2024). Evidence-based implementation of the family-centered model and the use of tele-intervention in early childhood services: A systematic review. *Health Care*, *12*(1), 112. Advance online publication. DOI: 10.3390/healthcare12010112 PMID: 38201017

Jobling, J. M., Teutsch, S. M., Eslick, G. D., & Elliott, E. J. (2025). Impact on the family of a child's rare disease: A large cross-sectional study. *Rare : Open Research in Rare Diseases*, *3*, 100066. DOI: 10.1016/j.rare.2025.100066

Johnson, M. H. (2011). Interactive specialization: A domain-general framework for human functional brain development? *Developmental Cognitive Neuroscience*, *1*(1), 7–21. DOI: 10.1016/j.dcn.2010.07.003 PMID: 22436416

Jomova, K., Alomar, S. Y., Alwasel, S. H., Nepovimova, E., Kuca, K., & Valko, M. (2024). Several lines of antioxidant defense against oxidative stress: Antioxidant enzymes, nanomaterials with multiple enzyme-mimicking activities, and low-molecular-weight antioxidants. *Archives of Toxicology*, *98*(5), 1323–1367. DOI: 10.1007/s00204-024-03696-4 PMID: 38483584

Jordan, T. L., Bartholomay, K. L., Lee, C. H., Lightbody, A. A., & Reiss, A. L. (2023). Cognition, academic achievement, and adaptive behavior in school-aged girls with fragile X syndrome. *Research in Developmental Disabilities*, *143*, 104622. DOI: 10.1016/j.ridd.2023.104622 PMID: 37939495

Jose, C., Melser, S., Benard, G., & Rossignol, R. (2013). Mitoplasticity: Adaptation biology of the mitochondrion to the cellular redox state in physiology and carcinogenesis. *Antioxidants & Redox Signaling*, *18*(7), 808–849. DOI: 10.1089/ars.2011.4357 PMID: 22989324

Karmiloff-Smith, A. (1998). Development itself is the key to understanding developmental disorders. *Trends in Cognitive Sciences*, *2*(10), 389–398. DOI: 10.1016/S1364-6613(98)01230-3 PMID: 21227254

Kasprzyk-Pawelec, A., Tan, M., Rahhal, R., McIntosh, A., Fernandez, H. R., Mosaoa, R. M., Jiang, L., Pearson, G. W., Glasgow, E., Vockley, J., Grabczyk, E., Grunwald, D. J., & Kasznica, J. M. (2024). Inactivation of the SLC25A1 gene during embryogenesis induces a unique senescence program controlled by p53. *Cell Death and Differentiation*, *32*(8), 818–836. PMID: 39733217

Katsarou, D. (2022). Fragile X syndrome and language skills. In Katsarou, D., & Zisi, V. (Eds.), *Disability and mental health* (pp. 133–149). Gutenberg.

Katsarou, D. (2023). Difficulties in locating discrete diagnostic categories: The examples of Down Syndrome and Williams Syndrome and Developmental Language Disorders and Dyslexia. In Katsarou, D. (Ed.), *Developmental Language Disorders in Childhood and Adolescence* (pp. 31–46). IGI Global. DOI: 10.4018/979-8-3693-0644-4.ch003

Katsarou, D., & Andreou, G. (2017). Receptive and Expressive Semantic Skills in Children with Down Syndrome. *International Education and Research Journal, 3*(3), 135–136.

Katsarou, D., & Andreou, G. (2022a). Phonological patterns in Greek language in toddlers and children with Down Syndrome and language impairment. *British Journal of Special Education, 49*(3), 420–237. DOI: 10.1111/1467-8578.12410

Katsarou, D., & Andreou, G. (2022b). Morphosyntactic abilities in young children with Down Syndrome: Evidence from the Greek language. *International Journal of Language & Communication Disorders, 57*(5), 937–947. DOI: 10.1111/1460-6984.12730 PMID: 35689466

Katsarou, D., Argyriadis, A., Sofologi, M., Argyriadi, A., Kougioumtzis, G., Megari, K., Mantsos, E., & Theodoratou, M. (2025a). Edwards Syndrome: Neurocognitive and linguistic profile, diagnosis, overlaps and treatment. *Polski Merkuriusz Lekarski, 54*(4), 540–545. DOI: 10.36740/Merkur202504116 PMID: 40929546

Katsarou, D., Theodoratou, M., Sofologi, M., Kougioumtzis, G., Efthymiou, E., Argyriadis, A., Patsiaouras, A., Mantsos, E., Argyriadi, A., & Papadopoulou, S. (2025b). Angelman Syndrome: Neurocognitive and linguistic profile, overlaps, interventions and quality of life. In Megari, K. (Ed.), *Clinical applications of pediatric neuropsychology from infancy to adolescence* (pp. 143–156). IGI Global. DOI: 10.4018/979-8-3693-9689-6.ch007

Katsarou, D., & Zisi, V. (2022). Down syndrome: Verbal short-term memory from early childhood to old age. *Archives of Hellenic Medicine, 39*(1), 54–59.

Kaye, D. K. (2023). Addressing ethical issues related to prenatal diagnostic procedures. *Maternal Health, Neonatology and Perinatology, 9*(1), 1. DOI: 10.1186/s40748-023-00146-4 PMID: 36737803

Khaliulin, I., Hamoudi, W., & Amal, H. (2024). The multifaceted role of mitochondria in autism spectrum disorder. *Molecular Psychiatry, 30*(3), 629–650. PMID: 39223276

Khan, R., Naseer, M., Hayat, M., & Khan, F. (2023). A transfer learning approach for multiclass classification of Alzheimer's disease using MRI images. *Frontiers in Neuroscience, 16*, 1050777. DOI: 10.3389/fnins.2022.1050777 PMID: 36699527

King, S., Teplicky, R., King, G., & Rosenbaum, P. (2004). Family-centered service for children with cerebral palsy and their families: A review of the literature. *Seminars in Pediatric Neurology, 11*(1), 78–86. DOI: 10.1016/j.spen.2004.01.009 PMID: 15132256

Klein-Tasman, B. P., Young, B. N., Levine, K., & Mohanty, E. (2023). Addressing fears of children with Williams syndrome: Therapist and child behavior in the context of a novel play-and humor-infused exposure therapy approach. *Frontiers in Psychology, 14*, 1098449. DOI: 10.3389/fpsyg.2023.1098449 PMID: 37599735

Knudsen, E. I. (2004). Sensitive periods in the development of the brain and behavior. *Journal of Cognitive Neuroscience, 16*(8), 1412–1425. DOI: 10.1162/0898929042304796 PMID: 15509387

Kodra, Y., Cavazza, M., De Santis, M., Guala, A., Liverani, M.-E., Armeni, P., Masini, M., & Taruscio, D. (2020). Social economic costs, health-related quality of life and disability in patients with cri du chat syndrome. *International Journal of Environmental Research and Public Health, 17*(16), 5951. DOI: 10.3390/ijerph17165951 PMID: 32824402

Komal, R., Dhavakumar, P., Rahul, K., Jaswanth, B., & Preeth, R. (2025). Hybrid deep learning framework for MRI-based Alzheimer's classification. *Brain Network Disorders, 1*(4), 239–249. DOI: 10.1016/j.bnd.2025.06.002

Kothinti, R. R. (2024). Artificial intelligence in healthcare: Revolutionizing precision medicine, predictive analytics, and ethical considerations in autonomous diagnostics. *World Journal of Advanced Research and Reviews, 19*(3), 3395–3406.

Kouznetsov, R., Angelopoulos, P., Moulinos, S., Dimakos, I., Gourzis, P., & Jelastopulu, E. (2023). Epidemiological study of autism spectrum disorders in greece for 2021: Nationwide prevalence in 2–17-year-old children and regional disparities. *Journal of Clinical Medicine, 12*(7), 2510. DOI: 10.3390/jcm12072510 PMID: 37048594

Kowalczyk, P., Sulejczak, D., Kleczkowska, P., Bukowska-Ośko, I., Kucia, M., Popiel, M., Wietrak, E., Kramkowski, K., Wrzosek, K., & Kaczyńska, K. (2021). Mitochondrial oxidative stress—A causative factor and therapeutic target in many diseases. *International Journal of Molecular Sciences, 22*(24), 13384. DOI: 10.3390/ijms222413384 PMID: 34948180

Kozel, B. A., Barak, B., Kim, C. A., Mervis, C. B., Osborne, L. R., Porter, M., & Pober, B. R. (2021). Williams syndrome. *Nature Reviews. Disease Primers*, *7*(1), 42. DOI: 10.1038/s41572-021-00276-z PMID: 34140529

Kuhlthau, K., Payakachat, N., Delahaye, J., Hurson, J., Pyne, J. M., Kovacs, E., & Tilford, J. M. (2014). Quality of life for parents of children with autism spectrum disorders. *Research in Autism Spectrum Disorders*, *8*(10), 1339–1350. DOI: 10.1016/j.rasd.2014.07.002

Kui, X., Dai, Y., Zou, B., Zhu, C., Li, Y., Ji, Z., Chen, L., & Bordallo López, M. (2026). Alzheimer's disease classification based on multimodal consistent distribution and trusted fusion. *Neural Networks*, *195*, 108245. DOI: 10.1016/j.neunet.2025.108245 PMID: 41172802

Kumar, H. V. K., A., & Kumar, S. (2025). Converging Realms of Social Health, Domestic Workers and Telemedicine Landscape: Challenges and Prospects. In P. Thaichon, P. K. Dutta, A. K. Haghi, & S. Dutta (Eds.), *Digital Disruption in Hospitality, Sustainable Hospitality* (pp. 213–228). Emerald Publishing Limited. DOI: 10.1108/978-1-83662-360-120251010

Kumari, L. K., Anusuya, V., & Ramalakshmi, K.. (2024). Edge enhanced densely connected convolutional network for liver tumor segmentation. In *ICACCS* (pp. 1136–1139). IEEE. DOI: 10.1109/ICACCS60874.2024.10717318

Kurnat-Thoma, E. (2020). Educational and Ethical Considerations for Genetic Test Implementation Within Health Care Systems. *Network and Systems Medicine*, *3*(1), 58–66. DOI: 10.1089/nsm.2019.0010 PMID: 32676590

La Valle, C., Johnston, E., & Tager-Flusberg, H. (2022). A systematic review of the use of telehealth to facilitate a diagnosis for children with developmental concerns. *Research in Developmental Disabilities*, *127*, 104269. Advance online publication. DOI: 10.1016/j.ridd.2022.104269 PMID: 35636261

Lachiewicz, A. M., Stackhouse, T. M., Burgess, K., Burgess, D., Andrews, H. F., Choo, T. H., Kaufmann, W. E., & Kidd, S. A. (2024). Sensory symptoms and signs of hyperarousal in individuals with fragile X syndrome: Findings from the FORWARD registry and database multisite study. *Journal of Autism and Developmental Disorders*, *54*(11), 4259–4277. DOI: 10.1007/s10803-023-06135-y PMID: 37840096

Lai, J., Li, A., Jiang, J., Yuan, X., Zhang, P., Xi, C., Wu, L., Wang, Z., Chen, J., Lu, J., Qiu, P., & Xu, Y. (2022). Metagenomic analysis reveals gut bacterial signatures for diagnosis and treatment outcome prediction in bipolar depression. *Psychiatry Research*, *307*, 114326. DOI: 10.1016/j.psychres.2021.114326 PMID: 34896845

Lalitsuradej, E., Sirilun, S., Sittiprapaporn, P., Sivamaruthi, B. S., Pintha, K., Tantipaiboonwong, P., Khongtan, S., Fukngoen, P., Peerajan, S., & Chaiyasut, C. (2022). The effects of synbiotics administration on stress-related parameters in Thai subjects—A preliminary study. *Foods, 11*(6), 759. DOI: 10.3390/foods11050759 PMID: 35267392

Lei, Z., Yuan, K., Xu, J., Miao, Y., Dai, Y., Wang, J., & Chang, J. (2025). Effects of physical exercises on balance in children with down syndrome: A systematic review and meta-analysis. *BMC Sports Science, Medicine and Rehabilitation, 17*(1), 165. DOI: 10.1186/s13102-025-01222-2 PMID: 40604949

Lenroot, R. K., & Giedd, J. N. (2011). Annual research review: Developmental considerations of gene by environment interactions. *Journal of Child Psychology and Psychiatry, and Allied Disciplines, 52*(4), 429–441. DOI: 10.1111/j.1469-7610.2011.02381.x PMID: 21391998

Li, F., Tang, Y., Li, F., Fang, S., Liu, X., Tao, M., Wu, D., & Jiang, L. (2022). Psychological distress in parents of children with autism spectrum disorder: A cross-sectional study based on 683 mother-father dyads. *Journal of Pediatric Nursing, 65*, e49–e55. DOI: 10.1016/j.pedn.2022.02.006 PMID: 35249769

Li, J. (2016). Genetic Information Privacy in the Age of Data-Driven Medicine. *2016 IEEE International Congress on Big Data (BigData Congress)*, 299–306. DOI: 10.1109/BigDataCongress.2016.45

Lim, Y., Hong, I., & Han, A. (2025). Health-related quality of life and family functioning in parents of children with Barth syndrome: An application of the Double ABCX model. *Orphanet Journal of Rare Diseases, 20*(1), 120. DOI: 10.1186/s13023-025-03636-0 PMID: 40075507

Li, X., Wu, K., Zeng, S., Zhao, F., Fan, J., Li, Z., Yi, L., Ding, H., Zhao, M., Fan, S., Liu, Y., & Zeng, L. (2021). Viral infection modulates mitochondrial function. *International Journal of Molecular Sciences, 22*(8), 4260. DOI: 10.3390/ijms22084260 PMID: 33923929

Lockhart, M., Chaux, R., Chevin, M., Celle, M., Raia-Barjat, T., Patural, H., Chabrier, S., & Giraud, A. (2023). Classification performance of the Ages and Stages Questionnaire: Influence of maternal education level. *Children (Basel, Switzerland), 10*(3), 449. Advance online publication. DOI: 10.3390/children10030449 PMID: 36980009

Lord, C., Brugha, T. S., Charman, T., Cusack, J., Dumas, G., Frazier, T., Jones, E. J. H., Jones, R. M., Pickles, A., State, M. W., Taylor, J. L., & Veenstra-VanderWeele, J. (2020). Autism spectrum disorder. *Nature Reviews. Disease Primers*, *6*(1), 5. DOI: 10.1038/s41572-019-0138-4 PMID: 31949163

Lorenzo, D., Esquerda, M., Bofarull, M., Cusi, V., Roig, H., Bertran, J., Carrera, J., Torralba, F., Cambra, F. J., Vila, M., Garriga, M., & Palau, F. (2023). The reuse of genetic information in research and informed consent. *European Journal of Human Genetics : EJHG*, *31*(12), 1393–1397. DOI: 10.1038/s41431-023-01457-y PMID: 37699995

Louzada, E. R., & Ribeiro, S. M. L. (2020). Synbiotic supplementation, systemic inflammation, and symptoms of brain disorders in elders: A secondary study from a randomized clinical trial. *Nutritional Neuroscience*, *23*(2), 93–100. DOI: 10.1080/1028415X.2018.1477349 PMID: 29788823

Lummer-Aikey, S., & Goldstein, S. (2021). Sibling adjustment to childhood chronic illness: An integrative review. *Journal of Family Nursing*, *27*(2), 136–153. DOI: 10.1177/1074840720977177 PMID: 33305651

Lv, L., Long, Z., Tan, X., Qin, L., Yan, W., Zhang, H., Ren, F., & Wang, C. (2024). Bidirectional two-sample Mendelian randomization analysis identifies causal associations between oxidative stress and Parkinson's disease. *Frontiers in Aging Neuroscience*, *16*, 1423773. DOI: 10.3389/fnagi.2024.1423773 PMID: 39026990

Maeder, J., Schneider, M., Bostelmann, M., Debbané, M., Glaser, B., Menghetti, S., Schaer, M., & Eliez, S. (2016). Developmental trajectories of executive functions in 22q11. 2 deletion syndrome. *Journal of Neurodevelopmental Disorders*, *8*(1), 10. DOI: 10.1186/s11689-016-9141-1 PMID: 27018204

Maenner, M. J., Shaw, K. A., Baio, J., Washington, A., Patrick, M., DiRienzo, M., Christensen, D. L., Wiggins, L. D., Pettygrove, S., Andrews, J. G., Lopez, M., Hudson, A., Baroud, T., Schwenk, Y., White, T., Rosenberg, C. R., Lee, L.-C., Harrington, R. A., Huston, M., & Dietz, P. M. (2020). Prevalence of autism spectrum disorder among children aged 8 years—Autism and developmental disabilities monitoring network, 11 sites, United States, 2016. *MMWR. Surveillance Summaries*, *69*(4), 1–12. DOI: 10.15585/mmwr.ss6904a1 PMID: 32214087

Maenner, M. J., Warren, Z., Williams, A. R., Amoakohene, E., Bakian, A. V., Bilder, D. A., Durkin, M. S., Fitzgerald, R. T., Furnier, S. M., Hughes, M. M., Ladd-Acosta, C. M., McArthur, D., Pas, E. T., Salinas, A., Vehorn, A., Williams, S., Esler, A., Grzybowski, A., Hall-Lande, J., & Shaw, K. A. (2023). Prevalence and characteristics of autism spectrum disorder among children aged 8 years—Autism and developmental disabilities monitoring network, 11 Sites, United States, 2020. *MMWR. Surveillance Summaries*, *72*(2), 1–14. DOI: 10.15585/mmwr.ss7202a1 PMID: 36952288

Malagelada, J. R. (2020). The brain-gut team. *Digestive Diseases (Basel, Switzerland)*, *38*(4), 293–298. DOI: 10.1159/000505810 PMID: 32114574

Malik, I., Ashraf, M. W., Saleem, M. A., & Ahmad, M. (2024). Deep learning for Alzheimer's disease prediction: A comprehensive review. *Diagnostics (Basel)*, *14*(12), 1281. DOI: 10.3390/diagnostics14121281 PMID: 38928696

Manickam, K., McClain, M. R., Demmer, L. A., Yu, T. W., & Hisama, F. M. (2021). Exome and genome sequencing for pediatric patients with congenital anomalies or intellectual disability: An evidence-based clinical guideline of the American College of Medical Genetics and Genomics (ACMG). *Genetics in Medicine*, *23*(11), 2029–2037. DOI: 10.1038/s41436-021-01242-6 PMID: 34211152

Mann, S., Spiric, J., Mitchell, C., & Hilgenkamp, T. I. M. (2023). Development of a physical therapy-based exercise program for adults with Down syndrome. *International Journal of Environmental Research and Public Health*, *20*(4), 3667. DOI: 10.3390/ijerph20043667 PMID: 36834362

Marsh, A., Spagnol, V., Grove, R., & Eapen, V. (2017). Transition to school for children with autism spectrum disorder: A systematic review. *World Journal of Psychiatry*, *7*(3), 184–196. DOI: 10.5498/wjp.v7.i3.184 PMID: 29043156

Martens, M. A., Wilson, S. J., & Reutens, D. C. (2008). Research Review: Williams syndrome: a critical review of the cognitive, behavioral, and neuroanatomical phenotype. *Journal of Child Psychology and Psychiatry, and Allied Disciplines*, *49*(6), 576–608. DOI: 10.1111/j.1469-7610.2008.01887.x PMID: 18489677

Martin, G. E., Losh, M., Estigarribia, B., Sideris, J., & Roberts, J. (2013). Longitudinal profiles of expressive vocabulary, syntax and pragmatic language in boys with fragile X syndrome or Down syndrome. *International Journal of Language & Communication Disorders*, *48*(4), 432–443. DOI: 10.1111/1460-6984.12019 PMID: 23889838

Mason-Apps, E., Stojanovik, V., Houston-Price, C., & Eadie, P. (2020). Early language development in Down syndrome: A longitudinal study. *Journal of Child Language*, *47*(3), 543–569.

Masten, A. S., & Cicchetti, D. (2010). Developmental cascades. *Development and Psychopathology*, *22*(3), 491–495. DOI: 10.1017/S0954579410000222 PMID: 20576173

McCarthy, E., & Guerin, S. (2022). Family-centred care in early intervention: A systematic review of the processes and outcomes of family-centred care and impacting factors. *Child: Care, Health and Development*, *48*(1), 1–32. DOI: 10.1111/cch.12901 PMID: 34324725

McCubbin, H. I., & Patterson, J. M. (1983). The Family Stress Process: The Double ABCX Model of adjustment and adaptation. *Marriage & Family Review*, *6*(1-2), 7–37. DOI: 10.1300/J002v06n01_02

McDuffie, A., & Abbeduto, L. (2009). Language disorders in children with mental retardation of genetic origin: Down syndrome, Fragile X syndrome, and Williams syndrome. *Handbook of child language disorders*, 44-66.

McMullan, J., Crowe, A. L., Bailie, C., Moore, K., McMullan, L. S., Shamandi, N., McAneney, H., & McKnight, A. J. (2020). Improvements needed to support people living and working with a rare disease in Northern Ireland: Current rare disease support perceived as inadequate. *Orphanet Journal of Rare Diseases*, *15*(1), 315. DOI: 10.1186/s13023-020-01559-6 PMID: 33168042

Merikhipour, M., Khanmohammadi-Doustani, S., & Abbasi, M. (2025). Spatial attention-based LSTM for classification. *Expert Systems with Applications*, *267*, 126196. DOI: 10.1016/j.eswa.2024.126196

Mertz, L. G., Thaulov, P., Trillingsgaard, A., Christensen, R., Vogel, I., Hertz, J. M., & Østergaard, J. R. (2014). Neurodevelopmental outcome in Angelman syndrome: Genotype-phenotype correlations. *Research in Developmental Disabilities*, *35*(7), 1742–1747. DOI: 10.1016/j.ridd.2014.02.018 PMID: 24656292

Mervis, C. B., & Klein-Tasman, B. P. (2004). Methodological issues in group-matching designs: A levels for control variable comparisons and measurement characteristics of control and target variables. *Journal of Autism and Developmental Disorders*, *34*(1), 7–17. DOI: 10.1023/B:JADD.0000018069.69562.b8 PMID: 15098952

Milla, L. A., Corral, L., Rivera, J., Zuñiga, N., Pino, G., Nunez-Parra, A., & Cea-Del Rio, C. A. (2023). Neurodevelopment and early pharmacological interventions in Fragile X syndrome. *Frontiers in Neuroscience*, *17*, 1213410. DOI: 10.3389/fnins.2023.1213410 PMID: 37599992

Mohammed, E. M. (2024). Detection of Alzheimer's disease using deep transfer learning models: A review. *Archives of Computational Methods in Engineering*, *31*(7). Advance online publication. DOI: 10.1007/s11831-024

Mohsen, S., Abdalla, M., & Hussein, M. (2025). Alzheimer's disease detection using deep learning and machine learning: A review. *Artificial Intelligence Review*, *58*(9), 262. DOI: 10.1007/s10462-025-11258-y

Molenaar, P. C. M. (2004). A manifesto on psychology as idiographic science. *Measurement*, *2*(4), 201–218.

Moore, D. S. (2016). *The developing genome: An introduction to behavioral epigenetics* (2nd ed.). Oxford University Press.

Morales, J. S., Valenzuela, P. L., Pareja-Galeano, H., Rincón-Castanedo, C., Rubin, D. A., & Lucia, A. (2019). Physical exercise and Prader-Willi syndrome: A systematic review. *Horumon To Rinsho*, *90*(5), 649–661. DOI: 10.1111/cen.13953 PMID: 30788853

Moran, G., Seymour, H., Walsh, N., O'Leary, N., & Gallagher, A. L. (2025). The Optimal Service for Children and Young People With Complex Neurodevelopmental Disabilities: Findings From an Integrative Literature Review. *Advances in Communication and Swallowing*, *28*(2), 87–101. DOI: 10.1177/27725383251339604

Morris, S., Farran, E. K., & Gilligan-Lee, K. A. (2024). Examining the prevalence and type of technology-use in people with Down syndrome: Perspectives from parents and caregivers. *Journal of Intellectual Disabilities*, *28*(3), 808–827. DOI: 10.1177/17446295231176121 PMID: 37201287

Morris, S., Hudson, E., Bloom, L., Chitty, L. S., Chitty, L., Fulop, N. J., Fulop, N., Hunter, A., Jones, J., Kai, J., Kerecuk, L., Kokocinska, M., Leeson-Beevers, K., Ng, P. L., Ng, P., Parkes, S., Ramsay, A. I., Ramsay, A., Simpson, A., & Walton, H. (2022). Co-ordinated care for people affected by rare diseases: The CONCORD mixed-methods study. *Health and Social Care Delivery Research*, *10*(05), 1–220. DOI: 10.3310/LNZZ5321 PMID: 35312266

Muhle, R., Trentacoste, S. V., & Rapin, I. (2004). The genetics of autism. *Pediatrics*, *113*(5), e472–e486. DOI: 10.1542/peds.113.5.e472 PMID: 15121991

Musick, K., Meier, A., & Flood, S. (2016). How parents fare: Mothers' and fathers' subjective well-being in time with children. *American Sociological Review*, *81*(5), 1069–1095. DOI: 10.1177/0003122416663917

Nadeem, A., Ahmad, S. F., Al-Harbi, N. O., Al-Ayadhi, L. Y., Sarawi, W., Attia, S. M., Bakheet, S. A., Alqarni, S. A., Ali, N., & AsSobeai, H. M. (2022). Imbalance in pro-inflammatory and anti-inflammatory cytokines milieu in B cells of children with autism. *Molecular Immunology*, *141*, 297–304. DOI: 10.1016/j.molimm.2021.12.009 PMID: 34915269

Nejad, A. R., Salimi, F. S. S., & Hemmasian, M.. (2026). Multi-class Alzheimer's disease classification using Swin Transformer and GWO. *Intelligence-Based Medicine*, *13*, 100362. DOI: 10.1016/j.ibmed.2026.100362

Neri, G., Marini, R., Cappa, M., Borrelli, P., & Opitz, J. M. (2013). Simpson-Golabi-Behmel syndrome: An X-linked encephalo-tropho-schisis syndrome. 1988. *American Journal of Medical Genetics. Part A*, *161A*(11), 2697–2703. DOI: 10.1002/ajmg.a.36317 PMID: 24166811

Neumärker, K.-J. (2003). Leo Kanner: His Years in Berlin, 1906-24. The roots of autistic disorder. *History of Psychiatry*, *14*(2), 205–218. DOI: 10.1177/0957154X030142005 PMID: 14518490

Nibali, L., Donos, N., & Henderson, B. (2009). Periodontal infectogenomics. *Journal of Medical Microbiology*, *58*(10), 1269–1274. DOI: 10.1099/jmm.0.012021-0 PMID: 19528161

Nie, Y., Chu, C., Qin, Q., Shen, H., Wen, L., Tang, Y., & Qu, M. (2024). Lipid metabolism and oxidative stress in patients with Alzheimer's disease and amnestic mild cognitive impairment. *Brain Pathology (Zurich, Switzerland)*, *34*(1), e13202. DOI: 10.1111/bpa.13202 PMID: 37619589

Ni, P., Ma, Y., & Chung, S. (2022). Mitochondrial dysfunction in psychiatric disorders. *Schizophrenia Research*, *250*, 122–129. PMID: 36175250

Nisbet, A. F., Hathaway, E. R., & Kalish, J. M. (2024). Simpson-Golabi-Behmel syndrome type 1. In Adam, M. P., Bick, S., & Mirzaa, G. M. (Eds.), *GeneReviews®* [Internet]. University of Washington.

Norlin, D., & Broberg, M. (2013). Parents of children with and without intellectual disability: Couple relationship and individual well-being. *Journal of Intellectual Disability Research*, *57*(6), 552–566. DOI: 10.1111/j.1365-2788.2012.01564.x PMID: 22533701

O'Brien, B. C., Harris, I. B., Beckman, T. J., Reed, D. A., & Cook, D. A. (2014). Standards for reporting qualitative research: A synthesis of recommendations. *Academic Medicine, 89*(9), 1245–1251. DOI: 10.1097/ACM.0000000000000388 PMID: 24979285

O'Neill, L. A., Kishton, R. J., & Rathmell, J. (2016). A guide to immunometabolism for immunologists. *Nature Reviews. Immunology, 16*(9), 553–565. DOI: 10.1038/nri.2016.70 PMID: 27396447

O'Neill, O. (2001). Informed Consent and Genetic Information. *Studies in History and Philosophy of Science Part C Studies in History and Philosophy of Biological and Biomedical Sciences, 32*(4), 689–704. DOI: 10.1016/S1369-8486(01)00026-7

Obaid, A. J., Kumar Shukla, V., Dutta, S., Bhattacharya, A., & Chakraborti, S. (Eds.). (2025). *Blockchain Technology for Healthcare Applications: Challenges, Privacy, and Securing of Data.* Nova Science Publishers, Inc., DOI: 10.52305/AUFT8731

Olszewski, A. K., Kikinis, Z., Gonzalez, C. S., Coman, I. L., Makris, N., Gong, X., Rathi, Y., Zhu, A., Antshel, K. M., Fremont, W., Kubicki, M. R., Bouix, S., Shenton, M. E., & Kates, W. R. (2017). The social brain network in 22q11. 2 deletion syndrome: A diffusion tensor imaging study. *Behavioral and Brain Functions : BBF, 13*(1), 4. DOI: 10.1186/s12993-017-0122-7 PMID: 28209179

Orphanet. (2023). *Simpson-Golabi-Behmel syndrome.* https://www.orpha.net/en/disease/detail/ 373

Oztenekecioglu, B., Mavis, M., Osum, M., & Kalkan, R. (2021). Genetic and epigenetic alterations in autism spectrum disorder. *Global Medical Genetics, 8*(4), 144–148. DOI: 10.1055/s-0041-1735540 PMID: 34877571

Page, M. J., McKenzie, J. E., Bossuyt, P. M., Boutron, I., Hoffmann, T. C., Mulrow, C. D., Shamseer, L., Tetzlaff, J. M., Akl, E. A., Brennan, S. E., Chou, R., Glanville, J., Grimshaw, J. M., Hróbjartsson, A., Lalu, M. M., Li, T., Loder, E. W., Mayo-Wilson, E., McDonald, S., & Moher, D. (2021). The PRISMA 2020 statement: An updated guideline for reporting systematic reviews. *BMJ (Clinical Research Ed.),* (71), n71. Advance online publication. DOI: 10.1136/bmj.n71 PMID: 33782057

Pagliuso, A., Cossart, P., & Stavru, F. (2018). The ever-growing complexity of the mitochondrial fission machinery. *Cellular and Molecular Life Sciences : CMLS, 75*(3), 355–374. DOI: 10.1007/s00018-017-2603-0 PMID: 28779209

Paleg, G. S., Hidalgo Robles, Á., Govender, P., & Livingstone, R. W. (2025). Occupational and Physical Therapy Interventions for Young Children with Developmental Central Hypotonia: An Overview of Systematic Reviews. *Disabilities*, *5*(1), 14. DOI: 10.3390/disabilities5010014

Palikara, O., Ashworth, M., & Van Herwegen, J. (2018). Addressing the educational needs of children with Williams syndrome: A rather neglected area of research? *Journal of Autism and Developmental Disorders*, *48*(9), 3256–3259. DOI: 10.1007/s10803-018-3578-x PMID: 29651682

Pallawi, S., & Singh, D. K. (2026). LEFF-ViT: A locally enhanced vision transformer framework for Alzheimer's disease classification. *Psychiatry Research: Neuroimaging*, *358*, 112155. DOI: 10.1016/j.pscychresns.2026.112155 PMID: 41653841

Palmer, C. S., Elgass, K. D., Parton, R. G., Osellame, L. D., Stojanovski, D., & Ryan, M. T. (2013). Adaptor proteins MiD49 and MiD51 can act independently of Mff and Fis1 in Drp1 recruitment and are specific for mitochondrial fission. *The Journal of Biological Chemistry*, *288*(38), 27584–27593. DOI: 10.1074/jbc.M113.479873 PMID: 23921378

Pandey, P. K., Srivastava, R. K., & Kumar, R. (2024). Enhancing healthcare recommendation: Transfer learning in deep convolutional neural networks for Alzheimer disease detection. *Frontiers in Medicine*, *11*, 1445325. DOI: 10.3389/fmed.2024.1445325 PMID: 39371344

Papadopoulou, S., Anagnostopoulou, A., Katsarou, D. V., Megari, K., Efthymiou, E., Argyriadis, A., Kougioumtzis, G., Theodoratou, M., Sofologi, M., Argyriadi, A., Pavlidou, E., & Toki, E. I. (2024). Enhancing Communication and Swallowing Skills in Children with Cri Du Chat Syndrome: A Comprehensive Speech Therapy Guide. *Children (Basel, Switzerland)*, *11*(12), 1526. DOI: 10.3390/children11121526 PMID: 39767955

Patel, R., Friedrich, B., Sanderson, S. C., Ellard, H., & Lewis, C. (2025). Anxiety and quality-of-life for parents of children with undiagnosed rare conditions: A multi-site quantitative survey study. *Journal of Genetic Counseling*, *34*(4), e70085. DOI: 10.1002/jgc4.70085 PMID: 40767117

Patel, T. A., Kevadiya, B. D., Bajwa, N., Singh, P. A., Zheng, H., Kirabo, A., Li, Y.-L., & Patel, K. P. (2023). Role of nanoparticle-conjugates and nanotheranostics in abrogating oxidative stress and ameliorating neuroinflammation. *Antioxidants*, *12*(10), 1877. DOI: 10.3390/antiox12101877 PMID: 37891956

Patterson, J. M. (2002). Understanding family resilience. *Journal of Clinical Psychology*, *58*(3), 233–246. DOI: 10.1002/jclp.10019 PMID: 11836706

Paxinos, I. (2022). Is there an "inspiration" of QOL in the field of clinical psychology and psychiatry? *Journal of Biomedical Engineering and Medical Imaging*, *9*(3). Advance online publication. DOI: 10.14738/jbemi.93.12415

Pelentsov, L. J., Fielder, A. L., & Laws, T. A. (2016). The supportive care needs of parents of children with rare diseases: A qualitative descriptive study. *Journal of Pediatric Nursing*, *31*(3), e207–e218. DOI: 10.1016/j.pedn.2015.10.022 PMID: 26651231

Pereira, R. C. M., Apis, A., Dos Santos, T. R., De Avó, L. R. D. S., Pilotto, R. F., Germano, C. M. R., & Melo, D. G. (2023). Quality of life of Brazilian families who have children with Williams syndrome. *Journal of Intellectual Disabilities*, *27*(3), 794–807. DOI: 10.1177/17446295221079583 PMID: 35543661

Pernas, L., & Scorrano, L. (2016). Mito-morphosis: Mitochondrial fusion, fission, and cristae remodeling as key mediators of cellular function. *Annual Review of Physiology*, *78*(1), 505–531. DOI: 10.1146/annurev-physiol-021115-105011 PMID: 26667075

Perochon, S., Di Martino, J. M., Carpenter, K. L. H., Compton, S., Davis, N., Eichner, B., Espinosa, S., Franz, L., Krishnappa Babu, P. R., Sapiro, G., & Dawson, G. (2023). Early detection of autism using digital behavioral phenotyping. *Nature Medicine*, *29*(10), 2489–2497. DOI: 10.1038/s41591-023-02574-3 PMID: 37783967

Picardi, A., Gigantesco, A., Tarolla, E., Stoppioni, V., Cerbo, R., Cremonte, M., Alessandri, G., Lega, I., & Nardocci, F. (2018). Parental burden and its correlates in families of children with autism spectrum disorder: A multicentre study with two comparison groups. *Clinical Practice and Epidemiology in Mental Health*, *14*(1), 143–176. DOI: 10.2174/1745017901814010143 PMID: 30158998

Pitchik, H. O., Tofail, F., Akter, F., Shoab, A. K. M., Sultana, J., Huda, T. M. N., Rahman, M., Winch, P. J., Luby, S. P., & Fernald, L. C. H. (2023). Concurrent validity of the Ages and Stages Questionnaire Inventory and the Bayley Scales of Infant and Toddler Development in rural Bangladesh. *BMC Pediatrics*, *23*(1), 93. Advance online publication. DOI: 10.1186/s12887-022-03800-6 PMID: 36859070

Prentice, C. M., Wehrli, S., Zahl, E., Orm, S., Botta, M., Vatne, T. M., Fredriksen, T., Kirchhofer, S., & Fjermestad, K. (2026). Parent-teacher discrepancies about the mental health of siblings of children with chronic disorders: A latent profile analysis. *Journal of Emotional and Behavioral Disorders*, •••, 1–11. DOI: 10.1177/10634266261417609

Priego-Ojeda, M., & Rusu, P. P. (2023). Emotion regulation, parental stress and family functioning: Families of children with disabilities vs normative families. *Research in Developmental Disabilities, 139*, 104548. DOI: 10.1016/j.ridd.2023.104548 PMID: 37320995

Prince, A. E. R., & Roche, M. I. (2014). Genetic Information, Non-Discrimination, and Privacy Protections in Genetic Counseling Practice. *Journal of Genetic Counseling, 23*(6), 891–902. DOI: 10.1007/s10897-014-9743-2 PMID: 25063358

Protic, D. D., Aishworiya, R., Salcedo-Arellano, M. J., Tang, S. J., Milisavljevic, J., Mitrovic, F., Hagerman, R. J., & Budimirovic, D. B. (2022). Fragile X syndrome: From molecular aspect to clinical treatment. *International Journal of Molecular Sciences, 23*(4), 1935. DOI: 10.3390/ijms23041935 PMID: 35216055

Pukeliene, V., & Starkauskiene, V. (2011). Quality of life: Factors determining its measurement complexity. *The Engineering Economist, 22*(2), 147–156. DOI: 10.5755/j01.ee.22.2.311

Punnett, H. H. (2000). *Simpson-Golabi-Behmel syndrome. Atlas of Genetics and Cytogenetics in Oncology and Haematology*. https://atlasgeneticsoncology.org/cancer-prone-disease/ 10038/ simpson-golabi-behmel-syndrome

Puri, D. V., Kachare, P. H., & Sangle, S. B.. (2026). Hybrid optimization for EEG channel selection. *Biomedical Signal Processing and Control, 112*, 108513. DOI: 10.1016/j.bspc.2025.108513

Quirke, A. M., Lugli, E. B., Wegner, N., Hamilton, B. C., Charles, P., Chowdhury, M., Ytterberg, A. J., Zubarev, R. A., Potempa, J., Culshaw, S., Guo, Y., Fisher, B. A., Thiele, G., Mikuls, T. R., & Venables, P. J. (2014). Heightened immune response to autocitrullinated Porphyromonas gingivalis peptidylarginine deiminase: A potential mechanism for breaching immunologic tolerance in rheumatoid arthritis. *Annals of the Rheumatic Diseases, 73*(1), 263–269. DOI: 10.1136/annrheumdis-2012-202726 PMID: 23463691

Rah, S. S., Jung, M., Lee, K., Park, J., Yoon, J. Y., & Hong, S. B. (2023). Systematic review and meta-analysis: Real-world accuracy of children's developmental screening tests. *Journal of the American Academy of Child and Adolescent Psychiatry, 62*(10), 1095–1109. DOI: 10.1016/j.jaac.2022.12.014 PMID: 36592715

Raina, P., O'Donnell, M., Rosenbaum, P., Brehaut, J., Walter, S. D., Russell, D., Swinton, M., Zhu, B., & Wood, E. (2005). The health and well-being of caregivers of children with cerebral palsy. *Pediatrics, 115*(6), e626–e636. DOI: 10.1542/peds.2004-1689 PMID: 15930188

Raj, A., & van Oudenaarden, A. (2008). Nature, nurture, or chance: Stochastic gene expression and its consequences. *Cell, 135*(2), 216–226. DOI: 10.1016/j.cell.2008.09.050 PMID: 18957198

Ramalakshmi, K., & Kumari, L. K. (2025). U-Net-based architecture with attention mechanisms and Bayesian optimization. *Computers in Biology and Medicine*, *195*, 110677. DOI: 10.1016/j.compbiomed.2025.110677 PMID: 40592172

Ramalakshmi, K., Rajagopal, S., Kulkarni, M. B., & Poddar, H. (2024). Hyperdimensional framework for brain tumor classification. *Biomedical Signal Processing and Control*, *96*, 106565. DOI: 10.1016/j.bspc.2024.106565

Ramalakshmi, K., Shukla, V. K., & Kumari, L. K. (2026). Transfer learning with CNNs for cancer detection. *Neural Computing & Applications*, *38*(8). Advance online publication. DOI: 10.1007/s00521-026-12091-2

Ramalakshmi, K., & Srinivasa Raghavan, V.. (2024). AI and segmentation methods in cancer recognition. *Biomedical Physics & Engineering Express*, *10*(4), 045046. DOI: 10.1088/2057-1976/ad555b PMID: 38848695

Reddy, V. P. (2023). Oxidative stress in health and disease. *Biomedicines*, *11*(11), 2925. DOI: 10.3390/biomedicines11112925 PMID: 38001926

Reilly, C., Senior, J., & Murtagh, L. (2015). A comparative study of educational provision for children with neurogenetic syndromes: Parent and teacher survey. *Journal of Intellectual Disability Research*, *59*(12), 1094–1107. DOI: 10.1111/jir.12210 PMID: 26780264

Rezq, K. A., Albalawi, H. M. H., & Alharbi, H. F. (2025). Exploring social support and quality of life among mothers of children with autism spectrum disorders: A Cross-sectional study. *Health Care*, *13*(2), 95. DOI: 10.3390/healthcare13020095 PMID: 39857122

Richards, C., Jones, C., Groves, L., Moss, J., & Oliver, C. (2015). Prevalence of autism spectrum disorder phenomenology in genetic disorders: A systematic review and meta-analysis. *The Lancet. Psychiatry*, *2*(10), 909–916. DOI: 10.1016/S2215-0366(15)00376-4 PMID: 26341300

Rimmer, J. H., Yamaki, K., Lowry, B. D., Wang, E., & Vogel, L. C. (2010). Obesity and obesity-related secondary conditions in adolescents with intellectual/developmental disabilities. *Journal of Intellectual Disability Research*, *54*(9), 787–794. DOI: 10.1111/j.1365-2788.2010.01305.x PMID: 20630017

Romski, M., Sevcik, R. A., Barton-Hulsey, A., Fisher, E., King, S., Albert, A., Kaldes, L., & Walters, C. (2023). Parent-implemented augmented communication intervention and young children with Down syndrome: An exploratory report. *Frontiers in Psychology, 14*, 1168599. DOI: 10.3389/fpsyg.2023.1168599 PMID: 37384179

Rose, S., Melnyk, S., Pavliv, O., Bai, S., Nick, T. G., Frye, R. E., & James, S. J. (2012). Evidence of oxidative damage and inflammation associated with low glutathione redox status in the autism brain. *Translational Psychiatry, 2*(7), e134–e134. DOI: 10.1038/tp.2012.61 PMID: 22781167

Rose, S., Niyazov, D. M., Rossignol, D. A., Goldenthal, M., Kahler, S. G., & Frye, R. E. (2018). Clinical and molecular characteristics of mitochondrial dysfunction in autism spectrum disorder. *Molecular Diagnosis & Therapy, 22*(5), 571–593. DOI: 10.1007/s40291-018-0352-x PMID: 30039193

Rossignol, D. A., & Frye, R. E. (2012). Mitochondrial dysfunction in autism spectrum disorders: A systematic review and meta-analysis. *Molecular Psychiatry, 17*(3), 290–314. DOI: 10.1038/mp.2010.136 PMID: 21263444

Rozensztrauch, A., Basiak, A., & Twardak, I. (2024). Rubinstein–Taybi Syndrome clinical characteristics from the perspective of quality of life and the impact of the disease on family functioning. *Journal of Clinical Medicine, 13*(17), 5210. DOI: 10.3390/jcm13175210 PMID: 39274423

Rozensztrauch, A., & Śmigiel, R. (2022). Quality of life in children with Prader–Willi syndrome and the impact of the disease on the functioning of families. *International Journal of Environmental Research and Public Health, 19*(23), 16330. DOI: 10.3390/ijerph192316330 PMID: 36498413

Rozensztrauch, A., Wieczorek, K., Twardak, I., & Śmigiel, R. (2023). Health-related quality of life and family functioning of primary caregivers of children with down syndrome. *Frontiers in Psychiatry, 14*, 1267583. DOI: 10.3389/fpsyt.2023.1267583 PMID: 38161724

Ruble, L. A., McGrew, J. H., Toland, M. D., & Findley, J. A. (2022). Individualized education program quality for transition-age students with autism. *Research in Autism Spectrum Disorders, 91*, 101900. DOI: 10.1016/j.rasd.2021.101900 PMID: 35096138

Saghazadeh, A., Ataeinia, B., Keynejad, K., Abdolalizadeh, A., Hirbod-Mobarakeh, A., & Rezaei, N. (2019). A meta-analysis of proinflammatory cytokines in autism spectrum disorders: Effects of age, gender, and latitude. *Journal of Psychiatric Research, 115*, 90–102. DOI: 10.1016/j.jpsychires.2019.05.019 PMID: 31125917

Sameroff, A. J. (2009). *The transactional model of development: How children and contexts shape each other*. American Psychological Association. DOI: 10.1037/11877-000

Sandbank, M., Bottema-Beutel, K., LaPoint, S. C., Feldman, J. I., Barrett, D. J., Caldwell, N., & Woynaroski, T. (2023). Autism intervention meta-analysis of early childhood studies (Project AIM): Updated systematic review and secondary analysis. *BMJ (Clinical Research Ed.)*, *383*, 383. DOI: 10.1136/bmj-2023-076733 PMID: 37963634

Sandin, S., Lichtenstein, P., Kuja-Halkola, R., Larsson, H., Hultman, C. M., & Reichenberg, A. (2014). The familial risk of autism. *Journal of the American Medical Association*, *311*(17), 1770–1777. DOI: 10.1001/jama.2014.4144 PMID: 24794370

Saoud, L. S., & AlMarzouqi, H. (2024). Explainable early detection of Alzheimer's disease using ROIs and an ensemble of 138 3D vision transformers. *Scientific Reports*, *14*(1), 27756. DOI: 10.1038/s41598-024-76313-0 PMID: 39532960

Saulnier, K. M., Cinà, M., Chan, B., Pelletier, S., Dorval, M., & Joly, Y. (2018). Communication of genetic information in the palliative care context: Ethical and legal issues. *Medical Law International*, *18*(4), 219–240. DOI: 10.1177/0968533218762239

Saunders, C. H., Sierpe, A., Von Plessen, C., Kennedy, A. M., Leviton, L. C., Bernstein, S. L., Goldwag, J., King, J. R., Marx, C. M., Pogue, J. A., Saunders, R. K., Van Citters, A., Yen, R. W., Elwyn, G., & Leyenaar, J. K. (2023). Practical thematic analysis: A guide for multidisciplinary health services research teams engaging in qualitative analysis. *BMJ (Clinical Research Ed.)*, *074256*, e074256. Advance online publication. DOI: 10.1136/bmj-2022-074256 PMID: 37290778

Savignac, H. M., Couch, Y., Stratford, M., Bannerman, D. M., Tzortzis, G., Anthony, D. C., & Burnet, P. W. J. (2016). Prebiotic administration normalizes lipopolysaccharide (LPS)-induced anxiety and cortical 5-HT2A receptor and IL1-β levels in male mice. *Brain, Behavior, and Immunity*, *52*, 120–131. DOI: 10.1016/j.bbi.2015.10.007 PMID: 26476141

Scarr, S., & McCartney, K. (1983). How people make their own environments: A theory of genotype–environment effects. *Child Development*, *54*(2), 424–435. PMID: 6683622

Schaefer, G. B., & Mendelsohn, N. J.Professional Practice Guidelines Committee. (2013). Clinical genetics evaluation in identifying the etiology of autism spectrum disorders: 2013 guideline revisions. *Genetics in Medicine*, *15*(5), 399–407. DOI: 10.1038/gim.2013.32 PMID: 23519317

Schieve, L. A., Gonzalez, V., Boulet, S. L., Visser, S. N., Rice, C. E., Van Naarden Braun, K., & Boyle, C. A. (2012). Concurrent medical conditions and health care use and needs among children with learning and behavioral developmental disabilities, National Health Interview Survey, 2006–2010. *Research in Developmental Disabilities, 33*(2), 467–476. DOI: 10.1016/j.ridd.2011.10.008 PMID: 22119694

Seager, E., Sampson, S., Sin, J., Pagnamenta, E., & Stojanovik, V. (2022). A systematic review of speech, language and communication interventions for children with Down syndrome from 0 to 6 years. *International Journal of Language & Communication Disorders, 57*(2), 441–463. DOI: 10.1111/1460-6984.12699 PMID: 35191587

Seruya, F. M., Feit, E., Tirado, A., Ottomanelli, D., & Celio, M. (2022). Caregiver coaching in early intervention: A scoping review. *The American Journal of Occupational Therapy, 76*(4), 7604205070. DOI: 10.5014/ajot.2022.049143 PMID: 35727822

Shahbazi, M., Abed, E. H., & Esmaili, S. K. (2026). Family-Centered Occupational Therapy Consultation for Children Under 18 Years Old: A Scoping Review. *Occupational Therapy International, 2026*(1), 1184326. DOI: 10.1155/oti/1184326 PMID: 41522633

Shah, S. M., Madhavan, S. P., Bowden, N., & Nedgungadi, P. (2026). Caregivers' experiences with autism from pre- to postdiagnosis: Multi-country perspectives using ecological systems theory. *Research in Autism, 132*, 202836. DOI: 10.1016/j.reia.2026.202836

Shaikh, M. G., Barrett, T. G., Bridges, N., Chung, R., Gevers, E. F., Goldstone, A. P., Holland, A., Kanumakala, S., Krone, R., Kyriakou, A., Livesey, E. A., Lucas-Herald, A. K., Meade, C., Passmore, S., Roche, E., Smith, C., & Soni, S. (2024). Prader–Willi syndrome: Guidance for children and transition into adulthood. *Endocrine Connections, 13*(8). Advance online publication. DOI: 10.1530/EC-24-0091 PMID: 38838713

Shields, N. (2021). Physiotherapy management of Down syndrome. *Journal of Physiotherapy, 67*(4), 243–251. DOI: 10.1016/j.jphys.2021.08.016 PMID: 34511385

Shikako-Thomas, K., Majnemer, A., Law, M., & Lach, L. (2008). Determinants of participation in leisure activities in children and youth with cerebral palsy: Systematic review. *Physical & Occupational Therapy in Pediatrics, 28*(2), 155–169. DOI: 10.1080/01942630802031834 PMID: 18846895

Shin, E., Ravichandran, C., Renzi, D., Pober, B. R., McDougle, C. J., & Thom, R. P. (2024). Diversity of participants in Williams syndrome intervention studies. *Journal of Autism and Developmental Disorders, 54*(10), 3888–3898. DOI: 10.1007/s10803-023-06088-2 PMID: 37584767

Shrout, P. E., Stadler, G., Lane, S. P., McClure, M. J., Jackson, G. L., Clavél, F. D., Iida, M., Gleason, M. E. J., Xu, J. H., & Bolger, N. (2018). Initial elevation bias in subjective reports. *Proceedings of the National Academy of Sciences of the United States of America, 115*(1). Advance online publication. DOI: 10.1073/pnas.1712277115 PMID: 29255039

Sideropoulos, V., Palikara, O., Burchell, E., Ashworth, M., & Van Herwegen, J. (2024). Anxiety during transition from primary to secondary schools in neurodivergent children. *JCPP Advances, 5*(2), e12262. DOI: 10.1002/jcv2.12262 PMID: 40519965

Silibello, G., Vizziello, P., Gallucci, M., Selicorni, A., Milani, D., Ajmone, P. F., Rigamonti, C., De Stefano, S., Bedeschi, M. F., & Lalatta, F. (2016). Daily life changes and adaptations investigated in 154 families with a child suffering from a rare disability at a public center for rare diseases in Northern Italy. *Italian Journal of Pediatrics, 42*(1), 76. DOI: 10.1186/s13052-016-0285-0 PMID: 27576488

Sim, A., Cordier, R., Vaz, S., & Falkmer, T. (2019). "We are in this together": Experiences of relationship satisfaction in couples raising a child with autism spectrum disorder. *Research in Autism Spectrum Disorders, 58*, 39–51. DOI: 10.1016/j.rasd.2018.11.011

Sirchia, F., Kalantari, S., Carli, D., Zadorozhna, M., Bassanese, F., Venti, E. T., Taft, R. J., Kesari, A., Sorasio, L., Antona, V., Guala, A., Feresin, A., Basile, A., Licciardi, F., Garau, J., Gasparini, P., Grosso, E., Mussa, A., Ferrero, G. B., & Giorgio, E. (2026). Advancing Neuropediatric Rare Disease Diagnosis Through Clinical Genome Sequencing. *Pediatric Neurology, 177*, 28–45. DOI: 10.1016/j.pediatrneurol.2026.01.004 PMID: 41619469

Skevington, S. M., Lotfy, M., & O'Connell, K. A. (2004). The World Health Organization's WHOQOL-BREF quality of life assessment: Psychometric properties and results of the international field trial. A Report from the WHOQOL Group. *Quality of Life Research: An International Journal of Quality of Life Aspects of Treatment, Care and Rehabilitation, 13*(2), 299–310. DOI: 10.1023/B:QURE.0000018486.91360.00 PMID: 15085902

Socransky, S., & Haffajee, A. (2012). Periodontal infections. In Lindhe, J., Lang, N., & Karring, P. (Eds.), *Clinical periodontology and implant dentistry* (pp. 207–267). Blackwell Munksgaard.

Spielberger, C. D., Gorsuch, R. L., & Lushene, R. E. (1970). *Manual for the State-Trait Anxiety Inventory (STAI)*. Consulting Psychologists Press.

Sroufe, L. A. (1997). Psychopathology as an outcome of development. *Development and Psychopathology*, *9*(2), 251–268. DOI: 10.1017/S0954579497002046 PMID: 9201444

Stake, R. E. (1995). *The art of case study research.* Sage Publications.

Steenbergen, L., Sellaro, R., van Hemert, S., Bosch, J. A., & Colzato, L. S. (2015). A randomized controlled trial to test the effect of multispecies probiotics on cognitive reactivity to sad mood. *Brain, Behavior, and Immunity*, *48*, 258–264. DOI: 10.1016/j.bbi.2015.04.003 PMID: 25862297

Stein, D. J., Phillips, K. A., Bolton, D., Fulford, K. W. M., Sadler, J. Z., & Kendler, K. S. (2010). What is a mental/psychiatric disorder? From DSM-IV to DSM-V. *Psychological Medicine*, *40*(11), 1759–1765. DOI: 10.1017/S0033291709992261 PMID: 20624327

Stojanovik, V., Pagnamenta, E., Sampson, S., Jarrold, C., & Burgoyne, K. (2024). Evaluating an early social communication intervention for young children with Down syndrome (ASCEND): Results from a feasibility randomised control trial. *Pilot and Feasibility Studies*, *10*(1), 127. DOI: 10.1186/s40814-024-01551-y PMID: 39369246

Stoner, J. B., Bock, S. J., Thompson, J. R., Angell, M. E., Heyl, B. S., & Crowley, E. P. (2005). Welcome to our world: Parent perceptions of interactions between parents of young children with ASD and education professionals. *Focus on Autism and Other Developmental Disabilities*, *20*(1), 39–51. DOI: 10.1177/10883576050200010401

Talukder, M. B., Kumar, S., & Das, I. R. (2024). Mindfulness of Digital Detoxification: Healthy Lifestyle in Tourism. In Kankaew, K., Chaudhary, S., & Widtayakornbundit, S. (Eds.), (pp. 56–71). Advances in Logistics, Operations, and Management Science. IGI Global., DOI: 10.4018/979-8-3693-1273-5.ch004

Tan, J., McKenzie, C., Potamitis, M., Thorburn, A. N., Mackay, C. R., & Macia, L. (2014). The role of short-chain fatty acids in health and disease. *Advances in Immunology*, *121*, 91–119. DOI: 10.1016/B978-0-12-800100-4.00003-9 PMID: 24388214

Tassone, F., Protic, D., Allen, E. G., Archibald, A. D., Baud, A., Brown, T. W., Budimirovic, D. B., Cohen, J., Dufour, B., Eiges, R., Elvassore, N., Gabis, L. V., Grudzien, S. J., Hall, D. A., Hessl, D., Hogan, A., Hunter, J. E., Jin, P., Jiraanont, P., & Hagerman, R. J. (2023). Insight and recommendations for fragile X-premutation-associated conditions from the Fifth International Conference on FMR1 Premutation. *Cells*, *12*(18), 2330. Advance online publication. DOI: 10.3390/cells12182330 PMID: 37759552

Telenga, M., Rozensztrauch, A., Giżewska-Kacprzak, K., & Śmigiel, R. (2024). From genotype to phenotype of polish patients with Pitt–Hopkins Syndrome concerning the quality of life and family functioning. *Journal of Clinical Medicine*, *13*(9), 2605. DOI: 10.3390/jcm13092605 PMID: 38731134

Teoli, D., & Bhardwaj, A. (2025 Jan). Quality of life. [Updated 2023 Mar 27] In *StatPearls* [Internet]. StatPearls Publishing., Available from https://www.ncbi.nlm.nih.gov/books/NBK536962/

Thelen, E., & Smith, L. B. (1994). *A dynamic systems approach to the development of cognition and action*. MIT Press. DOI: 10.7551/mitpress/2524.001.0001

Timimi, S., Milton, D., Bovell, V., Kapp, S., & Russell, G. (2019). Deconstructing diagnosis: Four commentaries on a diagnostic tool to assess individuals for autism spectrum disorders. *Autonomy (Birmingham, England)*, *1*(6), AR26. PMID: 31396391

Tremaroli, V., & Bäckhed, F. (2012). Functional interactions between the gut microbiota and host metabolism. *Nature*, *489*(7415), 242–249. DOI: 10.1038/nature11552 PMID: 22972297

Tsibidaki, A. (2021). Children with cerebral palsy: Family and parent demographic characteristics and family strengths in Greece and Italy. *Journal of Health Psychology*, *26*(12), 2071–2083. DOI: 10.1177/1359105319900276 PMID: 31918571

Turnage, D., & Conner, N. (2022). Quality of life of parents of children with autism spectrum disorder: An integrative literature review. *Journal for Specialists in Pediatric Nursing*, *27*(4), e12391. DOI: 10.1111/jspn.12391 PMID: 35986656

Turrisi, R., Saponaro, G., Vercelli, A., & Rossi, M. (2024). Deep learning approaches for Alzheimer's detection: Models, augmentation, and low-resolution MRI studies. *Frontiers in Computational Neuroscience*, *18*, 1360095. DOI: 10.3389/fncom.2024.1360095 PMID: 39371524

Tzinieri-Kokkosi, M. (2009). *Quality of life manual with the WHOQOL-100 questionnaire as its axis: Sections and content of topics* (Improved version.). *BETA Bulletin of Experimental Treatments for AIDS*.

UNICEF. (2021). *Good practice guide on building an inclusive playground*. UNICEF.

Urgesi, C., Butti, N., Ferrari, E., Oldrati, V., Strazzer, S., Biffi, E., Gagliardi, C., Foti, F., Menghini, D., Finisguerra, A., Vicari, S., & Borgatti, R. (2024). New insights into social cognition in Williams syndrome from a comprehensive assessment and a virtual reality task. *Scientific Reports, 14*(1), 23562. DOI: 10.1038/s41598-024-79289-z

Ursin, F., Timmermann, C., & Steger, F. (2021). Ethical Implications of Alzheimer's Disease Prediction in Asymptomatic Individuals through Artificial Intelligence. *Diagnostics (Basel), 11*(3), 440. DOI: 10.3390/diagnostics11030440 PMID: 33806501

Vale, A. R., De Avó, L. R. D. S., Pilotto, R. F., Germano, C. M. R., & Melo, D. G. (2022). Quality of life of Brazilian families who have children with Rubinstein–Taybi syndrome: An exploratory cross-sectional study. *American Journal of Medical Genetics. Part A, 188*(11), 3294–3305. DOI: 10.1002/ajmg.a.62914 PMID: 35913016

van der Sanden, B. P. G. H., Schobers, G., Corominas Galbany, J., Koolen, D. A., Sinnema, M., van Reeuwijk, J., Stumpel, C. T. R. M., Kleefstra, T., de Vries, B. B. A., Ruiterkamp-Versteeg, M., Leijsten, N., Kwint, M., Derks, R., Swinkels, H., den Ouden, A., Pfundt, R., Rinne, T., de Leeuw, N., Stegmann, A. P., & Vissers, L. E. L. M. (2023). The performance of genome sequencing as a first-tier test for neurodevelopmental disorders. *European Journal of Human Genetics : EJHG, 31*(1), 81–88. DOI: 10.1038/s41431-022-01185-9 PMID: 36114283

van Heyningen, V. (2024). Stochasticity in genetics and gene regulation. *Philosophical Transactions of the Royal Society B: Biological Sciences, 379*(1900).

van Niekerk, J., Gush, M., Moosa, S., & Pretorius, C. (2026). Coping with the challenges of caregiving: A qualitative exploration of the experiences of family caregivers of children with rare diseases in South Africa. *Journal of Genetic Counseling, 35*(2), 1–17. DOI: 10.1002/jgc4.70205 PMID: 41958204

Van Till, S. A. L., Bouman, A., Kleefstra, T., & Bunnik, E. M. (2025). Parental experiences and needs in Kleefstra Syndrome: A semi-structured interview study. *European Journal of Medical Genetics, 77*, 105037. DOI: 10.1016/j.ejmg.2025.105037 PMID: 40829731

Varni, J. W., Burwinkle, T. M., & Seid, M. (2005). The PedsQL™ as a pediatric patient-reported outcome: Reliability and validity of the PedsQL™ Measurement Model in 25,000 children. *Expert Review of Pharmacoeconomics & Outcomes Research, 5*(6), 705–719. DOI: 10.1586/14737167.5.6.705 PMID: 19807613

Varni, J. W., Burwinkle, T. M., & Seid, M. (2006). The PedsQLTM 4.0 as a school population health measure: Feasibility, reliability, and validity. *Quality of Life Research: An International Journal of Quality of Life Aspects of Treatment, Care and Rehabilitation, 15*(2), 203–215. DOI: 10.1007/s11136-005-1388-z PMID: 16468077

Varni, J. W., Burwinkle, T. M., Seid, M., & Skarr, D. (2003). The PedsQL™* 4.0 as a pediatric population health measure: Feasibility, reliability, and validity. *Ambulatory Pediatrics, 3*(6), 329–341. DOI: 10.1367/1539-4409(2003)003<0329:TPAAPP>2.0.CO;2 PMID: 14616041

Vasilopoulou, E., & Nisbet, J. (2016). The quality of life of parents of children with autism spectrum disorder: A systematic review. *Research in Autism Spectrum Disorders, 23*, 36–49. DOI: 10.1016/j.rasd.2015.11.008

Vears, D. F., Borry, P., Savulescu, J., & Koplin, J. J. (2021). Old Challenges or New Issues? Genetic Health Professionals' Experiences Obtaining Informed Consent in Diagnostic Genomic Sequencing. *AJOB Empirical Bioethics, 12*(1), 12–23. DOI: 10.1080/23294515.2020.1823906 PMID: 33017265

Verdugo, M. A., Schalock, R. L., Keith, K. D., & Stancliffe, R. J. (2005). Quality of life and its measurement: Important principles and guidelines. *Journal of Intellectual Disability Research, 49*(10), 707–717. DOI: 10.1111/j.1365-2788.2005.00739.x PMID: 16162115

Verma, M., Lizama, B. N., & Chu, C. T. (2022). Excitotoxicity, calcium and mitochondria: A triad in synaptic neurodegeneration. *Translational Neurodegeneration, 11*(1), 3. DOI: 10.1186/s40035-021-00278-7 PMID: 35078537

Vernhet, C., Michelon, C., Dellapiazza, F., Rattaz, C., Geoffray, M.-M., Roeyers, H., Picot, M.-C., Baghdadli, A., Baghdadli, A., Chabaux, C., Chatel, C., Cohen, D., Damville, E., Geoffray, M.-M., Gicquel, L., Jardri, R., Maffre, T., Novo, A., Roxane, R., & Vespérini, S.ELENA study group. (2022). Perceptions of parents of the impact of autism spectrum disorder on their quality of life and correlates: Comparison between mothers and fathers. *Quality of Life Research: An International Journal of Quality of Life Aspects of Treatment, Care and Rehabilitation, 31*(5), 1499–1508. DOI: 10.1007/s11136-021-03045-3 PMID: 34822048

Viswan, V., Shaffi, N., Mahmud, M., Subramanian, K., & Hajamohideen, F. (2024). Explainable artificial intelligence in Alzheimer's disease classification: A systematic review. *Cognitive Computation, 16*(1), 1–44. DOI: 10.1007/s12559-023-10192-x von der Lippe, C., Neteland, I., & Feragen, K. B. (2022). Children with a rare congenital genetic disorder: A systematic review of parent experiences. *Orphanet Journal of Rare Diseases, 17*(1), 375. Advance online publication. DOI: 10.1186/s13023-022-02525-0 PMID: 36253830

Walkowiak, D., Pospieszyńska-Martysiuk, K., Dianow, H., Węgrzyn, J., & Domaradzki, J. (2026). Measuring economic burden in families of individuals with Angelman Syndrome in Poland: A caregivers' survey. *Orphanet Journal of Rare Diseases, 21*(1), 24. DOI: 10.1186/s13023-025-04183-4 PMID: 41469742

Walsh, F. (2016). *Strengthening family resilience* (3rd ed.). Guilford Press.

Walton, H., Hudson, E., Simpson, A., Ramsay, A. I. G., Kai, J., Morris, S., Sutcliffe, A. G., & Fulop, N. J. (2020). Defining Coordinated Care for People with Rare Conditions: A Scoping Review. *International Journal of Integrated Care, 20*(2), 14. Advance online publication. DOI: 10.5334/ijic.5464 PMID: 32607101

Wandin, H., Lindberg, P., & Sonnander, K. (2023). Aided language modelling, responsive communication and eye-gaze technology as communication intervention for adults with Rett syndrome: Three experimental single case studies. *Disability and Rehabilitation. Assistive Technology, 18*(7), 1011–1025. DOI: 10.1080/17483107.2021.1967469 PMID: 34455895

Wang, K., & Chen, X. (2024). Protective effect of flavonoids on oxidative stress injury in Alzheimer's disease. *Natural Product Research, 38*(22), 4107–4134. PMID: 38910339

Wang, Y., Guo, X., Hong, X., Wang, G., Pearson, C., Zuckerman, B., Clark, A. G., O'Brien, K. O., Wang, X., & Gu, Z. (2022). Association of mitochondrial DNA content, heteroplasmies, and inter-generational transmission with autism. *Nature Communications, 13*(1), 3790. DOI: 10.1038/s41467-022-30805-7 PMID: 35778412

Warreman, E. B., Lloyd, S. E., Nooteboom, L. A., Leenen, P. J. M., Terry, M. B., Hoek, H. W., Van Rossum, E. F. C., Vermeiren, R. R. J. M., & Ester, W. A. (2023). Psychological, behavioural, and physical aspects of caregiver strain in autism-caregivers: A cohort study. *EClinicalMedicine, 64*, 102211. DOI: 10.1016/j.eclinm.2023.102211 PMID: 37767192

Watson, W. H. (2012). Family systems. In *Encyclopedia of Human Behavior* (pp. 184–193). Elsevier., DOI: 10.1016/B978-0-12-375000-6.00169-5

Weaver, I. C., Cervoni, N., Champagne, F. A., D'Alessio, A. C., Sharma, S., Seckl, J. R., Dymov, S., Szyf, M., & Meaney, M. J. (2004). Epigenetic programming by maternal behavior. *Nature Neuroscience*, *7*(8), 847–854. DOI: 10.1038/nn1276 PMID: 15220929

Wen, J., Thibeau-Sutre, E., Diaz-Melo, M., Samper-González, J., Routier, A., Bottani, S., Dormont, D., Durrleman, S., Burgos, N., & Colliot, O. (2020). Convolutional neural networks for classification of Alzheimer's disease: Overview and reproducible evaluation. *Medical Image Analysis*, *63*, 101694. DOI: 10.1016/j.media.2020.101694 PMID: 32417716

Westermann, G., Mareschal, D., Johnson, M. H., Sirois, S., Spratling, M. W., & Thomas, M. S. (2007). Neuroconstructivism. *Developmental Science*, *10*(1), 75–83. DOI: 10.1111/j.1467-7687.2007.00567.x PMID: 17181703

Wheeler, A. C., Gantz, M. G., Cope, H., Strong, T. V., Bohonowych, J. E., Moore, A., & Vogel-Farley, V. (2023). Age of diagnosis for children with chromosome 15q syndromes. *Journal of Neurodevelopmental Disorders*, *15*(1), 37. Advance online publication. DOI: 10.1186/s11689-023-09504-x PMID: 37936142

Whiting, M., Nash, A. S., Kendall, S., & Roberts, S. A. (2019). Enhancing resilience and self-efficacy in the parents of children with disabilities and complex health needs. *Primary Health Care Research and Development*, *20*, e33. DOI: 10.1017/S1463423619000112 PMID: 32799971

Wieckowski, A. T., Williams, L. N., Rando, J., Lyall, K., & Robins, D. L. (2023). Sensitivity and specificity of the Modified Checklist for Autism in Toddlers (original and revised): A systematic review and meta-analysis. *JAMA Pediatrics*, *177*(4), 373–383. DOI: 10.1001/jamapediatrics.2022.5975 PMID: 36804771

Winarni, T. I., Schneider, A., Borodyanskara, M., & Hagerman, R. J. (2012). Early intervention combined with targeted treatment promotes cognitive and behavioral improvements in young children with fragile X syndrome. *Case Reports in Genetics*, *280813*, 1–4. Advance online publication. DOI: 10.1155/2012/280813 PMID: 23074686

Wongkittirungrueang, S., & Cheausuwantavee, T. (2025). Developing a systematic plan to enhance transitions for autistic youth in Thailand: Applying Bronfenbrenner's ecological systems theory. *Journal of Social Studies Education Research*, *16*(1), 172–200. https://files.eric.ed.gov/fulltext/EJ1478321.pdf

World Health Organization. (2007). *International classification of functioning, disability, and health: Children & youth version: ICF-CY*. World Health Organization.

World Health Organization. (2020). *WHO guidelines on physical activity and sedentary behaviour*. World Health Organization.

World Health Organization. (2023). *Stress*. https://www.who.int/news-room/questions-and-answers/item/stress

Xu, S., Tang, C., & Shi, L.. (2026). Multi-modal deep-layer fusion for Alzheimer's classification. *Neurocomputing*. Advance online publication. DOI: 10.1016/j.neucom.2026.133697

Xu, Y., Jin, M.-Z., Yang, Z.-Y., & Jin, W.-L. (2021). Microglia in neurodegenerative diseases. *Neural Regeneration Research*, *16*(2), 270–280. DOI: 10.4103/1673-5374.290881 PMID: 32859774

Yin, R. K. (2018). *Case study research and applications: Design and methods* (6th ed.). Sage Publications.

Yoonjeong, L. (2023). Impact of raising children with rare diseases on parental quality of life and family functioning. *International Journal of Rare Diseases & Disorders*, *6*(1). Advance online publication. DOI: 10.23937/2643-4571/1710053

Zablotsky, B., Bradshaw, C. P., & Stuart, E. A. (2013). The association between mental health, stress, and coping supports in mothers of children with autism spectrum disorders. *Journal of Autism and Developmental Disorders*, *43*(6), 1380–1393. DOI: 10.1007/s10803-012-1693-7 PMID: 23100053

Zhang, X., Gao, L., Wang, Z., Yu, Y., Zhang, Y., & Hong, J. (2024). Improved neural network with multi-task learning for Alzheimer's classification. *Heliyon*, *10*(4), e26405. DOI: 10.1016/j.heliyon.2024.e26405 PMID: 38434063

Zhang, Y., Chen, H., Li, R., Sterling, K., & Song, W. (2023). Amyloid β-based therapy for Alzheimer's disease: Challenges, successes and future. *Signal Transduction and Targeted Therapy*, *8*(1), 248. DOI: 10.1038/s41392-023-01484-7 PMID: 37386015

Zhao, T., Allan, K., Taylor, J., Thorburn, D. R., White, S. M., Tan, T. Y., Christodoulou, J., Tan, N. B., & Stroud, D. A. (2025). Functional characterization of a novel GPC3 missense variant in Simpson-Golabi-Behmel Syndrome. *American Journal of Medical Genetics. Part A*, *200*(3), 632–641. DOI: 10.1002/ajmg.a.64287 PMID: 41122961

Zhou, J., Li, X., Zhang, Y., & Chen, W. (2025). A deep learning model for early diagnosis of Alzheimer's disease. *Scientific Reports*, *15*, 22421. DOI: 10.1038/s41598-025-22421 PMID: 40603911

Zia-ur-Rehman, A., Naeem, M., Tariq, M., & Hussain, A. (2024). Deep learning techniques for Alzheimer's disease detection in 3D imaging: A systematic review. *Health Science Reports*, *7*(9), e70025. DOI: 10.1002/hsr2.70025 PMID: 39296636

Ziegler, A., Koval-Burt, C., Kay, D. M., Suchy, S. F., Begtrup, A., Langley, K. G., Hernan, R., Amendola, L. M., Boyd, B. M., Bradley, J., Brandt, T., Cohen, L. L., Coffey, A. J., Devaney, J. M., Dygulska, B., Friedman, B., Fuleihan, R. L., Gyimah, A., Hahn, S., & Chung, W. K. (2025). Expanded newborn screening using genome sequencing for early actionable conditions. *Journal of the American Medical Association*, *333*(3), 232–240. DOI: 10.1001/jama.2024.19662 PMID: 39446378

Zimmer, M., Desch, L., Rosen, L. D., Bailey, M. L., Becker, D., Culbert, T. P., McClafferty, H., Sahler, O. J. Z., Vohra, S., Liptak, G. S., Adams, R. C., Burke, R. T., Friedman, S. L., Houtrow, A. J., Kalichman, M. A., Kuo, D. Z., Levy, S. E., Norwood, K. W.Jr, Turchi, R. M., & Wiley, S. E.Section On Complementary And Integrative Medicine. (2012). Sensory integration therapies for children with developmental and behavioral disorders. *Pediatrics*, *129*(6), 1186–1189. DOI: 10.1542/peds.2012-0876 PMID: 22641765

Zuna, N. I., Turnbull, A., & Summers, J. A. (2009). Family quality of life: Moving from measurement to application. *Journal of Policy and Practice in Intellectual Disabilities*, *6*(1), 25–31. DOI: 10.1111/j.1741-1130.2008.00199.x

Zuna, N., Summers, J. A., Turnbull, A. P., Hu, X., & Xu, S. (2010). Theorizing about family quality of life. In Kober, R. (Ed.), *Enhancing the quality of life of people with intellectual disabilities: From theory to practice* (Vol. 41, pp. 241–278). Springer., DOI: 10.1007/978-90-481-9650-0_15

Zurynski, Y., Deverell, M., Dalkeith, T., Johnson, S., Christodoulou, J., Leonard, H., & Elliott, E. J. (2017). Australian children living with rare diseases: Experiences of diagnosis and perceived consequences of diagnostic delays. *Orphanet Journal of Rare Diseases*, *12*(1), 68. DOI: 10.1186/s13023-017-0622-4 PMID: 28399928

About the Contributors

Dimitra V. Katsarou is a tenured Assistant Professor at the Department of Sciences in Preschool Education and Educational Design of the University of the Aegean, holding the chair of Developmental Psychopathology and Language Disorders. She studied Philology at the School of Philosophy of the Aristotle University of Thessaloniki. She holds four postgraduate degrees, PhD in "Language Development and Linguistic Abilities of Children with Down Syndrome" from the Department of Special Education of the University of Thessaly and two postdoctoral research projects at the University of Thessaly and the Aristotle University of Thessaloniki. Her scholarly work includes more than 50 articles in peer-reviewed indexed journals, 50 chapters in edited academic volumes, three books, ten international edited books, five Greek edited volumes, more than 100 conference presentations, and eleven children's books.

Assimina T. Tsibidaki is an Associate Professor of Special Education with the discipline "Special education: Psychopedagogical dimensions in family and school" in the Department of Primary Education (PTDE) at the University of the Aegean (Greece). Her research interests focus on the following areas: Students with special educational needs and disabilities (SEND), families raising a child with SEND, home-school collaboration, social support networks, technology and inclusive education, disability in children's literature and cinema. Her published work includes two books, editing and articles in Greece and abroad, as well as various participations in Greek and international conferences.

***

Ismagilova Madina Faridovna is a faculty member in the Department of Philology at Urgench State Pedagogical Institute, Urgench, Uzbekistan. She is involved in teaching and scholarly activities related to language, literature, and philological studies. Her academic interests include linguistics, literary analysis, language pedagogy, and the development of communicative competence in educational contexts. She actively contributes to curriculum development and student mentoring, with a focus on strengthening language education and critical reading skills. Her work supports the advancement of philological research and effective language instruction in higher education.

Deepak Gupta is a distinguished academician with over 20 years of teaching experience and expertise in Computer Science and Engineering. He holds a Ph.D. in Computer Engineering and has an extensive research portfolio, including many international journal papers, multiple conference proceedings, and several books. His research interests span machine learning, artificial intelligence, and data mining. Currently, Dr. Gupta serves as an Associate Professor and Head of Department of CSE (Emerging Branches) at ITM Gwalior, MP, India. He has also contributed significantly to the field through patents and copyrights and actively engages as a reviewer, conference chair and editor.

Nasiba Jumaniyazova is a faculty member in the Department of Psychology at Mamun University, Khiva, Uzbekistan. She is engaged in teaching and academic activities related to psychological science, human behavior, and educational psychology. Her academic interests include cognitive and developmental psychology, student mental well-being, and the application of psychological principles in educational settings. She is committed to fostering students' analytical thinking, emotional intelligence, and academic growth through learner-centered instruction. Nasiba Jumaniyazova actively contributes to academic and institutional initiatives aimed at strengthening psychology education and promoting research-informed teaching practices in higher education.

Christina Krystamtsi is a PhD candidate at the Department of Primary Education at the University of the Aegean, Greece. She is trained in Special Education and works as a kindergarten teacher in special education settings. She has been professionally engaged in the care and support of children and adolescents with special health care needs within community and special education contexts. Her doctoral research focuses on families of children with rare genetic syndromes, particularly Cri du Chat and Angelman syndromes, examining Family Quality of Life (FQoL), resilience, positive psychology, and marital satisfaction. Her broader research interests include family-centered care, psychosocial adjustment in rare conditions, and systemic approaches to disability and inclusion. Through both research and practice, she aims to contribute to the development of holistic and strengths-based support models that enhance long-term well-being for families of children with complex health and developmental needs

Ashok Kumar has completed his Bachelor's degree in Electronics and Communication Engineering from Government College of Technology, Coimbatore in 2008 and Master Degree in Computer Science and Engineering from Government College of Technology in 2011 . He has completed Doctor of Philosophy from College of Engineering, Guindy, Anna University, Chennai in 2025. He is currently acting as a Research Fellow of INTI International University, Malaysia.

Pardeep Kumar Assistant Professor, Department of Mathematics, Lovely Professional University, Phagwara, Punjab, India Dr. Pardeep Kumar holds a Ph.D. in Mathematics from Lovely Professional University (2021). His research expertise lies in Stochastic Processes, with a specialized focus on Markov Models, Engineering System Reliability, and Reliability Theory. He actively contributes to the modeling and reliability analysis of IoT-enabled and sensor-integrated systems for next-generation engineering applications. Dr. Kumar has a profound command of Stochastic Modelling, Reliability Testing, and advanced analytical methods for complex system behavior under uncertainty. His work emphasises practical implementations in smart technologies and cyber-physical systems. He has an exceptional academic track record, having qualified the prestigious CSIR-UGC NET twice, securing All India Ranks (AIR) of 15 and 32, respectively. To date, Dr. Kumar has published 26 high-quality research papers in reputed national and international journals, reflecting his continued contribution to the advancement of mathematical reliability and its engineering applications.

Sanjeev Kumar Is a Professor in Lovely Professional University Punjab India. He received Undergraduate in Hotel Management from Osmania University, Postgraduate in Tourism Management from Madurai Kamaraj University. He completed Doctor of Philosophy in Hospitality Management in 2019 from Amity University Jaipur India. His research areas lies in food Service Industry, his research focuses on Alcoholic beverages, Event management and Sustainable Management Practices, Metaverse, AI Machine Learning and Artificial Intelligence. He published more than 80 research papers, articles and chapters in Scopus Indexed, UGC Approved and peer reviewed Journals and books. Dr. Sanjeev Kumar participated and acted as resource person in various National and International conferences, seminars, session chair, research workshops and industry talks and his work has been widely cited. Dr. Sanjeev also edited more than 20 books with various International Publishers such as IGI Global, Cambridge Scholars, Emerald, CABI, Bentham Science, Taylor & Francis. Dr Sanjeev is an active researcher and has published numerous research articles in prestigious National and International journals and books.

Evangelos Mantsos is a Postdoctoral Researcher in the Department of Occupational Therapy at University of Western Macedonia. He holds a PhD in Physical Education, Sport Science and Dietetics from University of Thessaly with a dissertation entitled "Recreational Movement Activities for Holistic Wellness and Successful Aging in Individuals with Down Syndrome and Their Caregivers." He also holds an MSc from University of Nicosia and University of Patras, an Interdepartmental MSc in Exercise and Quality of Life from Democritus University of Thrace and the University of Thessaly, as well as a BA (Hons) in Early Childhood Studies from University of Derby. Dr. Mantsos has published extensively in peer-reviewed journals, edited volumes, and international conference proceedings on topics related to neurodevelopmental disorders, psychomotor development, mental health, therapeutic interventions, and inclusive practices.

SaranrajP. holds a Ph.D. in Microbiology from Annamalai University, Chidambaram, India, and is NET (ASRB–ICAR) qualified in Microbiology. He is currently serving as Assistant Professor and Head, Department of Microbiology, at Sacred Heart College (Autonomous), Tirupattur, Tamil Nadu, India. In addition, he is the Proprietor and Managing Director of JPS Scientific Publications, contributing actively to academic publishing and research dissemination. Dr. Saranraj has over 15 years of research experience and 10 years of teaching experience in the fields of Environmental Microbiology, Agricultural Microbiology, Industrial Microbiology, Bioremediation, Microbial Biotechnology, and Sustainable Ecosystem Management. His research work has focused on Microbial degradation of pollutants, Effluent treatment, Soil health improvement, Plant–microbe interactions, and Applied environmental sustainability. He has an extensive publication record, with more than 240 international research articles, over 90 books (international and national), and 70+ book chapters published with reputed academic publishers.

Yannis Paxinos is a clinical psychologist and holds a PhD from the National and Kapodistrian University of Athens. His doctoral dissertation focused on the assessment of quality of life among former patients of the Leros Psychiatric Hospital. He studied Clinical Psychology at the University of Leuven, Belgium, where he also completed his postgraduate studies specializing in family therapy and sexual disorders. He has worked at the Leros Psychiatric Hospital and at the Pain Clinic of Patission General Hospital. He currently works in the Child and Adolescent Psychiatry Department of the Children's Hospital, where he is primarily engaged in family therapy. He is a member of the Hellenic Psychological Society and teaches in higher education at both undergraduate and postgraduate levels.

Ilxom Sayfiddinov is affiliated with the Department of Bank Accounting and Auditing at Tashkent State University of Economics, Tashkent, Uzbekistan. He is an academic professional engaged in teaching, research, and scholarly activities in the areas of banking, accounting, and auditing. His work supports the development of students' knowledge of financial reporting, banking operations, audit procedures, and the role of accounting systems in modern economic institutions. He is committed to promoting academic excellence through a balanced approach that combines theoretical understanding with practical relevance. His academic interests may include bank accounting, financial analysis, auditing standards, corporate governance, and financial management. Through his role at Tashkent State University of Economics, he contributes to creating a strong learning environment that encourages analytical thinking, ethical awareness, and professional competence among students. His professional profile reflects dedication to quality education, research engagement, and the broader advancement of accounting and auditing studies in Uzbekistan.

Styliani Tziaferi is an Associate Professor in Community and Occupational Health Nursing at the University of Peloponnese, Greece, with over two decades of combined academic, clinical, and leadership experience. She holds a PhD in Occupational Health Risk Assessment, an MSc in Public Health, and is a Fellow of the European Academy of Nursing Science (FEANS). Dr. Tziaferi has led and coordinated major national and international research initiatives, including Erasmus+ and WHO-EURO–linked projects, with a strong focus on occupational health, community nursing, patient safety, and interprofessional pharmaceutical care. She has authored more than 85 peer-reviewed publications and several academic book chapters. A recognized leader in nursing education and policy, she has served in senior academic roles, governmental advisory committees, and European professional bodies, contributing significantly to the advancement of nursing practice, education, and workforce development across Europe.]

Index

A

B

C

D

N

O

P

Q

R

S

T

www.ingramcontent.com/pod-product-compliance
Lightning Source LLC
LaVergne TN
LVHW080906300926
849162LV00003B/575

* 9 7 9 8 3 3 7 3 8 4 8 5 6 *